THE MULTIPLE CRISES OF MARITAL SEPARATION AND DIVORCE

SEMINARS IN PSYCHIATRY

Series Editor
Milton Greenblatt, M.D.
Director, Neuropsychiatric Institute Hospital and Clinics
Professor and Executive Vice Chairman
Department of Psychiatry and Biobehavioral Sciences
University of California, Los Angeles
Los Angeles, California

Other Books in Series:

Psychiatric Aspects of Neurologic Disease, edited by D. Frank Benson, M.D., and
   Dietrich Blumer, M.D.
Borderline States in Psychiatry, edited by John E. Mack, M.D.
Topics in Psychoendocrinology, edited by Edward J. Sachar, M.D.
Consultation-Liaison Psychiatry, edited by Robert O. Pasnau, M.D.
Drugs in Combination with Other Therapies, edited by Milton Greenblatt, M.D.
Suicidology: Contemporary Developments, edited by Edwin S. Shneidman, Ph.D.
Alcoholism Problems in Women and Children, edited by Milton Greenblatt, M.D., and
   Marc A. Schuckit, M.D.
Ethological Psychiatry: Psychopathology in the Context of Evolutionary Biology, edited
   by Michael T. McGuire, M.D., and Lynn A. Fairbanks, Ph.D.
The Family in Mourning: A Guide for Health Professionals, edited by Charles E.
   Hollingsworth, M.D., and Robert O. Pasnau, M.D.
Clinical Aspects of the Rapist, edited by Richard T. Rada, M.D.
Sex Education for the Health Professional: A Curriculum Guide, edited by Norman
   Rosenzweig, M.D., and F. Paul Pearsall, Ph.D.
Psychopharmacology Update: New and Neglected Areas, edited by John M. Davis,
   M.D., and David Greenblatt, M.D.
Methods of Biobehavioral Research, edited by E.A. Serafetinides, M.D., Ph.D.
Alcohol and Old Age, by Brian L. Mishara, Ph.D., and Robert Kastenbaum, Ph.D.
Psychiatric Research in Practice: Biobehavioral Themes, edited by E. A. Serafetinides,
   M.D., Ph.D.
Family Therapy and Major Psychopathology, edited by Melvin R. Lansky, M.D.
The Afro-American Family: Assessment, Treatment, and Research Issues, edited by
   Barbara Ann Bass, M.S.W., Gail Elizabeth Wyatt, Ph.D., and Gloria Johnson
   Powell, M.D.
Mental Health and Hispanic Americans: Clinical Perspectives, edited by Rosina M.
   Becerra, Ph.D., Marvin Karno, M.D., and Javier I. Escobar, M.D.
Teaching Psychiatry and Behavioral Science, edited by Joel Yager, M.D.
Psychiatric Aspects of Neurologic Disease, Volume II, edited by D. Frank Benson,
   M.D., and Deitrich Blumer, M.D.

THE MULTIPLE CRISES
OF MARITAL SEPARATION AND
DIVORCE

Gerald F. Jacobson, M.D., Ph.D., *1922-*

Executive Director
Didi Hirsch Community Mental Health Center

Associate Clinical Professor of Psychiatry
School of Medicine
University of Southern California
Los Angeles, California

GRUNE & STRATTON
A Subsidiary of Harcourt Brace Jovanovich, Publishers
New York   London
Paris   San Diego   San Francisco   São Paulo
Sydney   Tokyo   Toronto

Library of Congress Cataloging in Publication Data

Jacobson, Gerald F. 1922–
    The multiple crises of marital separation and divorce.
    (Seminars in psychiatry)
    Bibliography
    Includes index.
    1. Divorce—Psychological aspects.   I. Title.
II.   Series: Seminars in psychiatry (Grune & Stratton)
HQ814.J32   1983   306.8'9   82-15766
ISBN 0-8089-1483-9

Grune & Stratton, Inc.
111 Fifth Avenue
New York, NY 10003

Distributed in the United Kingdom by
Academic Press Inc. (London) Ltd.
24/28 Oval Road, London NW 1

Library of Congress Catalog Number 82-15766 ⌐|‾‾83
International Standard Book Number 0-8089-1483-9

Printed in the United States of America

With love to
Doris
and
Eric, Lisa, and Julia

Contents

Acknowledgments

Much of the book is based on Research Grant R 12863 from the National Institute of Mental Health, of which the present author was Principal Investigator. This support is greatly appreciated.

I also wish to thank the following for their contributions: Stephen H. Portuges, Ph.D., as Research Associate on this project, made important contributions in a number of areas, including instrument development, data collection, and the first phase of data analysis. Dr. Kenneth Sirotnik was methodological consultant during this .phase. Margaret Bonnefil, A.C.S.W., and Kenneth Wurtz, Ph.D., were clinical raters. Professor Wayne A. Alves was consulted extensively on methodology during the writing of the book; additional consultation was obtained from Professor Wilfrid J. Dixon. The responsibility for the final version is, of course, my own. Sandra Frith spent many hours in computer programming and data processing.

My colleagues at the Didi Hirsch Community Mental Health Center/ Los Angeles Psychiatric Service, and especially at the Benjamin Rush Center where the work was conducted, worked closely with the research staff in subject recruitment. Lillian Stewart, Charlotte Cavataio, and Rebecca Slaughter carried out the demanding work of typing and revising the manuscript.

Very special thanks are due to Milton Greenblatt, M.D., who went beyond the call of duty in his role as Series Editor to encourage me to persist in a long and sometimes difficult project. Thanks are also due to the publishing staff of Grune & Stratton, who worked diligently with me during the process of preparing the manuscript for publication.

In addition, I would like to express my thanks to a group of people who provided support and inspiration throughout the period of conducting the research and writing the book: The Board of Directors of the Didi Hirsch Community Mental Health Center/Los Angeles Psychiatric Service have for many years helped to create an atmosphere in which research and scientific inquiry was encouraged. This work also owes a debt to the pioneers and researchers in the field of marital separation and divorce whose work is cited and on whose contributions I have tried to build.

I want to thank my wife, Professor Doris Jacobson, Ph.D., of the University of California at Los Angeles School of Social Welfare, for her emotional support and encouragement and for the opportunity to share ideas. I also want to thank my children, Eric, Lisa, and Julia for their continuing warm encouragement during the years that this work was in progress.

Foreword

Unlike other volumes in the *Seminars in Psychiatry* series, this book is by a single author. Dr. Gerald F. Jacobson has labored long years in the field of marital separation and divorce, applying highly sophisticated methodology in areas heretofore colored by considerable speculation and opinion. I am profoundly impressed by Dr. Jacobson's mastery of his field, and especially delighted that he has allowed us to publish his seminal study, a truly distinguished work!

Dr. Jacobson's findings illuminate the intimate relationships on which we depend for stability and happiness. His work gives us the basis from which to assess the damage done to families by separation and divorce, and outlines a strategy to help society emerge from its most private troubles.

Dr. Jacobson's contribution is important to several groups of readers. To the clinician it offers new insights into the world of persons whose marriages are dissolving. There are now more individuals who have experienced the end of a marriage than ever before, and these formerly married people seek clinical help to deal with their problems more often than do persons in other marital categories. Clinicians need to understand the experiences, perils, and opportunities that accompany marital separation and divorce. Dr. Jacobson's work explores these factors in depth, and will be a valuable resource to anyone working with individuals and families.

Of particular interest to researchers are the summaries of existing empirical studies, and Jacobson's new data from his well-designed three-year study. His research employed statistical methods to identify aspects of post-marital status and experience that correlate with measures of mental health. The study significantly increases our understanding of the connection between interpersonal relationships and psychopathology.

Dr. Jacobson also offers a new explanation of the known relationship between separation and divorce and severe psychiatric disturbance. He suggests that a combination of responses to loss and continued disturbed interaction with a former spouse may contribute to causing psychiatric symptoms.

Finally, this book is of interest to *all* behavioral scientists because it utilizes an important new method of investigation that bridges the gap between clinical phenomena and statistically oriented research. Attachment, conflict, hostility, and grief are assessed by means of structured questionnaires that can be analyzed statistically. This approach enables researchers to formulate more precisely clinical concepts, and to test more rigorously their relevance and realtionships to psychopathology.

Milton Greenblatt, M.D.
Series Editor
Seminars in Psychiatry

THE MULTIPLE CRISES OF
MARITAL SEPARATION AND DIVORCE

1

The Importance of Marital Separation and Divorce

Marital separation is one of the most profound experiences that a human being can undergo. Marriage is one of three milestones marking a lifetime: birth, marriage, and death. Most people in our civilization do marry, and for all but a very few, marrying is associated with fundamental changes in their view of themselves, their partners, and the world. The marriage ceremony marks the transition from the family of origin to a new family consisting of the two marital partners and possibly their children.

An individual entering into marriage undergoes transitions in intrapsychic, interpersonal, and social spheres. He or she usually directs inner drives for need satisfaction toward a unique other to a greater extent than most nonmarried adults do.

• The marital partner may be the object of a full range of intrapsychic drives, ranging from various infantile components to sublimated drives to mature adult sexuality. A marital partner may fulfill needs to nurture or be nurtured, to control or be controlled, to give or be given to, to gratify or be gratified sexually, and to express anger or be the target of another's anger.

• Where the intrapsychic viewpoint focuses on the inner psychic life of one person, the interpersonal approach considers interactions between two or more people. Viewing marriage from this perspective, a couple interacts in many aspects of life. These include common living arrangements, legal and financial contracts, numerous role assignments involving outside work and income, maintenance of the home and child-raising, and sexual and emotional interactions.

• Marital status is a key determinant, along with gender, age, occupation, and socioeconomic status, in defining a person's social status and role within society. Formally sanctioned by society, marriage affects patterns of relating to family of origin, friends, and such institutions as churches and schools. Commonly, social relations of married couples are mainly with other marrieds. Despite the recent phenomena of "open marriage" and "swinging," a married person tends to be viewed as committed primarily to one partner and therefore is not seen as a rival by other persons of the same sex. Married couples are often viewed as a unit when socializing. As a legal contract, marriage affects property rights; this issue assumes great significance if the marriage is dissolved.

One aspect of marriage that involves intrapsychic, interpersonal, and social dimensions is the common residence of a married couple. Coupling that does not involve sharing the same address is qualitatively different from that which involves living together. Marriage is the most common adult relationship in which a committed couple lives together, and it is the living arrangement that has the broadest social and legal sanctions. There are other relationships that involve sharing the same home, of course: children living with their families; persons sharing a domicile out of convenience or friendship; heterosexual and homosexual couples living together. However, none of these, except for children in families, involves sharing a residence as uniformly as in marriage. There is a deep psychological meaning attached to the concept of "a place to live." The terminology alone suggests the intimate association of domicile and life itself. The roots of this association lie with the original family in childhood, when the home becomes associated with the gratification, and also frustration, of the most profound wishes.

These characteristics of marriage have been reviewed because they form a basis for the understanding of the process of marital separation and divorce. If a complete dissolution is to occur—and as will be seen, this is by no means a foregone conclusion—all of the intrapsychic, interpersonal, and social processes are affected. It is self-evident that the separation cannot proceed without pain. The pain may be less than the sustained pain of an unhappy marriage; it may be diminished if the marriage was of short duration or if there was a gradually increasing separation between the spouses that had progressed to the point where formal dissolution of the marriage simply recognized an existing fact. But the marital dissolution that can occur without some degree of suffering is rare, if not nonexistent.

The existence of this pain is an important reason for the relative disregard of separation and divorce in the popular and scientific literature. The topic of marital separation and divorce tends to be avoided by all, including mental health professionals. Those who have not experienced separation or divorce do not wish to be reminded of the fact that it happens to others and may happen to them as well. This avoidance is similar to that relating to other areas of human unhappiness, such as fatal illness, severe trama, and in spite of its recent vogue, death. Avoidance—which is not necessarily conscious—takes a number of forms: Divorce may be treated as wholly or mainly the result of psychological illness. The implication of this approach is that divorce happens only to the "sick," not to those who are well or who get adequate help. Bergler[1] exemplifies this avoidance by stating that divorce is an attempt to resolve neurotic problems, which could and should instead be treated psychoanalytically. A parallel approach stressing pathology among the divorced was taken, among others, by Blumenthal.[2] While the recent increase in divorce has focused greater attention on its potentially adaptive aspects, many studies, as Westman[3] pointed out, stress only the destructive aspects and give little constructive information about divorce. Divorce in fact is painful, but it is not wholly or mainly an indicator of preexisting pathology.

Avoidance is also manifested by the attempt to see divorce as a single occurrence. Clinicians not familiar with this phenomenon are often surprised by the importance of the aftermath of divorce in persons who have dissolved their marriages months or years ago. The attitude, spoken or implied, is, "But this all happened a long time ago; it cannot be related to today's problems."

Another way in which the realities of divorce may be avoided is by focusing only on the children of divorcing couples. Of all subjects related to divorce, those relating to children are relatively the safest and least threatening. The message here is, Let us not think very much about the marriage that is no more; let us instead think about the parenting that remains.

Although we do not wish to deny the extreme importance of the impact of divorce on children, it is nonetheless true that emphasis on this aspect has been disproportionate. For example, an organization that clearly functions primarily as a social and mutual support group for formerly married adults chooses to define itself as "*Parents* Without Partners" (emphasis mine), although parenting-oriented activities make up only a small portion of its overall program. The professional literature shows the same tendency to overemphasize the otherwise legitimate topic of maintaining the parenting role while discontinuing the marital one. In practice, we have seen this lead to indiscriminate invitations for divorced parents to join in counseling sessions on behalf of the child, suggesting an undivided family unit when such a unit does not in fact exist. The pretense of its existence can be very disturbing to parent and child alike.

Though avoidance has deferred detailed consideration of marital separation and divorce as a process, the growing incidence of this phenomenon has made its careful examination inevitable. This volume is intended as an overview of the key issues encountered in marital dissolution. It is dedicated to the proposition that nothing is as destructive as the persistent denial of reality and to the corollary that better understanding and acceptance of the realistic and emotional issues of marital separation and divorce can strengthen those undergoing this process as well as help the professionals who propose to assist them.

The book is based on both clinical and research data. The clinical data include my experience in a very active crisis clinic, the Benjamin Rush Center for Problems of Living. The center, a division of the Los Angeles Psychiatric Service,* was established in 1962 under the direction of the author. Approximately 16,000 cases have been seen on a walk-in, brief-treatment basis for a maximum of six sessions. The crisis of marital separation and divorce is a major subgroup of the cases seen at the center. Other aspects of the Rush Center have been described elsewhere. [4-7]

This work also draws heavily on the findings of a research project funded by the National Institute of Mental Health.† Lastly, the presentation draws on my theoretical orientation, which is based on both psychoanalytic and community mental health frameworks.

REFERENCES

1. Bergler E: Conflict in Marriage: The Unhappy Divorce. New York, Harper Bros, 1949

---

*The Los Angeles Psychiatric Service is now known as the Didi Hirsch Community Mental Health Center/Los Angeles Psychiatric Service.

†NIMH Grant No. RO1 MH 21863, Relation of Suicide to Marital Separation and Divorce.

2. Blumenthal M: Mental health among the divorced. Arch Gen Psychiatry 16:603–608, 1967
3. Westman JC, Kline DW, Swift WJ, et al: Relation of child psychiatry and divorce. Arch Gen Psychiatry 23:416–420, 1970
4. Bonnefil M: Crisis intervention with children and families, in Jacobson GF (Ed): New Direction in Mental Health Services. Crisis Intervention in the 1980s. San Francisco, Jossey-Bass, 1980, pp 23–34
5. Jacobson GF, Wilner DM, Morley WE, et al: The scope and practice of an early-access brief treatment psychiatric center, in Barton HH (Ed): Brief Therapies. New York, Behavioral Publications Inc, 1971
6. Jacobson GF: Programs and techniques of crisis intervention, in Caplan G (Ed): American Handbook of Psychiatry, vol 2. New York, Basic Books, 1974, pp 810–825
7. Morley WE: Crisis intervention with adults, in Jacobson GF (Ed), New Directions in Mental Health Services. Crisis Intervention in the 1980s. San Francisco, Jossey-Bass, 1980, pp 11–21

2
Life Events, Crises, and the Crisis Matrix

We have always known that life events are important. Folk beliefs from time immemorial have included the idea that one can die of a broken heart or be driven mad by the loss of a lover. Yet until recently, psychological and social scientists have tended to disregard this subject, at times dismissing it as consisting of no more than outdated superstitions. Only in the last decade has there been a resurgence of scholarly interest in the adult life cycle. Yet even today the major theoretical approaches—biological, psychoanalytic, and sociological—emphasize long-term factors rather than discrete events. Genetic and biological framework stress those factors present at birth or those developing on a physiological or biochemical basis. Classic psychoanalysis focuses on the period from birth to age six, with relative disregard of later development. Sociocultural approaches deal with the impact of social class, poverty, and race, which tend to remain constant over a lifetime.

It should be noted that there is no conflict between the view that life events are important and other (physiological and psychological) approaches. Rather, psychological and physical functioning can be viewed as the result of the interaction of many factors, including genetic endowment, childhood development, sociocultural factors such as social class, and life events. While most scholars would agree with such a concept of multiple causality, the student of life events is still often treated with disinterest, if not suspicion. Brown[1] feels that in part the issue is political, that other approaches have vested interests in alternate explanations of physical and psychological health and therefore downplay life occurrences. Another psychological explanation is possible: scientists, like other human beings, experience life events that may be recalled with sadness or anticipated with apprehension. Many life events involve loss or threat of loss. It is often difficult to contemplate or recollect such losses as marital separation and divorce, bereavement, or related events. In teaching crisis intervention, I have found that students and even experienced mental health professionals use various defenses, including avoidance and minimizing, to deal with patients and clients who have undergone painful experiences. The more extreme the life event was, the greater the tendency of the professional to avoid it or downplay its importance. This is probably one of the reasons why victims of such tragedies as rape, confinement in concentration camps, and natural disasters report at times that mental health professionals have had difficulty listening to their experiences. Perhaps a similar avoidance in part explains the long delay in subjecting life events to scientific scrutiny: researchers are not above the same conflicts.

LIFE EVENTS

In spite of this reluctance to deal with life issues, catastrophic events including war, detention in prisoner-of-war and concentration camps, and major natural disasters have such obvious impact that their consequences are unmistakable. Even then the cause-and-effect relationship of event and disability is not always acknowledged. In addition, issues of financial compensation are sometimes involved. This problem was encountered by a team of psychiatrists, lawyers, and sociologists who worked with victims of the Buffalo Creek disaster, in which a tidal wave released by the collapse of a dam destroyed an entire community. Disastrous psychological consequences were found in the survivors, including traumatic neurotic reactions in 80 percent.[2] Nevertheless, it took litigation against the coal company that had operated the dam to bring about financial compensation for the victims.[3] Similar experiences have occurred with former inmates of Nazi concentration camps who suffered evident chronic psychological damage as a result of their confinement: German psychiatrists, contesting restitution claims made by victims, argued that constitutional factors or early childhood experiences, rather than the concentration camp trauma, resulted in the psychological disturbance seen in these patients.

In spite of the reluctance to admit their significance, there is an almost complete acceptance in the scientific community of the fact that severe enough life events can cause lasting psychological changes. In military parlance, this has been expressed as, "Everybody has a breaking point." It is not obvious, however, as Dohrenwend[4] pointed out, that less catastrophic although often clearly painful life events, such as marital separation, can also cause significant psychological changes.[4] Nevertheless, once we acknowledge that any life event can cause psychological changes, the principle of the relationship between events and psychological well-being is established. Further study now centers on which events under what circumstances will have such an impact. The following studies address this issue.

Life Events and Physical Illness

Studies regarding the association of life events and physical illness have been undertaken by several groups of workers,[1,5–12] and have been summarized by Dohrenwend and Dohrenwend.[13] Virtually all have taken the approach that a series of life events occurring over a period of time are related to subsequent physical or psychological illness. The reasoning is that one event, unless catastrophic, would not be sufficiently potent to affect psychiatric or physical well-being in a measurable way within a short time, but a cluster of such events would

Table 2-1
Social Readjustment Rating Questionnaire

Rank	Life Event	Mean Value
1	Death of spouse	100
2	Divorce	73
3	Marital separation	65
4	Jail term	63
5	Death of close family member	63
6	Personal injury or illness	53
7	Marriage	50
8	Fired at work	47
9	Marital reconciliation	45
10	Retirement	45
11	Change in health of family member	44
12	Pregnancy	40
13	Sex difficulties	39
14	Gain of new family member	39
15	Business readjustment	39
16	Change in financial state	38

Rank	Life Event	Mean Value
17	Death of close friend	37
18	Change to different line of work	36
19	Change in number of arguments with spouse	35
20	Mortgage over $10,000	31
21	Foreclosure of mortgage or loan	30
22	Change in responsibilities at work	29
23	Son or daughter leaving home	29
24	Trouble with in-laws	29
25	Outstanding personal achievement	28
26	Wife begin or stop work	26
27	Begin or end school	26
28	Change in living conditions	25
29	Revision of personal habits	24
30	Trouble with boss	23
31	Change in work hours or conditions	20
32	Change in residence	20
33	Change in schools	20
34	Change in recreation	19
35	Change in church activities	19
36	Change in social activities	18
37	Mortgage or loan less than $10,000	17
38	Change in sleeping habits	16
39	Change in number of family get-togethers	15
40	Change in eating habits	15
41	Vacation	13
42	Christmas	12
43	Minor violations of the law	11

From Rahe RH: Life crisis and health change, in May PRA, Wittenborn GR (Eds): Psychotropic Drug Response: Advances in Prediction. Springfield, Ill, Charles B. Thomas, 1969, 97. With permission.

have this effect. The unit of study thus becomes the number of events that have occurred during a given period of time. Such a cluster of events commonly occurs around marital separation and divorce.

Once it was agreed that *several* life events would be considered, the next step was to assign weights to each event. The first and most widely used instrument was the Social Readjustment Rating Scale (SRRS),[14] which is composed of 43 life events. Each event was given a numerical weight to indicate its intensity and the length of time necessary for its accommodation, regardless of its desirability. This scale is reproduced in Table 2-1.

The ratings were obtained by asking 394 subjects to complete a written questionnaire rating the life events by the readjustment required. Marriage was given an arbitrary value of 500 (later reduced to 50). Subjects were asked if each other event required a longer or shorter readjustment and to assign a proportionately larger or smaller number. Divorce and separation rank second and third, respectively. Only death of the spouse is rated as requiring more readjustment.

The numerical weights given to all events occurring within a given period of time were added together and the total was described as the Life Change Units (LCU) accumulated during that time. The LCU total was then compared with the appearance of illness or the application for medical treatment in the same or subsequent time periods. Most of the studies were retrospective.

There has been a rather large number of studies by Holmes, Rahe, and their associates as well as by others using either the original SRRS or derivatives. Although Holmes and Rahe are psychiatrists, their approach has been used mainly to deal with medical disorders rather than with purely psychiatric ones. This is because both of these authors originally were concerned with psychosomatic medicine and with the medical sequellae of stress. Rahe has applied the SRRS and subsequent versions to a number of groups. These included resident physicians;[14] a large group of Navy men;[15] survivors of myocardial infarction and victims of sudden coronary death;[16] and Norwegian Navy men.[8] An association of life changes with illness was reported in all of these groups. Other studies summarized by Holmes and Masada[6] have shown a relationship between LCU scores and the occurrence of fractures, the beginning of pregnancy, incarceration in a federal prison, and other events. Among the widely divergent factors found to be related to life events are health changes among officer training cadets,[17] juvenile rheumatoid arthritis,[18] and competitive performance in an Alaskan sled race.[19]

Rahe believes that a dividing line of 150 LCUs occurring within six months exists between persons who tend to become ill and those who do not. He postulated on the basis of his data that a gradual build-up of LCUs occurs in the two years preceding a health change, reaching a maximum level in the preceding six months. For this reason it is of interest to look at the life events that a person undergoing marital separation and divorce may experience within six months, as shown in the following list of events and their corresponding LCUs.

Thus a person who separates, then reconciles, and then divorces within a six-month period accumulates a score of 185 for these events

Divorce	73	Revision of personal	
Marital separation	65	habits	24
Marital reconciliation	45	Change in residence	20
Sex difficulties	39	Change in social	
Change in financial		activities	18
state	38	Change in sleeping	
Change in number		habits	16
of arguments		Change in number	
with spouse	35	of family	
Trouble with in-laws	29	get-togethers	15
Change in living		Change in eating	
conditions	25	habits	15

alone. (The Rahe scale does not differentiate between filing for divorce and obtaining a final decree.) It is likely that other events, such as changes in arguments with spouse, changes in financial state, changes in living arrangements and social activities, will also have occurred, so that the score may be much higher. The total LCUs of the events listed above is 457. While few if any persons will have a score of that magnitude, it is clear that marital separation and divorce may be associated with very high LCU levels.

It should be noted that Holmes and Rahe's approach is not beyond criticism. Problems that have been pointed out by various investigators include the presence in the SRRS of items that could be indicators of illness.[20] Another issue is that until now the majority of studies have been retrospective and therefore subject to unconscious falsification: people may be more likely to recall life events preceding an illness in order to explain its occurrence. A third problem is the difference between illness and illness behavior, the latter being identified as seeking a physician or health care provider. In spite of these reservations, the studies conducted are impressive and strongly suggest that some aspects of physical health are related to life changes.

Life Events and Psychological Disturbance

We now turn to the issue of the association of life events with psychological phenomena. This matter has been addressed by a number of investigators. One important center of relevant studies is Yale University in New Haven. The New Haven group uses a list of 61 life events that was generally derived from the work of Holmes and Rahe but differs somewhat. While Holmes and Rahe considered the *readjustment* required when a given event occurred, the New Haven group used the concept of *upset* as the criterion of the importance of a life

Table 2-2
Scaling Scores for Life Events

Rank	Event	Mean	SD
1	Death of child	19.33	2.22
2	Death of spouse	18.76	3.21
3	Jail sentence	17.60	3.56
4	Death of close family member (parent, sibling)	17.21	3.69
5	Spouse unfaithful	16.78	4.14
6	Major financial difficulties (very heavy debts, bankruptcy)	16.57	3.83
7	Business failure	16.46	3.71
8	Fired	16.45	4.20
9	Miscarriage or stillbirth	16.34	4.59
10	Divorce	16.18	4.95
11	Marital separation due to argument	15.93	4.55
12	Court appearance for serious legal violation	15.79	4.26
13	Unwanted pregnancy	15.57	5.18
14	Hospitalization of family member (serious illness)	15.30	4.15
15	Unemployment for one month	15.26	4.38
16	Death of close friend	15.18	4.55
17	Demotion	15.05	4.57
18	Major personal physical illness (hospitalization or one month off work)	14.61	4.44
19	Begin extramarital affair	14.09	5.40
20	Loss of personally valuable object	14.07	4.90
21	Law suit	13.78	5.02
22	Academic failure (important exam or course)	13.52	5.07
23	Child married against respondent's wishes	13.24	5.36
24	Break engagement	13.23	5.31
25	Increased arguments with spouse	13.02	4.91
26	Increased arguments with resident family member	12.83	5.15
27	Increased arguments with fiance or steady date	12.66	4.95
28	Take a large loan (more than one-half of a year's earnings)	12.64	5.43
29	Son drafted	12.32	5.75
30	Arguments with boss or co-worker	12.21	5.06
31	Argument with nonresident family member (in-laws, relatives)	12.11	5.09
32	Move to another country	11.37	6.05
33	Menopause	11.02	5.78

Rank	Event	Mean	SD
34	Moderate financial difficulties (bothersome but not serious, ie, Increased expenses, trouble from bill collectors)	10.96	4.98
35	Separation from significant person (close friend or relative)	10.68	5.18
36	Take important exam	10.44	5.03
37	Marital separation not due to argument	10.33	5.68
38	Change in work hours (much overtime, second job, much less than usual)	9.96	5.49
39	New person in household	9.71	5.45
40	Retirement	9.33	6.02
41	Change in work conditions (new department, new boss, big reorganization)	9.23	5.12
42	Change in line of work	8.84	5.38
43	Cease steady dating (of at least three months)	8.80	5.34
44	Move to another city	8.52	5.59
45	Change in schools	8.15	5.39
46	Cease full-time education (graduate or drop out)	7.65	5.73
47	Child leaves home (eg, college)	7.20	4.96
48	Marital reconciliation (after one partner left home)	6.95	5.91
49	Minor legal violation	6.05	4.78
50	Birth of live child (for mother)	5.91	5.70
51	Wife becomes pregnant	5.67	5.23
52	Marriage	5.61	5.67
53	Promotion	5.39	4.90
54	Minor personal physical illness (one that requires physician's attention)	5.20	4.29
55	Move in same city	5.14	4.49
56	Birth of a child (father) or adoption	5.13	5.45
57	Begin education (full time or half time)	5.09	4.48
58	Child becomes engaged	4.53	4.57
59	Become engaged	3.70	4.64
60	Wanted pregnancy	3.56	5.39
61	Child married with respondent's approval	2.94	3.75

From Paykel ES: Scaling of life events. Arch Gen Psychiatry 25:342–347, 1971. © 1971 American Medical Association. With permission.

event. The New Haven group felt that for psychiatric conditions the amount of upset brought about by a given event was more significant than the readjustment required. Therefore Paykel et al.[10] assigned weights to various events, using an approach similar to that of Holmes and Rahe but asking their raters to address the relevant amount of upset that various life events were likely to cause. Their scale is included in Table 2-2.

Divorce and marital separation ranked 10th and 11th out of 61 items, which is somewhat lower than in the Holmes and Rahe scale though still quite high. It is interesting that unfaithfulness of spouse ranked fifth, well ahead of either one. The ranking of events in this scale is surprising, since in my experience some of the items listed above divorce and separation, such as business failure, being fired, and major financial difficulties, do not have the impact of separation and divorce. One wonders if Paykel's raters, who were patients and their families, may have been somewhat inclined to rate conventionally acceptable life events ahead of separation and divorce, which in their view might carry a stigma.

In some studies by the New Haven group, the events listed were broken down into various categories,[12] including desirability, problem area, exits or entrances in the social sphere, intensity of upset, and control of the subject. Separation and divorce due to discord were characterized as undesirable, as exits from rather than entrances into the social sphere, and as bringing about a major rather than an intermediate or a minor upset. They were not included in either the controlled or uncontrolled groups. These categories were used in relating life events to both the onset of depression and to suicide attempts. It was found that depressed persons had significantly more exits from the social sphere than did the general population. They also had highly significantly more events in the marital area (including separation and divorce), and they experienced more intensely upsetting events. There was no difference in desirability or degree of control by the subject. Marital separation and divorce were components of all the subgroups associated with depression.

Compared to the general population, suicide attempters had more undesirable events at a highly significant level, more entrances into and more exits from the social sphere, highly significantly more events in the marital area and in other areas of activity (except work), more major upsets, more intermediate and minor upsets, and more uncontrolled events. Again, the clusters in which separation and divorce were included were associated with suicide attempts.

The occurrence of single events was also compared to depression and suicide. In most instances, not enough persons experienced any one event to make statistical comparison meaningful. One phenomenon, however, sometimes related to separation and divorce—serious arguments with spouse—proved to be highly significant in relation to both depression and suicide attempts. More suicide attempters and depressives experienced both marital separation and divorce than did the general population, but the numbers were not large enough to be statistically significant.

There is some evidence that life events are related to the onset of acute episodes of schizophrenia. Brown summarized the earlier work of Brown and Birley and flatly stated that his work "established the causal importance of life events in the onset of schizophrenic attacks."[1]

Jacobs and Myers[21] found that a group of 124 schizophrenics reported more recent life events than did an equal number of controls. They noted that the overall differences between schizophrenics and normals, however, appeared to be smaller than the differences between depressives and normals. They suggested a precipitating role of life events in schizophrenia, rather than a formative one. In the schizophrenic group there were six persons who had recently separated from their spouses, compared to two in the control group. Five schizophrenics and two controls reported recent changes with the spouse such as increase in number of arguments. In neither instance were the numbers large enough to be statistically significant.

Donovan et al.[22] reported on 23 non-schizophrenic and 16 schizophrenic patients who were hospitalized in a short-term crisis intervention ward. Both groups reported "great objective stress" prior to their crises. The crises of the schizophrenics seemed less likely to be concerned with loss than those of the non-schizophrenics and seemed to be concerned with situations in which closeness was once more not achieved.

Schwartz and Myers[23,24] compared 132 post-hospitalized schizophrenics with an equal number of community controls matched in age, race, sex, and social class. They found that the schizophrenics had greater impairment than their community counterparts and had experienced more life events. There was an association of life events with psychiatric impairment. The authors distinguished between those events that are under a person's control and those that are not, and found that both types of events correlated with disturbance in post-hospitalized schizophrenics. They concluded that schizophrenics experience more critical life events, both of their own and not of their own making. When the data were further subjected to regression analysis, it was found that life events contribute most to non-psychotic symptoms and make a lesser contribution to certain aspects of psychotic behavior. Although the data do not directly support the conclusion that life events trigger schizophrenic illness, the authors feel that the greater anxiety, depression, and somatic symptoms resulting from life events may increase vulnerability to the more severe and characteristically schizophrenic symptoms.

Dohrenwend[4] takes a somewhat cautious point of view on this matter and refers only to certain psychiatric disorders, such as acute episodes of schizophrenia, following life events. At any rate, the evidence relating life events to schizophrenia is most interesting because of the role of schizophrenia as a major cause of severe and long-term disability. It must be noted that the probable association of life events with acute schizophrenia does not necessarily imply an association with chronic schizophrenia. Future studies could raise the question of whether or not the development of chronic schizophrenia might be related to a succession of maladaptively resolved life experiences in conjunction with predisposing psychological and physiological factors as well as any effects of institutionalization that may occur.

In addition to studies associating life events with specific descriptive entities, a number of investigations deal with the relationships of life events to general indices of psychological dysfunction. Myers et al.[9] undertook a series of studies involving a group of adults (over age 18) selected at random from 720 households in a systematic sample of a mental health catchment area in New Haven. They compared an index of mental status that was adapted from instruments developed in prior survey studies with life crises that occurred during the previous year. Crises were identified as experiences involving a role transformation, a change in status or environment, or the imposition of pain. An association between life crises and the mental status schedule was found.

Mueller et al.[25] reported on interviews with 363 persons in Sacramento, California, drawn from a random sample of 930 households. Using a modified version of the Schedule of Recent Experience,[5] they found that undesirable events were associated with higher scores on psychiatric symptom scales.

MEDIATING FACTORS

The implication clearly emerges that a relationship of life events to psychiatric and physical symptomatology exists, and that a number of workers believe these events to be at least partly causative. A related and important issue will next be addressed: Why is it that not all individuals experiencing any given life event or any given number of life events develop the same degree of psychological disability? In other words, what are the factors that mediate between the experience of life events and the impact on psychological functioning? There are two general approaches to this question: one emphasizes sociological variables and another focuses on psychological variables.

SOCIOLOGICAL VARIABLES

The individual's place within society is significantly influenced by age, sex, marital status, social class, education, occupation, and income. Myers et al.[9] found the relationship between life events and psychiatric symptomatology to be mediated by what he called "social integration." This previously mentioned survey of 720 adults in New Haven revealed that the extent to which life events resulted in psychiatric symptoms was codetermined at three levels. The first of these involved the larger social stratification. The second level was termed the microsystem of the family. The third level involved the "instrumental role," namely satisfaction with job or role as homemaker. Factors at all three levels were found to mediate between life events and outcome. Those most affected by experiences are persons of lower socioeconomic status; those single, separated, widowed, or divorced; and those not satisfied with their job or homemaker role. Incidentally, it is interesting that in this analysis a recently divorced person would be considered at risk by virtue of both divorcing and being divorced. From a more general viewpoint, the general implication of the work of Myers et al. is, not surprisingly, that it is easier to cope with life changes when one is a member of a higher social class, is married, and is satisfied with one's occupation.

In a similar study Mueller et al.[25] found the same general relationship between life events and psychiatric symptomatology that others have observed. This relationship, however, did not hold with persons earning over $15,000 per year or with those over 60 years of age. The authors believed that for the older age group, factors other than life experiences assume a greater role in determining mental health.

Antonovsky[26] addressed the issue of resistance resources, which account for the fact that the same life event may cause some persons to experience less disturbance than others. He considered resistance resources to be homeostatic flexibility regarding social roles, values, and personal beliefs; ties to concrete others; and ties to the total community.

As focus of this book is the detailed understanding of the processes of marital separation and divorce and their crises, we shall not return to the sociological variables of social class and income. It is important to keep in mind—at least as a matter of conscience—that social class and income have a great deal to do with how well or poorly one copes with life problems, including those of marital separation and divorce. Whatever the stress and the psychological changes, it is easier to cope with them when one is economically well off than when one is poor. As we address the important and often subtle parameters of the separation of two marital partners, we need to keep in mind the powerful impact of social inequities on the ability to master this or any other life crisis.

PSYCHOLOGICAL VARIABLES

We now turn to the intervening psychological variables that help determine the impact of life events on psychological functioning. There are two aspects to this topic: the extent to which life events can be the result of psychological factors, and the psychological factors that, while not felt to cause the life occurrence, will affect the impact of the event on the psyche.

Can life events be the result, rather than the cause, of psychological processes? One possible answer—admittedly an extreme one but one that is sometimes proposed—is that with few exceptions all life events are under unconscious, if not conscious, control. There is some psychoanalytical thinking that could be interpreted along these lines. One important concept is that of the "repetition compulsion." This is a psychoanalytical construct that postulates that neurotics (and to some extent all people) experience a force that motivates them to relive situations that were important in childhood. Freud stated that both neurotics and some non-neurotics give the impression of "being pursued by a malignant fate . . . but psychoanalysis has always taken the view that their fate is for the most part arranged by themselves and determined by early infantile influence."[27] A frequently given example is the child of an alcoholic who then enters into repeated and unhappy marriages with alcoholics, apparently not learning from experience.

Some empirical studies deal with the possibility that events are brought about by the person experiencing them. Schwartz and Myers[24] divided 64 life events into 13 that were considered "uncontrolled" and 51 that were considered "controlled." In their view, marital separation and divorce were both seen as "controlled." As already mentioned, both controlled and uncontrolled events correlated with psychiatric impairment in post-hospital schizophrenics as well as in non-schizophrenic controls. Dressler et al.[28] studied 40 hospitalized patients in the emergency treatment unit of a mental health center. They found a high incidence of interpersonal stress-precipitating events and noted the so-called initiating role of the patient in provoking the emotional crisis.

No one who is familiar with unconscious forces can deny that repetition compulsion and other unconscious motivations play a large part determining the fate of human beings. It would be a mistake to conclude, however, that life events are nothing more than symptoms of deep-seated problems and therefore do not deserve further consideration. Such a conclusion is not warranted for three reasons:

- The trauma caused by an event is in no way diminished by the fact that the person experiencing it unconsciously may have brought it about. On the contrary, there is some reason to believe that an event may be *more* traumatic if it has been triggered by the person who experienced it. From a dynamic point of view, it is plausible that persons with at least a dim perception of having contributed to a distressing life event may feel more guilty and beset by a sense of failure than those who are obviously victims of a force beyond their control. This point is speculative at present. Pokorny and Kaplan,[29] however, found that defenselessness and life events together become predictive of suicide following psychiatric hospitalization, whereas neither circumstance alone was predictive. Defenselessness was defined on the Brief Psychiatric Rating Scale[30] as relating to guilt, introjection of blame, depressive mood, inferiority feeling, anxiety, suicidal ideation, and obsessive thoughts. Introjection of blame is defined as a general tendency to blame oneself for personal problems. There is an indication here that the extent to which individuals rightly or wrongly see themselves as having caused distressful events relates to guilt and introjection of blame, thus enhancing the negative effect of these events. Self-derogation, similar to self-blame, was found by Kaplan[31] to enhance the impact of life events on psychiatric disturbance.
- The fact that a life event may be brought about wholly or partially by oneself does not mean that all the consequences of this event were intended. For example, someone may have chosen for conscious or unconscious reasons to migrate from one country to another. This does not mean that the experience of grief over the loss of the prior home or the hardships of immigrant life were chosen, nor were the burdens significantly lightened by the fact that the move was intentional. Much of the same can be said of the person leaving a marriage.
- No one can claim that all life events are controlled. Some unquestionably are, in whole or in part, uncontrolled. Marital separation and divorce fall into this category for at least some individuals.

There is, therefore, no logical reason to take the viewpoint that life events are merely epiphenomena—mechanical aftereffects of other forces, such as preexisting psychological determinants. My view, based mainly on experiences with many persons in crises, is that a reciprocal interaction commonly exists between psychological factors and life events. A life event may eventuate in a psychological state, which in turn may contribute to other life events, which again may lead to psychological consequences. A common example is seen in the clinical setting when a therapist unilaterally terminates a patient, as occurs when a student therapist leaves a clinic. Sometimes the patient may then try to resolve the feeling of passively suffering abandonment by actively creating other separations, such as leaving a job or separating from a spouse. To repeat: *that a life event may be the result of psychological forces in no way changes the fact that it can also be the cause of a psychological state.*

Psychological factors may also mediate between life events and outcome. Here we are not talking about factors causing the event, but rather about the role they play in determining outcome, with the event as a given. Hudgens[20] is a self-proclaimed critic of some of the broader claims by life-events researchers regarding the supposed etiological role of such events in psychosis and depression. He nevertheless reported a study that shows a clear association between life events and depression in medically hospitalized adolescents, and further related the presence or absence of depression to psychiatric disorder in the parents of the adolescents and to the adolescents' medical prognosis. Of the youngsters who had both parents with psychiatric disorder and a serious medical condition, 50 percent were found to be depressed; of those for whom neither was true, only 9 percent were depressed. The latter findings introduce factors that mediate between the life event and the depression.

Researchers tend to look for mediating factors between life events and outcome that are relevant to their field of study. Organically oriented workers thus will look at genetically or biologically determined phenomena as likely mediators. Psychoanalysts search for earlier life experiences, particularly those of childhood, as laying down a pattern that, together with later life occurrences, determines the outcome. Data from clinical psychoanalysis suggest that the meaning of a given life event is strongly colored by early experience. Some ongoing research addresses one aspect of this question: the extent to which losses of parents in childhood predisposes to more severe reactions to losses in adult life. It will be interesting to follow the results of this emerging area of investigation.

MEANING OF LIFE EVENTS

It will be recalled that in the various scales used to study the relationships of life events, weights were assigned to events on the basis of the readjustment the event required or the upset it produced. Brown[1] pointed out that basic to the rating of either readjustment or upset is an understanding of the meaning of the event. He criticized other scales, particularly the Schedule of Recent Experience of Holmes and Rahe,[5] for describing events in such general terms that a variety of meanings is possible. For example, he pointed out that the item "changes in health in family members" is not specific regarding the type of change of health in family members or the family members that may be included. Since a number of methodological problems arise from this situation, he developed an alternative that initially consisted of interviews during which subjects were asked only about very specific events involving specific persons. The events so defined were those that in the opinion of the raters, would be expected to be stressful to the average person. Using this approach, Brown felt that he had "established the causal importance of life events in the onset of schizophrenic attacks." The problem is, however, that a wide range of events were treated as alike and were given the same weight.

In the London studies of depression,[1] events were rated as more or less stressful on the basis of "the configuration of factors surrounding a life event." For example, two women may learn that their husbands are terminally ill. One may be socially isolated except for the contact with the husband, may have no assurance of remaining in her home once he dies, and may have had no warning of his illness; whereas for the second woman the opposite may be true in all regards. The threat of the illness would be therefore be much greater for the first woman. The measure employed here is that of "contextual threat." From a research viewpoint, Brown's[1,32] is an ingenious approach. He has gone from the simple listing of an event, which assumes that it has the same meaning for everyone, to a consideration of the specific circumstances that contribute to that meaning. At the same time, Brown defined an event as that which an average individual in a given society at a particular time would experience. It is much easier to get rater agreement on this point than it is for raters to agree on the unique meaning of an event for a single person. However, the clinician, if not necessarily the researcher, must understand the specific meaning of each event to each person. Generally, this method can be used to make meaningful predictions about life events as causes of psychological illness.

Because he has elaborated on the concept of the meaning of life events, Brown's work will serve as a transition to a discussion of crisis theory, in which the meaning of a life event holds a central place.

CRISIS THEORY

Life-events research is most effective in studying the association between life events and outcome, whether that outcome is measured in terms of physical illness or psychological state. It is not greatly concerned with the processes that lie between the event and the outcome. When mediating factors are considered, they are described in general terms and are often measured statistically. Life-events research does not focus on the psychological processes by which people cope with life. The understanding of the processes involving events, coping, crisis, and outcome as well as their nature and interrelationship have become known as crisis theory.

The terms "crisis," "crisis theory," and "crisis intervention" are often loosely used. In this context, they have quite specific definitions and meanings, which are discussed below.

Lindemann's Bereavement Study

The late Erich Lindemann, who was both a psychoanalyst and a community psychiatrist, wrote what has become a classic paper, "Symptomatology and Management of Acute Grief,"[33] which will serve as an introduction to crisis theory.

During World War II, a sudden fire occurred in the Cocoanut Grove nightclub in Boston, as a result of which many young adults unexpectedly and tragically lost their lives. Lindemann and some collaborating psychiatrists made use of this unfortunate natural experiment by interviewing the surviving close relatives of the fire victims. Some survivors of persons who had died in the armed forces were also included. In all, 101 persons were given a series of psychiatric interviews. All therapeutic suggestions and interpretations to the bereaved individuals were avoided until a clear picture of the manifestations of grief emerged. As a result, Lindemann was able to conceptualize a normal grief process characterized by somatic (physical) distress, preoccupation with the image of the deceased, guilt, hostile reactions, and loss of usual patterns of conduct. The study also included a therapeutic aspect, which consisted of helping the individual accept the discomfort associated with these responses, which Lindemann eventually called "grief work." In instances where the grief work proceeded without interruption, relief of tension usually occurred in four to six weeks. Lindemann also described morbid grief reactions that involved delay or postponement in dealing with feelings of loss. This maladaptive coping was at various times associated with overactivity, acquisition of an illness related to the last illness of the deceased, development of psychosomatic illnesses such as asthma or colds, alterations in relationships with friends and relatives, avoiding activities and antagonizing people, difficulty in initiating social activity, and behavior detrimental to the self. Again, the first four to six weeks were found to be crucial in determining whether grief would be adaptively or maladaptively resolved.

The study is cited here for two reasons. First, some grief processes in marital separation and divorce are similar in certain respects to those associated with bereavement. Second, and more important in this context, Lindemann found that a crucial time period, lasting four to six weeks, follows a traumatic event. During this time, coping that is either adaptive or maladaptive occurs, and the degree of adaptiveness has a long-lasting impact on physical, psychological, and interpersonal functioning.

History and General Characteristics
of Crisis Theory

Crisis theory has developed primarily in the past 20 years, evolving from a number of sources, the most important of which are psychoanalysis and sociology. It may surprise the reader that psychoanalytic theory is included as one of the substrates of crisis theory, since it has previously been noted that some aspects of that theory, particularly that of the repetition compulsion, suggest that events of adult life may be no more than the results of predispositions derived from childhood.[27] However, Freud was clearly aware of the importance of life events. He warned against taking sides in the "unnecessary dispute whether neuroses were exogeneous or endogenous illnesses," that is, whether they were the results of life experiences or "whether the person would have fallen ill in any case, whatever they had experienced . . . "[34]

The psychoanalytic roots of crisis theory also include Erikson's concept of developmental crises.[35] He described various stages characteristic of the life span from birth to death, each of which is marked by what he termed an emotional crisis. How an individual deals with one stage significantly influences the way in which subsequent ones will be dealt with. Some of the stages or crises occur in childhood and are similar to Freud's psychosexual stages, whereas others relate to adolescence and adult life. Erikson discussed the conflicts and tasks of each crisis and described adaptive or maladaptive alternative solutions. For example, in young adulthood the ultimate outcome may be intimacy or isolation, whereas in adolescence it may be identity or role diffusion. As will be seen, our concept of crisis differs from that of Erikson. However, his theory is crucial to the understanding of the concept that psychological crises constitute turning points with the potential for adaptational failure or continued growth. What Lindemann described in regard to a single life event, bereavement, Erikson conceptualized in relation to stages of normal living.

Sociological theory contributed the concept of social role,[36] which is the expectation that an individual carry out roles defined by society. When there is a sudden or major change in social role, a crisis may ensue. As an example, from a sociological standpoint, separation and divorce are seen as the change from a spouse role to a former spouse role and possibly that of a single parent. Crises occur during the process of this rearrangement of social roles.

Caplan[37] defined crisis as being provoked when "a person faces an obstacle to important life goals that is for a time insurmountable through the utilization of customary methods of problem solving. A period of disorganization ensues, a period of upset, during which many different abortive attempts at a solution are made. Eventually some kind of adaptation is achieved, which may or may not be in the best interests of that person or his fellows."[37] In other words, each crisis state has inherent within it a potential for resolution for better or for worse. It has been noted in this connection that the Chinese character for crisis combines the pictograph for "danger" with that for "opportunity." Along the same lines, the German philosopher Friedrich Nietzsche said, "What does not kill you, will make you stronger." Or, as Benjamin Franklin put it, "Crosses and losses make us stronger and wiser."

More detailed discussions of crisis theory will be found in the work of Caplan,[37] Harris et al.,[38] Jacobson,[39-41] Kalis,[42] Langsley and Kaplan,[43] and Morley and Brown.[44]

The Crisis State

The crisis framework enables us to think about the psychological processes that intervene between a life event and its eventual outcome. This sequence is outlined in Figure 2-1.

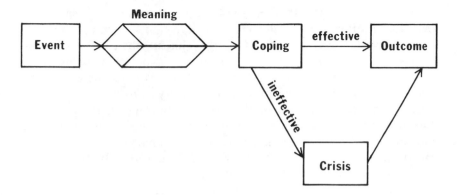

Figure 2-1. Variables intervening between events and outcome. Meaning is depicted as a prism because it determines the manner in which an event is perceived. (Adapted from Figure 55-1 in Jacobson GF: Programs and techniques of crisis intervention, in Arieti S (Ed): American Handbook of Psychiatry, vol 2 (ed 2). New York, Basic Books, Reproduced by permission. The diagram was originally based on Hill R: Generic features of families under stress. Social Casework, Nos. 2 and 3, 1958.)

THE EVENT

Unlike the work reviewed in the preceding section, crisis theorists do not use a specific list of life events. To understand this further, the types of populations whose crises are studied must be further described. There are two major kinds of studies. The first of these deals with homogeneous groups of people who have undergone a similar life experience. Lindemann's bereavement study is an example. Other events that have been studied in this framework include premature birth,[45] and engagement and marriage.[46] Since this type of research looks at each event and its sequellae in considerable depth, it has not yet been possible to study more than a few occurrences.

While this approach is limited to the intensive examination of homogeneous subgroups, others have used crisis theory to understand applicants to a walk-in clinic—a very heterogeneous group. This has been the approach at the Benjamin Rush Center in Los Angeles (see Chapter 1), where the study sample of the research described in this book was collected.

Any occurrence that has caused someone to ask for help urgently enough to come to a walk-in clinic is considered, by definition, an event that has precipitated a crisis. Details of the techniques of crisis intervention are beyond the scope of this book; suffice it to say, however, that it often requires detective work to find the life changes that have resulted in the application for help. This may be true because the events are painful and there is a tendency to avoid recognizing or revealing them. Furthermore, occurrences that took place the day or two before application for help may seem relatively trivial, but a major life event of the type appearing on the Holmes and Rahe[5] or Paykel et al.[12] lists has occurred a few weeks to a few months earlier. This is because the person used some emergency coping mechanism to deal with the initial trauma, which was effective for a period of time but then broke down as a result of a relatively minor matter that had a "last straw" effect. For instance, a patient came to the Benjamin Rush Clinic for help several weeks after a marital separation that had caused seemingly little disturbance. Immediately before going into crisis, however, he had gone to see the attorney, who was a friend of his wife's but whom both he and his wife had retained. He found to his surprise that the attorney was vigorously representing his wife's interests and not his own. This discovery shattered his fantasy that he could divorce his wife and still maintain a friendly relationship and, as gradually emerged on the basis of further material, that he could in fact be divorced and yet not have his relationship with his wife change too profoundly. This fantasy represented the emergency coping, which had become impossible to maintain, and he went into crisis as a result. Crisis theory applied in this type of setting refers to a series of events in a time line going back weeks, months, and sometimes years and culminating in the crisis.

THE MEANING OF THE EVENT

I will next address the prism ("meaning") in Figure 2-1. The meaning of a life event is unique to the person experiencing it. It is determined on the one hand by past history and on the other by the context of the current life situation. The death of a spouse for example may have none, one, or several of the following meanings: recapitulation of the death of or the separation from a parent; current loss of emotional support, of sexual gratification, of financial security, or of participation in a sado-masochistic exchange; or relief from the burden of a long illness or freedom to live with another partner. It is clear that knowing the event alone without knowing its emotional significance for the individual does not provide sufficient understanding. Unconscious fantasies also play a major part in determing this meaning. The life event together with its significance is usually termed the "hazard."

COPING

Coping is defined here in a particular way. It includes but is not limited to the usual intrapsychic defense mechanisms such as denial, repression, projection, and displacement. In addition, coping designates ways of behavior that are intended to diminish anxiety, such as seeking emotional support from a new person, drinking or taking drugs, or efforts to change a difficult reality situation to a more pleasant one. I would like to emphasize that coping as used here can be either adaptive or maladaptive. A crisis will be avoided when coping of either kind is sufficient to deal with the situation. When coping is effective, the outcome occurs without an intervening crisis, whether this outcome is desirable for the person's mental health or not (Figure 2-1). To repeat: avoidance of a crisis is not necessarily desirable, nor, conversely, is a crisis in and of itself undesirable.

CRISIS

If coping is not effective, a crisis ensues. Characterized by a state of acute, time-limited disorganization and upset, a crisis involves anxiety, usually depression, and rapidly alternating coping mechanisms. It usually occurs in the context of low self-esteem.

The psychoanalytic concept of regression may help clarify the term *crisis*. Regression literally means going backward. It is used here in the sense of reliving childhood experiences and conflict. This process, though not usually conscious, may be inferred by the trained observer on the basis of behavior more appropriate to childhood than to the present and by the same methods used for identifying conscious processes, such as reports of dreams, slips (of the tongue and otherwise) and, when available, free association. Regression can to a significant extent be made conscious through interpretation.

At the outset of a crisis, the individual is unable to cope with a current reality problem. A common response is regression to childhood patterns. In a defensive maneuver, the regression temporarily diverts attention from the difficult current issue. There is the danger, however, of a vicious circle. The current difficulties recede into the background and regression reactivates unresolved earlier conflicts. This sequence, rather than solving the present difficulty, makes its solution more difficult. For example, a bereavement or a divorce may be experienced as if it were an early traumatic separation that left the person in a state of helplessness and impotent rage. Under these circumstances, further maladaptive coping such as lashing out, withdrawal, and for some, psychotic decompensation or suicidal thoughts or actions may ensue.

On the other hand, adaptive resolution is entirely possible and in fact occurs frequently. With suitable support, possibly on the part of mental health professionals, the regression runs its course and terminates, and appropriate attention is again focused on solving the present dilemma. For some people, an even more rewarding development occurs: As a result of the crisis and the subsequent regression, new light is shed on the earlier conflict and progress in working through of these childhood conflicts may be made. This is qualitatively similar to what occurs in psychoanalytic therapy. In both, the reliving of childhood conflicts, whether generated by life—as in crises—or by the analysis, affords an opportunity for a new and better resolution. The person has a second chance to deal with old problems.

Crises as defined here do not last more than four to six weeks and then end spontaneously. They should not be confused with some seemingly chaotic life-styles characteristic of some people over long periods of time, perhaps for their entire lives. In observing such people closely, one finds that these apparently disjointed life-styles are actually quite consistent and follow a predictable pattern. They represent stable, though unusually maladaptive, coping styles. Persons with these styles are likely to precipitate crises in others without being in crisis themselves. True crisis, with its acute disorganization, cannot and does not go on indefinitely.

While crises invariably end, it has already been made clear that there is no such invariability as to outcome. Depending upon whether

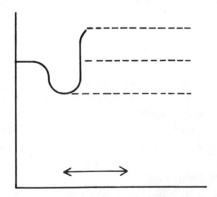

Figure 2-2.   The vertical axis represents the level of mental health, and the horizontal axis represents time. The dip reflects the lowering of functioning during the acute phase of the crisis. At the end of the crisis, adaptation may be at a lower level, higher level, or the same level as before the crisis began.

or not the outcome is adaptive, a crisis may result in functioning at a higher or lower level than before. An analogy may be made to the medical concept of a "crisis" in pneumonia, particularly before the days of antibiotics. At a given point in the illness, there was a period during which the patient was very ill and thereafter either recovered or died. Similarly, nature ends psychological crises after a limited period of time, but whether the result is for better or worse is not predictable. The possible outcomes of crises can be diagrammed in Figure 2-2.

The Crisis Matrix

When discussing life events, the time periods most frequently referred to are six months, one year, and two years. In relation to crises, the relevant time element is the length of the crisis, which is six weeks. Both time frames are based on sound theoretical considerations and on observation. On the one hand, it is both expected and true that major life changes such as divorce or bereavement have an impact lasting from several months to several years. At the same time, it is also true that the time elapsing between the occurrence of a clearly defined hazard and the restoration of a new level of equilibrium is no more than four to six weeks. It is therefore necessary to develop a concept that will bridge these findings. I have previously proposed[47] the concept of a crisis matrix to serve this unifying purpose. A crisis matrix is a period of several months to several years, during which an individual is particularly prone to experiencing several crises of the six-week type. Marital separation and divorce is such a crisis matrix and the multiple crises referred to in the title of this book are contained within this crisis matrix. When looked at in this way, the major life change, in our instance divorce, constitutes not a single occurrence, but a series of occurrences that are clustered in accordance with a common guiding principle but that have separate and unique characteristics.

Using this concept, each of the crises described by Erikson can be considered as a crisis matrix. For example; as a young person passes through adolescence we do not observe a single and uninterrupted period of turmoil, continuing at one level of intensity. Rather, we see briefer periods of crisis occurring in relation to a variety of life events, such as the onset of menses, the forming and dissolution of relationships with boy and girl friends, changes of school, problems in school, and often changes involving the parents, which might include marital separation and divorce. Little or no disturbance may occur between these points. What links these various potential crises is the special vulnerability that the adolescent has as a result of more prolonged and slower changes having biological, psychological, and social facets.

Bereavement seems to be an excellent example of an event that constitutes a single occurrence with a clear onset, namely, the death of an important person. On closer examination, however, bereavement can be considered a crisis matrix. Except in instances of sudden death, there is a more or less prolonged period of terminal illness, with potential crises relating to worsening of the illness. The death itself ushers in the six-week type of crisis so well described by Lindemann.[33] Numerous potential hazards remain, however, including settling the estate, moving, going to work, establishing new social and sexual relationships, and dealing with the adverse effects of the death on important relationships. The longer-term grief work goes on while several shorter crises are experienced. Each new hazard is another reminder of the bereavement. This reminder is painful and at the same time represents an opportunity to work through the loss in yet another context. The grief work is therefore an attribute of the crisis matrix. Another potential crisis matrix might be pregnancy. Crises may occur around diagnosis of pregnancy, change in or cessation of sexual activity, change in or termination of work or social patterns, childbirth itself, leaving the hospital, resumption of sexual activity, returning to work, and specific changes in living patterns or in the marital relationship. Other examples of a crisis matrices are retirement, change of occupation, or relocation to a different area, particularly in a different country. The crisis matrix of separation and/or divorce constitutes the subject matter for most of the remainder of this book and so will not be further detailed at this point.

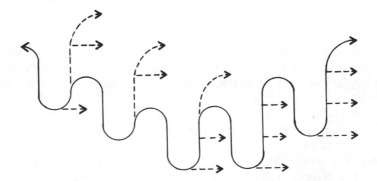

Figure 2-3.   Crisis matrix showing return to original level of functioning.

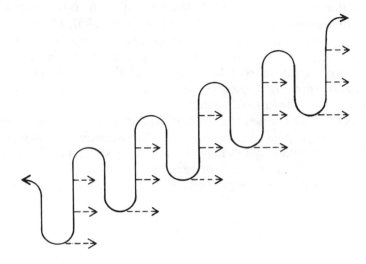

Figure 2-4.   Crisis matrix showing increase in level of functioning.

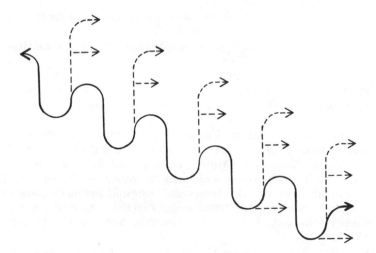

Figure 2-5.   Crisis matrix showing decrease in level of functioning.

Just as each crisis represents both danger and opportunity, the same is true of a crisis matrix. Each crisis within the crisis matrix has the previously described characteristics: it may result in a level of functioning that is lower, the same, or higher than that existing before the onset. Figures 2-3, 2-4, and 2-5 apply this concept to the crisis matrix. Each shows a crisis matrix consisting of five crises. In all diagrams the solid line represents the assumed actual outcome; the dotted lines are the alternative outcomes of each crisis.

It is clear, of course, that an endless combination of outcomes in multiple crises is possible. The manner of diagramming a crisis matrix should not be understood to mean that the only shifts during crises do occur in an upward or downward direction. More gradual movement is indeed common, but the largest and most dramatic changes occur during crises.

REFERENCES

1. Brown GW: Meaning measurement and stress of life events, in Dohrenwend BS, Dohrenwend BP (Eds): Stressfull Life Events: Their Nature and Effects. New York, John Wiley and Sons, 1974, pp 217–243
2. Tichener JL, Kapp FT: Family and character change at Buffalo Creek. Am J Psychiatry 133: 295–299, 1976
3. Stern GM: From chaos to responsibility. Am J Psychiatry 133:300–301, 1976
4. Dohrenwend BP: Sociocultural and social-psychological factors in the genesis of mental disorders. J Health Soc Behav 16:365–492, 1975
5. Holmes TR, Rahe RH: The social readjustment rating scale. J Psychosom Res 11:213–218, 1967
6. Holmes TH, Masada M: Life change and illness susceptibility, in Dohrenwend BS, Dohrenwend BP (Eds): Stressful Life Events: Their Nature and Effects. New York, John Wiley and Sons, 1974, pp 45–72
7. Rahe RH: The pathway between subjects' recent life changes and their near-future illness reports: Representative results and methodological issues, in Dohrenwend BS, Dohrenwend BP (Eds): Stressful Life Events: Their Nature and Effects. New York, John Wiley and Sons, 1974, pp 73–86
8. Rahe RH, Flistad I, Bergen T, et al: A model for life changes and illness research. Arch Gen Psychiatry 31:172–177, 1974
9. Myers JK, Lindenthal JJ, Pepper MP: Life events, social integration and psychiatric symptomatology. J Health Soc Behav 16:421–429, 1975
10. Paykel ES, Prusoff BA, Uhlenhuth EH: Scaling of life events. Arch Gen Psychiatry 25:342–347, 1971

11. Paykel ES: Life stress in psychiatric disorder: Applications of the clinical approach, in Dohrenwend BS, Dohrenwend BP (Eds): Stressful Life Events: Their Nature and Effects. New York, John Wiley and Sons, 1974, pp 135–150

12. Paykel ES, Prusoff BA, Myers JK: Suicide attempts and recent life events. Arch Gen Psychiatry 32:327–333, 1975

13. Dohrenwend BS, Dohrenwend BP: Stressful life events: Research issues, in Jacobson GF (Ed): New Directions in Mental Health Services. Crisis Intervention in the 1980s. San Francisco, Jossey Bass, 1980, pp 57–65

14. Rahe RH: Life crisis and health change, in May PRA, Wittenborn GR (Eds): Psychotropic Drug Response: Advances in Predictions. Springfield, Il, Charles C. Thomas, 1969, pp 92–125

15. Rahe RH, Mahan JL, Arthur RJ: Prediction of near-future health changes from subjects' preceding life changes. J Psychosom Res 14:401–406, 1970

16. Rahe RH, Bennett L, Romo M, et al: Subjects' recent life changes and coronary heart disease in Finland. Am J Psychiatry 130:1222–1226, 1973

17. Cline DW, Chosy JJ: A prospective study of life changes and subsequent health changes. Arch Gen Psychiatry 72:51–53, 1972

18. Heisel JS: Life changes as etiologic factors in juvenile rheumatoid arthritis. J Psychosom Res 16:411–420, 1972

19. Popkin MK, Stillner L, Pierce CM, et al: Recent life changes and outcome of prolonged competitive stress. J Nerv Ment Dis 163:302–306, 1976

20. Hudgens RW: Personal catastrophy and depression: A consideration of the subject with respect to medically ill adolescents, and a requiem for restrospective life-events studies, in Dohrenwend BS, Dohrenwend BP (Eds): Stressful Life Events: Their Nature and Effects. New York, John Wiley and Sons, 1974, pp 119–134

21. Jacobs S, Myers J: Recent life events and acute schizophrenic psychosis: A controlled study. J Nerv Ment Dis 162:75–87, 1976

22. Donovan JM, Dressler DM, Geller RA: Psychiatric crisis: Comparison of schizophrenic and non-schizophrenic patients. J Nerv Ment Dis 161:172–179, 1975

23. Schwartz CD, Myers JK: Life events and schizophrenia. II. Impact of life events on symptoms configuration. Arch Gen Psychiatry 34:1242–1245, 1977B

24. Schwartz CD, Myers JK: Life events and schizophrenia. I. Comparison and schizophrenics with a community sample. Arch Gen Psychiatry 34:1238–1241, 1977A

25. Mueller DP, Edwards DW, Yarvis RM: Stressful life events and psychiatric symptomatology: Change or undesirability? J Health Soc Behav 18:307–317, 1977

26. Antonovsky A: Conceptual and methodologic problems in the study of resistance resources and stressful life events, in Dohrenwend BS, Dohrenwend BP (Eds): Stressful Life Events: Their Nature and Effects. New York, John Wiley and Sons, 1974, pp 245–258

27. Freud S: Standard Edition of the Complete Psychological Work of Sigmund Freud, vol 18. London, Hogarth Press, 1955, p 21

28. Dressler DM, Donovan JM, Geller RA: Life stress and emotional crisis: The idiosyncratic interpretation of life events. Compr Psychiatry 17:549–558, 1976

29. Pokorny AD, Kaplan HB: Suicide following psychiatric hospitalization. The interaction affects of defenselessness and adverse life events. J Nerv Ment Dis 162:119–125, 1976

30. Overall JE, Gorham DR: The brief psychiatric rating scale. Psychol Rep 10:799–812, 1962

31. Kaplan HB: Self-derogation and adjustment of recent life experiences. Arch Gen Psychiatry 22:324–347, 1970

32. Birley JLT, Brown GW: Crises and life changes preceding the onset of relapse of acute schizophrenia: Clinical aspects. Br J Psychiatry 116:327–333, 1970

33. Lindemann E: Symptomatology and management of acute grief. Am J Psychiatry 101:141–148, 1944

34. Freud S: Standard Edition of the Complete Psychological Work of Sigmund Freud, vol 16. London, Hogarth Press, 1963, pp 346–347

35. Erikson E: Identity and the life cycle. Psychol Issues 1:1, 1959

36. Johnson HM: Sociology: A Systematic Introduction. New York, Harcourt, Brace, 1960, pp 16–19

37. Caplan G: An Approach to Community Mental Health. New York, Grune & Stratton, 1961, p 18

38. Harris MR, Kalis BL, Freeman EH: Precipitating stress: An approach to brief therapy. Am J Psychother 17:465–471, 1963

39. Jacobson GF: Crisis theory and treatment strategy: Some socio-cultural and psychodynamic considerations. J Nerv Ment Dis 141:2, 1965

40. Jacobson GF: Crisis oriented therapy, in Sloane BR, Staples FR (Eds): Proceedings of the Symposium on Brief Psychotherapy. Psychiatr Clin North Am, vol 2: pp 39–54, April 1979

41. Jacobson GF: Crisis theory, in Jacobson GF (Ed): New Directions for Mental Health Services. Crisis Intervention in the 1980s. San Francisco, Jossey Bass, 1980, pp 1–10

42. Kalis BL: Crisis theory: Its relevance for community psychology and directions for development, in Adelson D and Kalis BL (Eds): Community Psychology and Mental Health: Perspectives and Challenges. Scranton, Pa, Chandler, 1970

43. Langsley DG, Kaplan D: The Treatment of Families in Crisis. New York, Grune & Stratton, 1968, 1–15

44. Morley WE, Brown VB: The crisis-intervention group: A natural mating or a marriage of convenience? Psychotherapy: Theory, Research and Practice 6:1, 1969

45. Kaplan D: Study and treatment of an acute emotional disorder. Am J Orthopsychiatry 35:69–77, 1964

46. Rapoport R, Rapoport RN: New light on the honeymoon. Hum Relations 17:33–56, 1964

47. Jacobson GF, Portuges SH: An investigation of marital separation and divorce life crisis and its relation to suicide: Concepts, rationale and pilot study (unpublished paper, 1974).

3

Separation, Divorce, and the Failing Marriage: General Considerations

Marriage and divorce rates have been rising substantially since 1960. Between then and 1980 (provisional rate), the rate of divorce in the United States has risen from 2.2 to 5.3 per 1000 population, an increase of 241 percent.[1] There are indications that divorce increased at a less rapid rate in the second half of the 1970s than in the previous decade: The rate doubled between 1966 and 1976, rising from 2.5 to 5.0 per 1000 population, but between 1976 and 1980 the rate rose only from 5.0 to 5.3. The provisional rate nationally for 1980 is 5.3, the same as that for 1979. Even so, there were an estimated 1,182,000 divorces reported for 1980, a record high. Glick and Norton in 1973[2] projected that eventually 25 to 29 percent of young women in their late twenties and early thirties were likely to end their first marriage in divorce. Besides the increases in total numbers, there are also important qualitative changes in the kinds of people who become separated and divorced compared to the past. For example, there is an increase in divorce among the better educated and more affluent. As is true of many social problems, the amount of attention paid to the issue by concerned professionals and the general public increases in direct proportion to the extent to which the problem becomes associated with the middle and upper social classes.

For these reasons, there has been a rapid increase in the popular and scientific literature on the subject of marital separation and divorce in recent years. This increased concern, taken as a whole, has a constructive effect: it catalyzes the formation of new attitudes and value judgments, and tends to bring about new definitions of social role and conduct applicable to the divorced. Such a development is beneficial, since the absence of socially accepted guidelines represents one of the most difficult problems for the separated and divorced. Our society is currently engaged in the modification of the social institutions of marriage and the family to provide new ground rules for marital separation and divorce and, in many instances, remarriage.

Marital separation and divorce cannot be explained solely on the basis of either individual or social pathology. Pathology may indeed play a role in some cases, and this question is discussed further in Chapter 11 and Appendix II. Separation and divorce, however, occur to a cross–section of people differing widely in their psychological and social assets and limitations. It is therefore not meaningful to explicate it solely or mainly as "sick" behavior. Furthermore, without needing to assume any preexisting sickness, the divorce process requires a profound readjustment that in many instances produces a picture indistinguishable from that of more deep-seated psychopathology.

Separation and divorce are of interest to psychiatrists and other mental health professionals for several reasons. First, as members of and leaders in society, they are expected to be informed and knowledgeable about major social trends. Second, the distress of marital separation and divorce is a common reason for consulting a mental health specialist. Understanding the phenomena specific to this process helps the professional distinguish them from pathology of other origins and increases the potential for effective treatment.

This chapter will deal with four topics: (1) the number of separated and divorced people; (2) the length of separation and divorce and its importance for mental health; (3) demographic and socioeconomic characteristics of individuals most likely to be divorced, which are discussed not to recite dry statistics but to draw some tentative conclusions about the reasons why some persons are more likely to undergo marital dissolution than others; (4) some aspects of the failing marriage and of those who are or will at some point become the "formerly married."[3]

THE NUMBER OF SEPARATED AND DIVORCED

In part because we are experiencing rapid changes in divorce rates, there are some limitations in the reporting of both vital and census statistics.[4] The data available can give us a reasonable approximation of the real situation, but they should not be viewed as invariably precise. It is interesting to note that such a seemingly obvious datum as whether or not a person is currently married is not consistently reported by identical respondents on successive occasions, and an even greater margin of error exists in reporting one's own status as either separated or divorced.[4] Perhaps the emotionally charged nature of this question introduces some inaccuracies. In any event, research in the divorce area must take into account the fact that marital separation status cannot be defined without ambiguity in each instance. We do know enough, however, to obtain an overview of the characteristics of the separated and divorced.

Recent publications reflect the continuing increase in the number of separated and divorced. In March 1976, U.S. Bureau of Census figures quoted by Hunt and Hunt[5] put the total number of separated and divorced persons in the United States at 10,960,000, of whom 3,771,000 were separated and 7,189,000 were divorced. Two years prior, there were 5,944,976 divorced and 3,446,188 separated persons in the United States, or a total of 9,391,164.[4] The separated then accounted for 1.5 percent of U.S. males 14 years and over and for 2.7 percent of females. The divorced represented 3.1 percent of men and 4.4 percent of women.

If the sets of figures for 1974 and 1976 are comparable, the number of separated and divorced increased by 16.7 percent between 1974 and 1976. In both years, there were significantly more women than men in both the separated and divorced groups. In 1974, there were 2,220,588 separated women compared to 1,125,600 men, while divorced women outnumbered divorced men by 3,618,736 to 2,326,240. The combined totals were 5,839,324 separated and divorced women compared to 3,451,840 men. In other words, approximately twice as many women as men (197 percent) were separated at the same point in time in 1974, and somewhat more than one-and-a-half times as many (156 percent) were divorced; there were approximately 70 percent more women than men (169 percent) in the combined categories. Similar relationships prevailed in 1976, when 65 percent more women than men were separated and divorced. According to Glick,[6] the most likely explanation of the greater number of separated women than men is that some women, especially those with children, will describe themselves as separated when in fact they were never married. An additional possibility is that some men who are in fact separated may be reported as single, especially if they are living with a woman to whom they are not married. The discrepancy between divorced men and women may be due in part to the same factors. We will come back later to other possible reasons for the differential.

Because remarriage is so common, the total number of persons ever divorced is much larger than those divorced at any one time. In 1971, about one in every six women had been divorced at one time or was then divorced.[4] By the mid-1970s, there was for every nine married people one separated or divorced person and three persons who had remarried.[5]

LENGTH OF SEPARATION AND DIVORCE AND ITS IMPORTANCE FOR MENTAL HEALTH

Psychiatrists and related professionals working in the area of marital separation and divorce are, of course, interested in what statistical data can tell us about the total numbers of separated and divorced persons in the population. But also of interest is the possibility that there may be differences in mental health levels depending upon the length of time that has elapsed since the beginning of the separation/divorce process. Seen from the perspective of a lifetime, the entire period of separation and divorce is a transitional one between marriages for most persons: All but one sixth of the men and one fourth of the women eventually remarry.[4] It is possible that there is a difference in the mental health of those in the early phases of the transition from marriage to separation and divorce and those in the later stages, who, as length of time divorced increases, will encompass more and more of those persons who will never remarry.

For this reason we now turn to the available data on the averages and ranges of duration of separation and divorce. Although this information is still incomplete, it is to be hoped that it will be collected more extensively in the future. One set of data deals with the relationship of the separated to the divorced. The former group, virtually by definition, are in an interim phase of their marital lives, although in rare instances the separated status becomes permanent without divorce ever occurring. As noted previously, there are more divorced than separated persons in the population at any one time. In 1974, the ratio of divorced to separated persons was 2.07 for men, 1.63 for women, and 1.73 for men and women combined.[4] These figures suggest that women tend to remain separated longer than men—a situation perhaps related to their lower probability of remarriage. There has been a trend, however, toward an increase in women who proceed toward divorce: Between 1960 and 1974, while the number of separated women increased by 35 percent, the number of divorced women grew by 52 percent.[4] Carter and Glick interpreted this to mean that more couples are ending their marriage completely, "rather than lingering in a state of separation."[4] Two years later, in 1976, the ratio of divorced to separated of both sexes had risen further to 1.91, indicating that almost twice as many formerly married were divorced than were separated.[5] In recent years, in at least some parts of the country, the ratio of divorced to separated has continued to increase sharply. The Los Angeles County Department of Health Services[7] reports in data used for 1977–1978 planning that the ratio of divorced to separated in the western portion (coastal region) of Los Angeles County is 3.05 for men and 4.46 for women. These figures represent not only a sharp increase of the divorce/separation ratio over the earlier national figures, but also a reversal of the findings regarding women and men: women now have the higher ratio.[7]

We next turn to the length of separation before divorce. Generally, the divorcing couple separates before filing for the divorce. With very few exceptions, they separate when the decree becomes final. Carter and Glick[4] reported that among persons who become divorced 71 percent separate one year or less prior to the divorce, and 12 percent are separated for two years before divorcing. While the median separation lasts 0.7 years prior to divorce, only 2.4 percent are separated 10 years or more before divorce; a small but unknown number remain separated for the remainder of their lives without reconciling or divorcing.

The duration of divorce is shown in Table 3-1. It can be seen that for those persons who do remarry, the median length of the divorce is three years. A more precise approach to the average number of years that have elapsed since divorce may be found in the June 1975 Current Population Reports published by the U.S. Bureau of the Census.[8] This information is available for women 14 to 75 years old. The total number of divorced women surveyed in June 1975 was 3,083,000. The number of years that elapsed between the divorce and the report is shown in Table 3-2. The median number of years elapsed since divorce was 4.7.

Table 3-1
Median Intervals (in Years)

	Men	Women
Between first marriage and divorce	6.7	7.3
Between divorce and remarriage	3.1	3.2
Between remarriage and redivorce	5.1	5.5

From Glick PC, Norton AJ: Marrying, Divorcing, and Living Together in the U.S. Today. Population Bulletin 32(5):8. Reprinted courtesy of the Population Reference Bureau, Inc., Washington, DC, 1977.

Table 3-2
Years Elapsed Since Divorce

Years Since Divorce	Women (%)
0–1	26.7
2–3	18.5
4–5	12.9
6–7	8.5
8–9	5.3
10–14	11.1
15 or more	17.0

Data from Current Population Reports 1977.[8] The data include only women who were divorced at the time of the survey.

For women 14 to 29 years of age, the median was 3.4 elapsed years. For ages 30 to 39 it was 5.8 years, and for ages 40 to 75 it was 6.5 years.[8]

With this information at hand, it should be possible to analyze divorced persons admitted to mental health facilities to determine whether the average length of their time divorced coincides with or differs from national data. Naturally, any such comparison would be an approximation, so long as we do not have a national sample for comparison that was drawn in the same year as the census data. At least in principle, however, we should be able to add a classification by length of time divorced to our customary analysis of marital status for admissions to psychiatric hospitals and other facilities. Such an analysis will provide valuable information on whether the newly or long-term divorced are at greater risk of becoming psychiatric casualties or whether indeed the liability of each subgroup to be admitted to a mental health facility is the same.

DEMOGRAPHIC AND SOCIOECONOMIC CHARACTERISTICS OF THE SEPARATED AND DIVORCED

Sex and Age

One important fact that is not immediately evident is that there are far more separated and divorced women than men. In 1976, the figures stood at 6,826,000 women and 4,138,000 men, a ratio of about 5 to 3.[5]

Since more divorced men eventually remarry than do women, more divorced men marry women who were never married than divorced women marry never-married men. In some instances, a man may marry and divorce two or more women. In addition, mortality rates are higher for men than women in the older age groups, which accounts for more women than men remaining in the divorced state for more extended periods.

There is considerable information regarding the ages of the formerly married. The average age at divorce is decreasing: In 1971 it was estimated to be 29 or 30 years for women born between 1930 and 1934, compared to age 33 for women born between 1900 and 1914; in 1960–1962 the median age of the husband at divorce was about 34 years and the wife 31 years. However, one fourth of all divorced women were over 40 years of age and one fourth of divorced men were over 44 years old.

Hunt and Hunt[5] stated that there is, contrary to popular belief, no current divorce boom in middle age; divorces in that period increase simply because of the overall increase in divorce. However, Plateris[9] reported that divorces are increasing for longer-married persons. For example, of persons married in 1950, 3.9 percent were divorced at a marriage interval of 10 to 14 years, but for those married in 1960 the corresponding figure was 7.7 percent—close to twice as many.

Another way of looking at this issue is to consider the age of those separated or divorced at any one point in time. In 1974, men and women separated and divorced clustered in the age group 25 to 54, with a peak in the 35 to 44 range. In this group, 2.4 percent of the men were separated and 4.7 percent were divorced; among women the rates were 4.7 percent separated and 6.9 percent divorced.[4]

Ethnicity, Education, and Income

Ethnicity, income, and education and the related variable of social class have long been known to be clearly associated with health and general well-being in the physical as well as the psychological spheres.[10-15] This association raises the important question of the extent to which the relationship of separation and divorce to psychological disability is in turn related to the high proportion of financially and educationally disadvantaged among those dissolving their marriages.

Ethnicity (race) is a major factor in determining who will separate or divorce. The chances of being separated or divorced are far greater for the Hispanic and black population than for non-Hispanic whites. In June 1971, the percentage of all black women born in 1930 to 1934

known to have ever been divorced was 24.3, while for the corresponding group of white women it was 16.7.[4] Similarly in 1970, 83.6 percent of
non-Hispanic white women 35 to 44 years old were married with husband present, for 3.5 percent the husband was absent, 2.5 percent were
widowed, and 5.1 percent were divorced. The remainder were never
married. For black women of the same age group, 58.5 percent were
married with husband present, 17.6 percent reported husband absent,
6.6 percent were widowed, and 8.3 percent were divorced. The proportions for Hispanic women in five southwestern states were 77.9 percent married with husband present, 6.5 percent husband absent, 3.1
percent widowed, and 6.0 percent divorced.[4]

The relationship between divorce and educational level is an interesting one. Persons who are "high school dropouts" (having completed
9 to 11 years of schooling) have the greatest likelihood of divorce. The
rate drops for high school graduates, rises again for college dropouts,
and falls for college graduates. For women but not for men, and most
clearly for black women, there is another rise for those who have one
or more years of postgraduate education. In general, the highest rates
are for those who did not complete high school. Carter and Glick linked
this finding to personality and to experiences that cause a person to
complete a broad level of school. Carter and Glick felt that these factors also "tend to have a significant bearing on the chance that the
marriage . . . will last."[4]

As with education, there are significant relationships between income and divorce. For white men ages 25 to 44, the chance of ever
having been divorced becomes successively smaller at each higher level of income. Strikingly, however, for white women the opposite is
true: the higher the woman's income, the greater the likelihood of her
having been divorced. The relation is linear in both cases but in the
opposite direction. A man 35 to 44 years old without income in 1970
was three times as likely to have been divorced as his relatively affluent counterpart earning $20,000 or more. But a woman earning $15,000
and more (the highest level reported in the 1970 census) is three times
as likely to be divorced than is a woman without her own income.[4]

Income patterns differ between blacks and whites in several aspects: (1) There is less variation among income levels. (2) The largest
proportions ever divorced occur both at the highest and at the lowest
income levels. (3) When incomes for white and black men are compared, the higher the income the higher the divorce rate for blacks. The
reverse is true for women, however: The higher the income, the lower
the rate of divorce compared to whites. There is a tendency to divorce
more frequently among *affluent* black men and *poor* black women

than compared to whites with similar incomes. The highest rates overall in this group were for white women earning maximum income, and
the lowest rates were for white women with no income.

The reasons for these relationships are not clear, but some possibilities may be considered. Carter and Glick[4] believe that families with
relatively few worries about providing material necessities have more
freedom to tackle other problems. This is no doubt an important factor.
Grinding anxiety about financial matters strains all personal relationships, particularly those in a marriage. But this explanation addresses
neither the reverse association of income and divorce for women nor
the findings for blacks. Some other factors may therefore be considered: It is possible that marriages among whites in which the man has a
relatively high income and which available data suggest are rather stable, are those in which husband and wife follow more traditional sex
roles. The husband is the main earner and the wife wholly or in major
part is homemaker and mother. The assumed stability of such marriages may be because they afford a greater degree of satisfaction. It
may also be, in at least some instances, that even if they do not afford
greater satisfaction, the financial price of dissolution is great. A single
income—the man's, typically—will now need to be divided up to support two households and the standard of living of both parties will be
meaningfully changed. Furthermore, the wife after divorce is dependent to a significant extent on the husband's willingness to support her
and her children; that willingness is not always there. Given this, a
couple may tolerate a greater degree of marital stress before breaking
up the marriage than would a couple for whom the material penalties
are smaller.

White households with a low husband's income and/or a high
wife's income are likely to be those in which the financial contribution
of both spouses is closer to equal, and in some instances, the wife earns
more than the husband. In the case of the very low-earning husband,
public support is an important factor; under these circumstances, neither spouse has much to lose materially by divorce. Generally, for
lower-income men, spousal and child support are often minimal to non-
existent, and the working wife may do as well or better on her own. In
instances where the wife has a high income, particularly if the husband
does not, she will not be dependent on her husband's willingness or
ability to support her. It may well be that high-income black men are
married to high-income black or white women and that husband and
wife may therefore be reasonably well off separately.

Psychiatrists and other mental health professionals do not tend to
think often about the impact that such a "crude" consideration as

money has on people's lives. Yet it is essential to be aware of its real importance, not only directly as a source of satisfaction and material comfort but also indirectly as a factor that impacts on life decisions such as those to separate or not to separate. Pointing out that the risk of material loss holds some couples together was not meant to be cynical. Financial interdependence is a powerful emotional force that has links with issues of psychological dependence and independence and with the manner in which these issues have been resolved over the course of a lifetime. If two people married to each other share the same expectations in regard to their respective roles in providing and consuming income, the marriage is more likely to be stable than if they do not. This is true whether the marriage is traditional, or whether both partners contribute to the household. There are, however, usually fewer agreed-upon ways to work out the latter arrangement, and this absence of known patterns may increase the tendency to discrepant expectations, disharmony, and divorce.

Closely related to education and income is social class, which is derived as an index from educational and occupational characteristics. Contrary to a belief that may still linger, divorce is not mainly characteristic of the rich and glamorous. There is, however, some historical reason for this widely held view. Divorce rates in western nations were in fact once higher for high-income marriages.[16] Divorce first became respectable in the highest social classes.[17] In Edith Wharton's novel "Autre Temps," which takes place in the second decade of the 20th century, a woman who had lost her social position as a result of being divorced found that her divorced daughter's standing in society was no longer adversely affected by her divorce. Some time shortly thereafter, however, the association between divorce rates and income became inverted. As Levinger[16] noted, it is likely that greater general and marital unhappiness have always existed among the relatively lower social classes, probably because of the greater stresses of daily living.* When divorce became more readily obtainable and perhaps also when the availability of public financial support for the formerly married wife became greater, this unhappiness was translated into increased divorce rates.

Data from 1970 for men aged 45 to 54 indicate that men with high socioeconomic status (SES) who "had everything going for them" in

---

*There is an alternative explanation that downward drift of persons genetically or psychologically predisposed to malfunction explains the greater instance of various forms of social and psychological problems among the lower social classes. In my view such a process, if it exists, does not completely explain this phenomenon.

regard to education, occupation, and earnings were married in a very high proportion of cases—95 percent for white men and 92 percent for black men.[4] Ten percent of the high SES white men and 22 percent of the high SES black men were known to have been divorced at one time. The corresponding figures for low SES white men and black men are almost identical at 19 percent. The fact that earnings of all men known to have been divorced are higher than those currently divorced indicates that greater earnings are a factor in fostering remarriage.

Other Factors Related to Separation and Divorce

Other factors that have been investigated in regard to their possible association with marital separation and divorce are religion, urban versus rural location, regional location, and whether or not the couple has children.

Contrary to generally held beliefs, according to Hunt and Hunt[5] there is no longer any significant difference in divorce rate among the major American religious groups. They stated that prior to 1960, the Roman Catholic divorce rate was very low, but citing reports from sociologists and public-opinion researchers, concluded that Catholic and Protestant divorce rates are converging. They also indicated that there is no longer a significant difference between the divorce rates of the devout and the non-devout.

Census data cited by Hunt and Hunt[5] show that somewhat smaller percentages of rural and village dwellers than urban dwellers are separated and divorced, but their own survey data and interviews have led them to believe that this may be because suburban and rural people migrated to the city when their marriages began to fail. The data on this point are inconclusive at this time.

There are some variations in separation and divorce rates between different states and regions in the United States. In 1960, the highest percentage of divorced white men was in the north central United States, followed closely by the west. For white women, the west had by far the highest rates.[4] In Los Angeles County, data gathered for the preparation of 1977–1978 mental health plan reported 7.8 percent of the men as separated or divorced, compared to 10.7 percent of the women.[7] According to Hunt and Hunt,[5] in 1975 the divorce rate in Nevada was more than six times as high as that in New Jersey, North Dakota, or Pennsylvania.

In spite of the sometimes-held assumption that children hold marriages together, about 60 percent of all divorcing people in 1973 had children.[5] Childless marriages do have a higher divorce rate, however, particularly in the age group of women 35 to 39 years old.[5]

Summary

The separated and divorced make up a significant and increasing percentage of the population, though there are indications that the rate of increase is slackening. The ratio of divorced to separated persons is rising, indicating a tendency to proceed more rapidly from the separated to the divorced state. Nationally, the average person is separated 0.7 months before divorcing, and the median divorced woman, whether or not she eventually remarries, has been divorced 4.7 years. All but one sixth of men and one fourth of women eventually remarry. There are significantly more women than men separated and divorced, due to the tendency of men to marry single women and to the greater longevity of women. The average age at divorce is around 30 years.

Blacks are significantly more likely to be separated or divorced than are whites. Low-income white men are less likely to remain married than high-income white men, but the reverse is true for white women—the higher the income, the greater the chances for divorce. The average separated or divorced person is somewhat more likely to live in an urban than a rural area, to be found in the western United States, and to be a parent. Neither religious preference nor devoutness appears to affect likelihood of divorce.

All of this information is important to mental health professionals. The relationship of separated and divorced status to various forms of psychiatric symptomatology is generally accepted. A better knowledge of the characteristics of persons who separate and divorce can help us understand whether psychiatric "casualties" are evenly distributed within the separated and divorced population or whether certain segments are more prone to experience difficulties than are others. This issue has been addressed in some detail in relation to the question of possible differences between individuals who have recently entered the separation and divorce process compared to those for whom more time has elapsed. Similar questions have been raised in regard to mental health differentials within the separated and divorced when grouped by age, sex, ethnicity, income, and other characteristics. If differences are found, the reasons for such differentials can be explored, and this understanding may contribute to our therapeutic armamentarium. While demographic characteristics are not the main focus of this book, some of these topics will be further considered.

THE FAILING MARRIAGE

As this is a book about what happens to people after they separate and/or divorce, its main thrust does not deal with the reasons marriages fail, a subject that could easily fill another volume. I will touch very briefly on this subject, however.

The issues in the failing marriage are complex, and no single dominant theory has emerged in the literature. Levinger[16] looked at the matter from the standpoint of the marital dyad. Forces holding together the marriage consist of positive attractions between the partners and barriers against competing attractions to others; forces tending toward dissolution are negative attractions (animosities) between the partners and weak barriers toward alternate attractions. Marriages with strong negative attractions between the partners but strong barriers against other involvements remain intact but as "empty shells."

So-called "causes" of divorce that have been emphasized widely include broad social trends such as the tendency toward younger marriage and the greater acceptability of divorce as an option—in Levinger's[16] terms a lowering of the barriers against marital dissolution. Some authors have raised the question as to what extent the feminist movement has contributed to the increase in divorce rates, but as yet there are no conclusive studies in this area. Economic factors have been touched on. The increase in divorce rates among the relatively poor probably relates to some improvement in their economic situation that has made the dissolution of unhappy marriages possible. Increased earning power for some women enable them to divorce, if they so desire, rather than needing to remain married because of dependence on their husbands.

An interesting approach is taken by Margaret Mead, who related the decrease in monogamous and permanent unions to the decline of the extended family, in which the child's security was safeguarded by many individuals. On the other hand, in the nuclear (couple and children only) family, "each American child learns, early and in terror, that his whole security depends on a single set of parents who, more often than not, are arguing furiously in the next room."[18] The burden on the parent and on the child growing up to be a parent constitutes an excessive strain that many marriages cannot withstand. Extended families, on the other hand, in which many persons share in child-caring tasks, promote greater marital stability, according to Mead.[18]

Remarkably little has been done in the way of systematic studies about the processes involved in the maintenance or deterioration of marriages. The literature of marital counseling does of course contain references to characteristics of good marriages, but it does not delineate the manner in which difficulties proceed stepwise to a solution that either maintains the marriage or results in divorce. What has been described are individual personality traits of either spouse, such as immaturity, alcoholism, or outright mental illness, but their identification does not tell us why some marriages continue in spite of these traits and others do not.

My own approach involves a focus on the gradual changes in mutual satisfaction and dissatisfaction experienced by each partner. There is a process occurring over time in which the ratio of satisfaction to dissatisfaction fluctuates. In direct correspondence, the ratio of loving feelings to angry feelings also fluctuates. There is a certain point of no return that occurs when dissatisfaction and angry feelings persistently outweigh satisfaction and loving feelings. If and when that point is reached, the marriage dissolves or becomes an empty shell.

All of the factors previously described enter into this process: early marriage with little preparation and perhaps magical expectations, alternative options, poverty, and such individual and maladaptive ways of coping, as alcoholism. Sometimes the process of marital estrangement is so slow and insidious that by the time it is identified the marriage has reached the point of no return.

There is another possibility, however. Certain specific changes may occur to alter the balance in what was previously a working marriage. One of these that has received attention in the literature is the serious illness or death of a child. Several contributions have dealt with the impact of cystic fibrosis and related diseases on marriages.[19-21] While there is no consensus, the indications are that serious illness in a child increases the tendency toward divorce in the parents. Similar increases in divorce rates have occurred in parents of children with leukemia.[22-23]

Changes need not be as drastic as the serious illness or death of a child. Any major reverses or successes of either partner may unbalance a previous marital equilibrium. Physical illness in one or both partners may have the same effect. In such instances, emotional demands by one partner on another may increase; blame for the misfortune may be attributed to one or both of the spouses. Although this process never identified as such, it can lead to marital deterioration. Timely intervention that accurately identifies the recent course of events may reestablish a mutually satisfactory marital interaction.

To summarize, societal factors, such as tendencies to early marriage and greater economic choices, interact with interpersonal ones to maintain or terminate a marriage. Ultimately, the fate of the marriage is determined by the extent of satisfaction or dissatisfaction of each partner. This in turn is often influenced by life events that may be extrinsic to the marital pair. In that instance, intervention may change the progression toward marital dissolution.

REFERENCES

1. Monthly Vital Statistics Report, vol 29, no 13. National Center for Health Statistics, US Department of Health and Human Services, Public Health Service, Office of Health Research, Statistics and Technology, 1981
2. Glick PC, Norton AJ: Perspective on the recent upturn in divorce and remarriage. Demography 10:301–314, 1973
3. Hunt M: The World of the Formerly Married. New York, McGraw Hill, 1966
4. Carter H, Glick PC: Marriage and Divorce: A Social and Economic Study. Cambridge and London, Harvard University Press, 1976
5. Hunt M, Hunt B: The Divorce Experience. New York, McGraw Hill, 1977
6. Glick PC: Personal communication, May 1981
7. Los Angeles County Department of Health Services: Plan for Mental Health Services, County of Los Angeles, 1977-78—1977-80. Breakdown of marital status based on all persons 13 years and older. Breakdown between separated and divorced categories by personal communication. Oct. 1978
8. Current Population Reports. U.S. Bureau of the Census, Current Population Reports, Series P-20, No. 312. Marriage, Divorce, Widowhood and Remarriage by Family Characteristics: June 1975. U.S. Government Printing Office, 1977
9. Plateris A: Divorces by marriage cohort, U.S. Department of Health, Education and Welfare, Public Health Service, Office of Health Research, Statistics and Technology, National Center for Health Statistics, Series 21, No. 34, DHEW Publication no. (PHS) 79-7912, 1979
10. Hollingshead AB, Redlich FC: Social Class and Mental Illness: A Community Study. New York, Wiley, 1958
11. Srole L, Langner TS, Michael ST, et al: Mental Health in the Metropolis. New York, McGraw Hill, 1961
12. Langner TS, Michael ST: Life Stress and Mental Health. Toronto, Free Press of Glencoe, Collier-Macmillan Canada, 1963
13. Leighton DC, Harding JS, Macklin DB, et al: The Character of Danger: Stirling County Study #3. New York, Basic Books, 1963
14. Myers JK, Bean LL: A Decade Later: A Follow-up of Social Class and Mental Illness. New York, John Wiley, 1968

15. Ilfeld FW: Psychologic status of community residents along major demographic dimensions. Arch Gen Psychiatry 35:716–724, 1978
16. Levinger G: A social psychological perspective on marital dissolution. J Soc Issues 32:21–47, 1976
17. Bernard J: No news, but new ideas, in Bohannan P (Ed): Divorce and After. New York, Doubleday, 1970, pp 1–29
18. Mead M: Anomalies in American post-divorce relationships, in Bohannon P (Ed): Divorce and After. New York, Doubleday, 1970, pp 107–125
19. Tew BJ, Payne H, Laurence KM: Must a family with a handicapped child be a handicapped family? Med Child Neurol (Supp 32) 16:95–98, 1974
20. Tew BJ, Laurence KM, Payne H, et al: Marital stability following the birth of a child with spina bifida. Br J Psychiatry 131: 79–82, 1977
21. Begleiter ML, Burry UF, Harris DJ: Prevalence of divorce among parents of children with cystic fibrosis and other chronic diseases. Soc Biol 23:261–264, 1976
22. Lansky SB: Childhood leukemia. The child psychiatrist as a member of the oncology team. J Am Acad Child Psychiatry 13:499–508, 1974
23. Lansky, SB quoted in Clin Psychiatry News, April 1978, p 36

4

Mental Health Implications of Divorce or Death of Partner

My treatment of bereavement is based only on a careful study of a limited number of key contributions to the literature and on personal clinical experience working with bereaved patients. Undoubtedly those more expert in the field of bereavement will have justifiable criticism of this exposition. I hope, however, that I have presented the key issues of bereavement with sufficient clarity to lay the groundwork for the concepts used in this volume in discussing marital separation and divorce.

One further note: marital separation and divorce are here defined as including any stage of the process. To avoid repetitive use of this term, "separation," "divorce," "dissolution," and "M.S.D." will all be used interchangeably with "marital separation and divorce," unless otherwise stated.

MENTAL HEALTH AND MARITAL STATUS

There is considerable evidence in the literature that married people are better off in terms of psychological functioning and physical health than those not married. There are also indications that among the unmarried, the never-married are best off, followed by the widowed, divorced, and separated. The evidence has been well summarized by Gove,[1] who used mortality rates in men and women for five conditions he related to psychological factors: suicide, homicide, motor vehicle accidents, cirrhosis of the liver, and lung cancer. The last two are included because of their association with excessive drinking and smoking, which Gove saw as being related to psychological disturbance. In all of these categories, a comparison of the mortality rates of the married and the various subgroups of the unmarried favors the married. The suicide rate, for example, for single women is one-and-a-half times that for married women, for widowed women the rate is more than twice as great, and for the separated and divorced it is the highest—almost three-and-a-half times the married rate. There is no difference in mortality for illnesses not related to psychological or social factors, such as leukemia.

The comparisons within the unmarried group are interesting. Gove[1] did not consider the separated as a separate category and therefore compared only the single, divorced, and widowed. In all cases, the single were better off than those whose marriages had terminated, and in 8 of the 10 categories the divorced were worse off than the widowed.

More recent studies generally confirm that marriage is more conducive to the maintenance of mental health than non-marriage, at least for men, and that the separated and divorced are worse off than the widowed. The place of the never-married in the mental health continuum is less clearly established. Ilfeld surveyed 2299 adult community residents in the Chicago area using the Psychiatric Symptom Index.[2] In general, the married showed the least symptomatology, with increasing symptomatology for the widowed, single, divorced, and separated, respectively. By far the greatest amount of symptomatology was noted in the separated. The significance remains when the data are controlled for sex and age but not for income level. Mellinger et al.[3] reviewed the incidence of high levels of psychic distress in a nationwide sample of 2552 adults. In men, the least distress was found in the married, with distress progressively increasing for the widowed, never-married, and separated or divorced. Theirs was the only study that indicated that among women the married are not best off. Lowest distress was found among the never-married, closely followed by the widowed and the married, with the separated or divorced reporting a much higher distress level than any of the others.

These findings clearly indicate that there are differentials in mental health related to marital status. There are a number of reasons for these differentials, including some related to the protection from psychological distress that the marital state provides, at least for men. Another facet—more directly related to the theme of this book—involves the reaction to the loss of a spouse, either by death or divorce. It is certain that the latter reason plays a role, at least in the early period after the termination of the marriage, and psychological reactions to loss may have long-term effects as well. This is of potential importance regarding the difference between the mental health of the divorced and the widowed, a difference strongly suggested by the evidence just cited. As we shall see, a differential pattern of loss response is one possible explanation for this difference.

In the following sections, therefore, I will discuss various explanations for the differences in mental health between marital status categories, particularly those between the widowed and the divorced. I will treat non-psychological explanations, including biological, sociological, and economic approaches, as well as a model suggesting that differences between the widowed and divorced may be more a function of the time that has elapsed since the end of the marriage than of marital status per se. I then will deal with psychological processes in greater detail, focusing on those related to coping with loss.

MENTAL HEALTH AND MARITAL STATUS
RELATIONSHIPS: NON-PSYCHOLOGICAL
CONSIDERATIONS

The biological viewpoint explains differences between the married and the single by assuming that getting married is a sign of mental health; therefore, mental health is etiologic to marital status, not vice versa. Regarding the differences between the widowed and the divorced, the simplest biological explanation begins with the premise that intentional marital separation and divorce is a symptom of pathology, while bereavement is not.

This viewpoint is held (not necessarily in its extreme form) by some psychoanalysts and some biologically oriented psychiatrists. Earlier psychoanalysts have stated that divorce is caused by unresolved earlier conflicts that must be dealt with in intensive therapy lest the neurotic problems also destroy a later marriage.[4] The biologically oriented viewpoint is exemplified by Briscoe and Smith,[5] who compared a group of divorced and bereaved depressives who were not matched for age and sex. They reported that the bereaved had significantly fewer episodes of depression than the divorced; that the bereaved showed no suicidal ideation, while it was present in 42 percent of the divorced; and that the divorced but not the bereaved tended to consult psychiatrists. Also, they reported significantly more affective illness in the relatives of the divorced than the relatives of the bereaved. Briscoe and Smith interpreted these findings to mean that the divorced more frequently suffer from at least partially biologically determined "depressive disease," whereas bereavement constitutes a separate category, not to be classified as illness. One criticism that can be made of the biological approach is that it does not account for the finding that widowed men consistently show more impairment in psychological health than married men, and that the difference in symptomatology between the widowed and divorced is one only of degree. This is difficult to translate into the assumption that one group has a disease and the other does not.

Gove[1] advanced a sociological explanation based on changes in the individual's position in society. Using the terminology of Parsons,[6] each person has a status that defines his or her position and rights in the social structure and a role that defines activities and obligations in relation to others. Together these make up the "status-role bundle." Marital status is one important component in defining both status and role: to be married involves certain commonly understood rights and obligations, while an entirely different set is characteristic of the widow(er), and still another characterizes the divorced individual. The transition from one status and role to the other is uniformly stressful. This constitutes, from the sociologist's viewpoint, one explanation of why those whose marriages have ended are more disturbed than those who are married. The difference between the single and the married is said by some sociologists to be due to Durkheim's concept of a "coefficient of protection" afforded by marriage.[1] This does not explain, however, why the divorced should be more disturbed than the widowed.

To explain this difference in degree of disturbance, one must assume that role transitions are more easily accomplished by the widow(er) than by the divorced individual. There are some reasons to believe this is so. Because widowhood has always characterized a large proportion of the population, widowhood has been institutionalized in the same manner as marriage has. There are specific patterns of responsibilities and prerogatives that pertain to a widowed person. For example, widow(er)s are frequently active and well accepted in religious groups; they also tend to be clearly defined as members of extended families. Unlike widowhood, marital separation and divorce has until quite recently involved only a very small portion of the total adult population. For this reason, definition of social position has lagged, and what definition there has been is ambiguous. One example of this confusion is found in a film used by Kessler to stimulate discussion groups.[7,8] The film shows a couple going over an invitation list for a social event. While doing so, they discuss a couple that has recently separated and debate whether to invite either the husband or the wife.

In the end they decide to invite neither, since they cannot find an acceptable way of inviting either one. In this instance, there is no social prescription that allows others to relate to the separated or divorced in expected ways.

The absence of a clearly defined role causes a serious strain on the individuals involved. One also can approach this same concept from the standpoint of ego psychology. The ability of the ego to integrate the inner and outer world depends to a significant degree on the availability of external guidelines. In the absence of such guidelines, internal conflicts fail to be resolved adaptively, and symptomatic disturbances, such as anxiety and depression, result.

Another major theory for the differences between marital status categories is the economic one. We have already noted that Ilfeld[2] reported that differences between marital status and psychiatric symptoms remain when the data are controlled for sex and age but not for income level. As a general rule, the married are economically better off than the unmarried, and this is particularly true for the widowed and divorced. (The general issues of the relationship of mental health to social class and income were discussed in Chapter 2.) Chapter 5 addresses this relationship as it emerged in my research, and some work specifically dealing with the relation of class and economic factors to divorce will be cited. For now, it is only necessary to state that economic status makes a contribution to mental health in various marital status categories.

Still another possible explanation for differences between the widowed and divorced has to do with the number of years spent widowed compared to the number of years spent separated or divorced. We have already noted that for most people divorce is not a permanent state, whereas considerably fewer widowed than divorced persons eventually remarry. In a cross-section of adults surveyed in 1970, the proportion of widowed persons who had remarried was only about half as large as that of divorced persons.[9] This difference is not simply a result of age, since it holds true when comparisons are made for the same age group. Clark and Glick[9] believed that their finding "is no doubt related to the fact that many persons obtain a divorce for the purpose of being free to marry someone else, whereas few persons become intentionally widowed in order to remarry!"[9]

It is possible that the separated and divorced as well as the widowed are more disturbed in the first few years after the end of the marriage than they are later on. Since the widowed are likely to remain widowed for a longer time than the divorced are likely to remain divorced, this difference could account for the lower level of disturbance among the widowed. In this model, the real explanation of the difference is the time elapsed since the end of the marriage, regardless of the cause of the dissolution. It is therefore important that future studies of mental health of those whose marriages have ended include as a parameter the length of time elapsed since the end of the marriage.

MENTAL HEALTH AND MARITAL STATUS RELATIONSHIPS: PSYCHOLOGICAL CONSIDERATIONS

As already mentioned, the explanations of the differences between the married and the unmarried groups of the population can be looked at from the standpoint of the protective function of marriage on the one hand and the reaction to loss on the other. When dealing with psychological variables, I will not go into any detail regarding the psychology of marriage but will instead focus on the phenomenon of loss and the processes involved in the adaptation to that loss. This section deals with general considerations on responses to the loss. Specific aspects of response to loss will be separately addressed.

"The uncoupling of associations," wrote Freud in 1895, "is always painful."[10] That simple statement encapsulates what might be the most profound and distressing experiences that humans encounter. One of the ways of dealing with the pain is to follow Shakespeare's advice to Macduff, who had just learned that his wife and children had been murdered: "Give sorrow words. The grief that does not speak whispers the over-fraught heart, and bids it break."[11] As Freud noted in his essay "On Transience," individuals "recoil from anything that is painful," and this results in "a revolt in their minds against mourning."[12] As Pollock[13] pointed out, there had been by 1961 "surprisingly few investigations" of the subject by psychoanalysts and other psychological researchers. He brought up the point that the paucity of writing on mourning may be related to the painful nature of the subject.

Although it is true that the subject of psychological responses to loss still has not received enough consideration, there has been a significant increase in work on this subject in the past two decades. Notable among these are the careful and comprehensive review of the subject of the grieving spouse by Greenblatt[14] and the works of Parkes[15,16] and Bowlby.[17,18] The ensuing discussion is based in significant part on the works of these authors, as well as the earlier and previously cited pioneer contribution of Lindemann,[19] the above-mentioned paper by Pollock,[13] and the work of Freud[10,12,27] which has influenced the thinking of all later writers on the subject.

Two basic psychological explanations of response to loss* were provided by Freud and Bowlby. The main difference between the two is that Freud viewed other people as important because they satisfy instinctual needs. The pain of the loss is due to the interruption of the gratification. It is not important who provides this gratification, and therefore Freud was not concerned with attachments to people as such. He said, "When people are absent, children do not miss them with any great intensity; many mothers have learned this to their sorrow."[21] However, Bowlby,[17] in tracing the development of the concept of the child's tie to the mother in psychoanalytic literature, pointed out indications that toward the end of his life Freud had begun to move in the direction of postulating a primary instinct of attachment of the child to the mother. Bowlby[17,18] took the position that the attachment of the child to its mother is fundamental to all attachments throughout life. Attachment is defined in terms of specificity, duration through a large part of the life cycle, engagement of emotion, ontogeny, learning, and organization.[18] Specific responses by the mother and later by others, rather than solely the gratification of instinctual drives, are important in attachment. Anxiety is a uniform response to separation, originally from the mother, but subsequently from important persons at any age. Pain and anger are associated with the dissolution of attachments.

These sketchy summaries of the views of Freud and Bowlby do not, of course, attempt to reflect the sum of the contributions of either. Nor is it within the scope of this book to even touch on a number of important workers whose writings have a bearing on the subject, including Fairburn, Klein, Mahler, Spitz, Robertson, and others. A possible synthesis of the approaches of Freud and Bowlby may be helpful: The attachment and separation processes can be looked at from an intrapsychic point of view. This approach need not be limited to considerations of instinctual drives but can deal with the ego and superego as well. This would allow us to consider not only the loss of instinctual gratification, but also ego factors that pertain to the extent to which an important other assists the ego in its synthetic function of integrating the demands of id, superego, and reality. Superego aspects relate to the role of such others in regulating value systems, particularly the sense of guilt. Seen from this standpoint, distress occurring when attachment is interrupted relates to all three psychological levels. This formulation provides a framework that allows the conceptualization of the differences between responses to divorce and grief.

---

*In general, discussion of loss relates to other human beings. The concept is sometimes used, however, in a broader sense, such as in Fried's work on grieving for a lost home.[20]

MANIFESTATIONS AND PSYCHOLOGICAL PROCESSES
IN LOSS OF SPOUSE BY DEATH

Many of the considerations relating to bereavement in general also apply to conjugal bereavement, and the works of Parkes[15] and Greenblatt[14] specifically address the loss of a spouse by death. There is general agreement that conjugal bereavement is more traumatic than the other commonly experienced bereavement, namely, the loss of one's parents, because such a loss is not anticipated. Only the loss of a child can be compared to the loss of a spouse in terms of the emotional impact. As has already been mentioned, Holmes and Rahe[22] list death of a spouse as the event having the highest weight in their Social Readjustment Rating Scale.

Grief as a Process

The term "bereavement" refers to being deprived (literally "robbed") of someone by death. Grief is the term usually applied to the psychological processes following bereavement. Grief is, as Parkes emphasizes, a process and not a state.[15] This process involves the readjustment of the individual to a changed life situation. Bereavement means that adaptation to a changed environment is required. From a psychoanalytical viewpoint, Hartmann[23] saw the ego as the psychic structure that furthers adaptation by maintaining or restoring an equilibrium between the external and internal worlds. Adaptation to a changing outside world may involve any one or more of three pathways: altering the environment (alloplastic changes), making appropriate changes in one's own psychophysical system (autoplastic changes), or selecting a new and more appropriate environment.[23] All three can come into play in relation to conjugal bereavement. Therefore, Pollock's statement that "the mourning process is . . . obviously intrapsychic, as the external loss cannot be undone"[13] is indeed true, but changes in one's relation to the outside world are a crucial aspect of the grief process. As Greenblatt[14] pointed out, "crystallization of new relationships" and/or "the development of a new role in life without the partner" are part of the final phase of the mourning process.

Duration of the Grief Process

There is no consensus on the duration of the grief process following the death of the spouse. Lindemann[19] suggested that the first six weeks determine whether or not the bereavement would be mastered adaptively or whether pathologic grief with lasting psychological or psychosomatic malfunction would ensue, although the total process clearly lasts much longer than six weeks. Parkes[15] expected that most of the acute grief of his subjects would have passed after 13 months, but found this was not so. He believed that follow-up after two or three years is in order to determine for how long decrement in features of grief continues. In my view also, major aspects of grief are observable for at least two to three years in many affected persons.

General Manifestations of Grief

Distinctions between manifestations (symptomatology) and psychological processes are not always clear in the literature. Manifestations may be defined as descriptions based on observations of behavior by the self and others, whereas models of psychological processes are one step removed from empirical observation.

Shock and denial constitute the most common first reaction to the death of a spouse. Parkes,[15,24] in a study of 22 widows who were patients of family practitioners, noted that even when a serious illness preceded the death, few of the women had accepted warnings of the impending demise and were thus unprepared. The women reported that the initial reaction was numbness[15] frequently accompanied by difficulty in accepting the fact that the husband was really dead, and sometimes by sudden panic responses including "shrieking, wailing and moaning".[13,15,24] According to Parkes these responses may last a few days to a month.

By definition, everything in the grief process relates to the death of the spouse. It is possible, however, to distinguish between relatively nonspecific changes and changes that clearly relate to responses toward the deceased person. To take the nonspecific reactions first: Summarizing various reports from the literature, Greenblatt[14] noted that widows during the first year of bereavement consult physicians more, use sedatives more frequently, and spend more time in hospitals than comparable non-widowed women of the same age. Health deterioration is common in the first year, and mortality is higher in widows during the first and even the second year following death of a spouse. There are also important general psychological changes. Greenblatt[14] noted anger, irritability, fear, sleeplessness, and weight loss. Parkes spoke of an "overall affective disturbance,"[15] which he defined as a general estimate of the amount of "negative emotional upset." This disturbance peaked after the initial stage of numbness but recurred throughout the first year in a number of his subjects and was still present in a third of the widows he studied at the end of 12 months.

Specific Manifestations of Grief Related to the Spouse

There are three psychological processes that clearly relate to the deceased person: pining and yearning, protest involving anger, and identification with the deceased.

Pining and yearning is described by all cited writers dealing with the subject. A specific phase called "yearning," originally based on responses of children separated from their mothers, has been identified by Bowlby and Parkes.[25] Bowlby believed that the bereaved person in this phase experiences a strong urge to recover the lost person. Parkes[15] noted the following components of this phase: pining and preoccupation with thoughts of the deceased person, direction of attention toward places and objects associated with him or her, development of a perceptual "set" for the deceased, and crying for the lost person. He saw thoughts of the deceased and the affect of pining as the central and pathognomonic features of grief.[15] Lindemann[19] also described how the mourner recalls one incident after another involving the deceased, and recognizes each time that the lost person will never again be encountered.

All writers agree that anger is a common and universal response to loss that may reach the intensity of rage. Nevertheless, anger, particularly rage, is an uncomfortable subject for us all. As mentioned earlier, any discussion of loss and grief evokes painful feelings, which is one reason why the subject has until recently received little emphasis. Today the taboo on at least some aspects of this topic has been lifted, yet the subject of rage still retains some of the qualities of a taboo, and even the literature on divorce treats anger as an unfortunate phenomenon. Shakespeare knew better. "Let's make us medicines of our great revenge—to cure this deadly grief. . . let grief convert to anger;/blunt not the heart, enrage it."[11] Shakespeare gave Macduff a realistic reason for rage. His wife and children have been murdered and the rage is to be put in the service of revenge. But on a deeper level, Shakespeare understood the importance of rage as part of the grief process and its resolution.

Anger is referred to by Parkes[15] as part of the protest stage, which occurs simultaneously with (or is another aspect of) the stage of yearning. This formulation is based on observation of the mother–child separation. The stage of protest is followed in the child separated from the mother by the stage of despair. Parkes saw both pining and protest mainly as characteristic of the earlier months of the grief process. Nevertheless, anger in the form of general irritability and bitterness, and the feeling that the world had become an insecure and dangerous place, persisted throughout the first year in over half of the women Parkes studied. Frank anger against the spouse was relatively rare. Pollock[13] noted that anger at being left typically comes out in an undisguised fashion in children. In adults, the anger may be displaced to others, as hostility to the dead is not easily tolerated by the mourning ego. Accusations may be made against physicians, hospital personnel, and relatives, among others. Indeed, Parkes found that anger against specific others, such as family members, clergy, and doctors, occurred in eight widows.[15] Manifestations of anger correlated with restlessness, tension, and overall affect, but not with the searching or yearning features.[15] Parkes also observed that negative aspects of the relationship with the husband were most easily forgotten and that "idealization of the dead" was very common.

Guilt about the deceased spouse is believed by Lindemann[19] to be a regular component of grief, along with sadness and anger. Parkes did find guilt among his psychiatrically normal widows, but he did not find this phenomenon as regularly as he did anger.[15] He reported that the guilt in the non-psychiatrically ill widows did not compare in intensity, frequency, or duration with that found in another group of 22 bereaved patients who developed a psychiatric illness subsequent to their bereavement.[26] In the non-psychiatrically ill widows, there was an association of anger with guilt in the first month after bereavement but not subsequently.[15]

The last aspect of the description of grief relates to conscious observable identification, as opposed to an unconscious or intrapsychic process. Parkes[15] found clear evidence of identification in 5 of 22 subjects and strongly suggestive indications in another 9. The most common occurrence was the reported tendency by the widow to behave more like the spouse. Less frequent were symptoms similar to those of the husband during his last illness, and perceiving the presence of husband in the widow or the children. Guilt or self-reproach was the only psychological feature studied that correlated with identification.[15]

Psychological Processes in Grief

When addressing psychological processes, we are no longer dealing with empirical data directly but rather with formulations based on theories as to the phenomena underlying the observations. These theories are derived mainly from the psychoanalytical framework. There are three main aspects to the intrapsychic grief process: reality testing, introjection and identification (now in its intrapsychic sense), and recathexis of objects in the outside world.

Reality testing involves a prolonged and painful process during which the fact of the death of the important other is gradually accepted. While in all but a few instances that fact is intellectually recognized almost from the beginning, the bereaved person initially feels and behaves as if the death had not taken place. In "Mourning and Melancholia" Freud stated, " . . . people never willingly abandon a libidinal position, [investment of another with loving feelings] not even, indeed, when a substitute is already beckoning to them."[27] The giving up, bit by bit, requires a great deal of energy. It is not, however, possible to complete the grief process unless reality testing prevails and the libidinal investment is withdrawn from the person who no longer exists.

There is some difference of opinion regarding the extent to which fantasy and daydreaming about the deceased are part of normal grief. Lindemann[19] felt that such preoccupation was a universal part of the grief process, and unless it was excessive or unduly prolonged, did not interfere with resolution. Pollock,[13] on the other hand, believed that fantasies and daydreams can interfere with the mourning work. The issue here is whether or not the person recognizes that the object of the fantasies is dead and uses the fantasies to give up the tie as opposed to maintaining the deceased individual indefinitely as a fantasy figure.

Freud believed that identification with the lost person was a fundamental way in which human beings deal with loss. In fact, he saw the ego (the integrating and coordinating part of the psychic apparatus) as consisting of the precipitate of abandoned object cathexis.[28] In other words, a major part of the personality is developed by our taking on attributes and traits of persons whom we have known but who are no longer in our lives. This concept is more readily understood when we keep in mind the experiences that all of us over time have, when we unconsciously take on many of the characteristics of parents, teachers, and so on.

When applied to bereavement, identification involves two stages. The first is that of introjection. During this stage there is a fantasy of "ingesting" the lost person whole and "undigested." This concept accounts for the above-cited clinical observation that Parkes' widows sometimes felt as if their husbands were literally inside of them. The phenomenon of feeling that someone is inside one is not an uncommon clinical observation, particularly in bereavement. The next step is identification, which no longer involves perceiving another as a separate entity inside of oneself, but rather is a gradual assimilation of various aspects of the other person's individuality. No longer is the other felt to be separate. Instead, his or her traits have become part of the survivor's new identity. Freud believed that in this manner the survivor preserved the lost one without ever denying the reality of the death. Identification is present—and alleviates grief—in the form of the survivor feeling lastingly enriched by the memory of having loved and having been loved. The survivor may also be enhanced by learning and integrating coping skills of the deceased into his or her repertory. In a broader sense, our cherishing of traditions has a similar purpose.

The last aspect in the psychic model of the grief process is the recathexis of the outside world. Loving feelings are once again directed outward to another person. Adaptive resolution of grief involves the cessation of the previously described phenomena. It also involves the establishment of new and different relationships. For those who have suffered conjugal bereavement, this may or may not involve a new dyadic love relationship. In all instances where grief has been successfully resolved, a new pattern of mutually satisfying interaction with family and friends is formed. As Pollock[13] noted, however, in later life other objects may not be as readily available, and thus older people may withdraw their libido to a greater degree into themselves. The result of excessive depletion of libidinal attachments to others may be death, as is seen when the death of one partner in a long marriage is shortly followed by the death of the other.

Pathological Grief

Greenblatt,[14] in reviewing pathological grief, surveyed the work of various authors including Volkan and Wahl. He mentioned anniversary reactions, failure to grieve, and grief that is excessive in length of intensity, including irrational despair and severe feelings of hopelessness, as indicators of pathological grief. Other indicators are protracted apathy, irritability without appropriate affect, thanatophobia, loss of identity or interest, and failure to plan for the future. Of special interest in light of psychopathological explanations of abnormal grief are self-blame for the death and the development of symptoms similar to those of the deceased. As already mentioned, Parkes[15] found that widows who subsequent to their bereavement developed a psychiatric illness reported guilt of greater intensity, frequency, and duration than did widows who were not patients. Ideas of guilt or self-blame in relation to the deceased were expressed by two thirds of the bereaved psychiatric patients.[24] Over half of the patients who expressed ideas of self-reproach also expressed marked hostility toward other individuals including doctors, nurses, and others who had been involved with the dying person. Parkes further stated that those who have worked clinically with bereaved psychiatric patients are likely to be impressed by the frequency with which "ambivalence toward the dead person is seen by the patient as an important problem, and such evidence as there is tends to confirm this impression."[24]

Ambivalence is a key to Freud's theory of pathological grief. Although anger was noted by Bowlby[24] and Lindemann[19] to be a normal component of grief, there does not seem to exist a description of the resolution of anger in non-pathological grief. Freud,[27] while acknowledging that ambivalence is universal and not pathological, discussed anger in terms of a "tendency to sadism" and stated that it is this tendency that makes "melancholia" (depression) "so interesting and so dangerous."[27] Ambivalence is defined as simultaneously existing loving and angry feelings. The angry component, as Freud saw it, mainly refers to feelings predating the loss of the person by death or other reasons. Such hostility may be associated with death wishes. Magical belief in the causality of death, together with great guilt, may be the major contributor to subsequent serious psychopathology.[13] Survival may also result in a feeling of triumph over the deceased.

Ambivalence further interferes with the normal progress of introjection to identification. The bereaved individual introjects the lost other without integrating the other's characteristics; instead, the lost person is located within the survivor. We must remember that we are talking about a concept of psychological functioning and not necessarily about a conscious perception. The bereaved person's symptoms and behavior suggest that he or she fantasizes having the lost person inside. The result is melancholia, or depression, as attacks upon the lost or dead person, now located within the depressed individual, become attacks against the self. Freud explained the self-reproaches of depressives and those showing pathological bereavement as being anger originally directed at the lost or dead one that is redirected toward the dead one within oneself and therefore toward oneself. Grief under these circumstances ends only when, as Freud stated, "the fury has spent itself."[27] It may also end when the survivor has found a new person with whom to act out a mutually angry relationship. This is an extreme picture; most bereavements contain some of the features just described, but to a lesser degree.

Ambivalence toward the lost or dead individual is not the only important factor in determining whether or not grief will be adaptively resolved. Other factors include the suddenness of the loss,[29] the intensity of the attachment, the availability of social supports,[14] experiences with previous losses, social class, changes in financial situation, and the preexisting psychological state. This discussion, however, focuses on ambivalence as a significant variable in regard to the post-loss level of mental health.

MANIFESTATIONS AND PSYCHOLOGICAL PROCESSES
IN MARITAL SEPARATION AND DIVORCE

The loss of a spouse by divorce has frequently been compared to loss of a spouse by death. According to Bohannon,[30] "emotional divorce results in the loss of a loved . . . person as fully—but by quite a different route of experience—as does the death of a spouse." Bohannon also referred to grief and mourning as a phase of the divorce process, as did Fisher.[31] Goode[32] believed that divorce and bereavement "appear to be structurally similar and both may be traumatic experiences." He qualified his position, however, by indicating that divorce, unlike bereavement, follows a reduction in attachment and stated, "We do not believe comparison is fruitful."[32] Wiseman[33] stated that "the divorce process can be seen as one of both grief and growth" and that "there are many characteristics of the grief process." She noted, on the other hand, that some processes are unique to divorce. Among authors emphasizing differences between the separated and bereaved is Weiss,[34] who indicated that while both groups are subjected to traumatic loss, "the experience of the bereaved and the separated differs in many ways and I would not try to equate them."

One key difference between divorce and death must be introduced at the very start. There is no doubt about the reality of the loss when a spouse dies. There is, on the other hand, a great range of possibilities about the loss when marital separation and divorce occur. A spouse may leave without warning, never to be seen again, or may reside in the same house and even sleep in the same bed for years after a legal divorce. The common picture is one of repeated distancing, followed by partial reconciliation, new withdrawal, and an eventual equilibrium, which may range from complete to partial to no loss of the interspouse relationship. This interaction allows rapprochement and distancing from a living spouse to be used as an important element of modulating psychological separation.

The second fundamental difference between divorce and death is that anger at the spouse before the marriage is ended is generally more frequent and more intense in separation or divorce than in bereavement. There are, of course, a few instances where a spouse dies during the course of a marital separation. But bereavement typically occurs at a time when both spouses are committed to the continuation of a marriage. As stated earlier, divorce takes place when angry feelings become predominant over loving ones. It is true that bereavement may occur at a time of great anger, but this is rare.

These two factors constitute the key differences between bereavement and divorce: the presence in divorce of both a living partner and the possibility of interacting with him or her, and pre-existing anger to a far greater degree than in bereavement.

General Manifestations of Response to Separation

There exists a continuum ranging from prolonged periods during which a separation is anticipated, on the one extreme, and the announced sudden departure of a spouse, on the other. There are probably fewer sudden separations than there are sudden deaths, but all of the phenomena of shock and denial that are observed in bereavement may also occur in separation. A manifestation that occurs in separation and not in bereavement is the effort to reverse the separation and bring about a reconciliation. Such intent is often accompanied by intense affect. If reconciliation does not ensue, the nonspecific manifestations are very similar to those seen in bereavement. We have already addressed the adverse health changes and increased mortality relating to the separated and divorced. Numerous reports have appeared describing the symptomatology among those dissolving their marriages. Weiss[34] described the occurrence of distress, including anxiety and depression. Hetherington et al.[35] reported that in the first year following divorce, divorced mothers and fathers feel more anxious, depressed, angry, resentful, and incompetent than married controls. Briscoe[5] noted in a divorced group the presence of suicide plans, death wishes, somatic complaints, weight loss, self-pity, and blaming of others. Chester,[36] in a study of 150 women 6 to 30 months after divorce, found that only 13 percent had no adverse health effects. Of the remainder, 80 percent had at least four of eight "stress indicators," the most common of which were crying and weight loss, followed by tiredness, difficulty in concentration, changes in smoking patterns, self-neglect, and increased drinking. Hunt[37] noted sleeplessness, loss of appetite, and depression.

Heiman,[38] in a review of recently available police suicide data from several cities in the United States and from the Metropolitan Police Department of London, concluded that the average policeman who committed suicide was either divorced or seeking divorce. Rose and Rosow[39] reported the tendency for men to commit suicide was highest among the divorced and lowest among the married. Divorced physicians were 13 times more likely to kill themselves than were their married colleagues, whereas the ratio in the general population was 3 to 1.

In his pioneering work, Goode[32] developed a "behavioral index of divorce trauma" that included difficulty in sleeping, poorer health, greater loneliness, low work efficiency, memory difficulty, increased smoking, and increased drinking. The first three of these variables were found in over 60 percent of his subjects. Using the index, he found that about 63 percent of the sample were high- or medium-trauma respondents. Chiriboga and Cutter[40] used a trauma and relief scale based on Goode's work, which will be discussed further in Chapter 5. The work of Gove,[1] Ilfeld,[2] and Mellinger et al.[3] all showed high rates of disturbance in the separated and divorced.

There are a few dissenting voices: Brown et al.,[41] writing from a feminist perspective, saw divorce as a "chance of a new lifetime." They interviewed 30 "non-systematically selected respondents" separated for one to five years and reported that 12 were happy or relieved only and another 6 were happy or relieved but had mixed feelings. White and Asher,[42] in a study of 30 divorced men, report that most of their subjects adjusted to divorce with little trauma. Those that did not adjust well had lower levels of self-esteem, confidence, and independence. Finally, Jaffe and Kanter[43] studied divorce occurring within the setting of a commune and stated that only a minority reported that separation was a negative experience. They attribute the difference between their findings and those of most others in the literature to the support of a household and friends.

The great majority of studies, then, associate separation and divorce with a high incidence of psychological disturbance. The general symptoms are quite similar to those in bereavement, with one notable addition: suicidal ideation, suicide attempts, and completed suicide receive far more frequent mention in relation to separation and divorce than they do to bereavement. Simon and Lumry[44] addressed this subject specifically under the heading of "suicide as a divorce substitute." Their study population was drawn from the Minneapolis Veterans Administration Hospital and involved 9 patients whose spouses committed suicide and 31 former patients who committed suicide two days to eight days after discharge. Of the total, 23 experienced serious marital discord: eight were divorced, ten were separated, and for five there was threat of divorce. Two patients murdered their spouses before committing suicide.

Specific Manifestations Involving the Spouse

Pining and yearning can be as intense in marital dissolution as in grief, though this is far from always the case. The most obvious manifestations are found in spouses who did not seek divorce and who feel abandoned, particularly if the separation was not anticipated. The feeling is captured in some of the vignettes used by Hunt.[37] One of these involves a woman whose husband has just left her and who said, "I am acting like a frightened child, a little girl who's lost her Mommy in the crowd." Another woman said, "I was relieved to have him gone, but also I felt dreadful anguish. It couldn't have been worse if he were dead. I had loved my life and loved him (when he wasn't drinking) and simply couldn't bear to have all that torn asunder. . . . " And a third woman illustrated pining and yearning even more clearly: "During the night I tossed fitfully . . . only to wake up flailing my arms frantically over the bed, looking for my lost companion . . . . I finally piled his side of the bed with boxes of things, pillows, so it would feel heavy, as if there were someone there."

Weiss,[34] who had previously collaborated with Glick and Parkes on the Harvard bereavement studies,[45] proposed that loss of attachment accounts for the distress seen in marital separation. Building on Bowlby,[17,18] Weiss related attachment back to infancy and usually to the mother. Attachment continues throughout life and is an important factor in marriage.[34] In this context Weiss describes separation distress as accompanying the interruption of attachment and indicates that it consists of "focusing of attention on the lost figure, together with intense discomfort because of the figure's inaccessibility."[34] These are virtually the identical terms that Parkes[24] used to describe searching behavior in the bereaved.

There are two important differences between separation and bereavement, however. First, pining and yearning are not universal in the separated. Relief and euphoria are noted by both Hunt[37] and Weiss[34] as the first reactions to separation, but most people subsequently experience pining and distress. Secondly, and of broader significance, in marital dissolution the pining can be assuaged, at least temporarily, by making contact with the living partner. Continuing and frequent contacts between the spouses are the rule in early separation, and it is not unusual for them to continue for months and years. The separated spouse has an option that the bereaved one lacks: There is no need to be limited to fantasizing about the spouse when that spouse can be contacted in person or by phone. Other risks, however, may attend the exercise of this option.

The next phase of grief involves anger and protest. This subject will receive more detailed attention in a subsequent chapter. For the moment, it may be said that anger is to be reasonably expected as a result of both the bitter disappointment in the failure of the marriage and the loss of the spouse. Fisher said of the separating couple: "Burning with feelings of anger and distrust, they are often told to be friendly and achieve an 'amicable divorce.' I believe there is no such thing as an amicable divorce."[31]

Concluding the earlier discussion of grief were comments on identification. There have been no references to this phenomenon in divorce. Complete identification in the sense of internalizing and integrating characteristics of the spouse do not usually play a significant role in dissolution. This is one of the important differences between separation and grief. On the other hand, introjection does play a role, though it is not yet described as a clinical phenomenon.

Psychological Processes in Separation and Divorce

Although psychological processes in separation and divorce are generally similar to those in grief (reality testing, introjection, identification, and recathexis of the outside world), there are some differences. Reality testing is an important part of the marital separation process. If the spouse is completely absent, which is rare, the characteristics of reality testing are identical to those in grief. More commonly, the reality being tested relates to whether a resumption of the marriage is possible and if not, what the extent of the separation will be. The difference between reality testing in dissolution and grief is that in dissolution, most of the reality testing is carried out through real contact with the spouse.

Introjection does occur when reality testing reveals that separation will be total or nearly so. If and when the spouse is no longer available for interaction, introjection will occur for the same reason that it does in bereavement. Now we have a situation where rage is frequent; this then is directed against the introject. Here we have an explanation within our psychological model for the frequent intense depression and the common suicidal preoccupation. To kill oneself is to kill the introject of the spouse within oneself. If the actual spouse is still living, however, another aspect is present: the conscious or unconscious attempt to punish that spouse. Simon[44] quoted Goldberg and Mudd as saying that suicide is the most hostile type of transaction any spouse can carry out. Once more we see how intrapsychic grief work is complicated in divorce by the existence of the living spouse.

The final stage of grief, if it is successfully worked through, is recathexis of the outside world with the establishment of new relationships. This is clearly the end result of a successful divorce as well. We have seen that the divorced, more frequently than the widowed, do remarry, and a successful remarriage is the optimal outcome of the divorce process. To accomplish this outcome, it is necessary to renounce the former spouse as the primary object of attachment and to carry on with work of mourning.

A MODEL OF DYADIC RELATIONSHIPS

One of the chief concerns of this book is the ongoing interaction between the spouses and the relationship between their transaction and their levels of mental health. A model that deals with intrapsychic management of responses to the end of the marriage, the ongoing interpersonal relations after separation or divorce, and the relationship between these two has been developed to help interpret these data.

A dyadic relationship affects the id, ego, and superego of both participants. This relationship may afford the id opportunities for discharge of instinctual drives and/or may frustrate the attempt to discharge them. A dyadic relationship also contributes to the environment within which the ego integrates the demands of id, superego, and reality. Responses from the other member of the dyad are important parts of that reality. Regarding the superego, a dyadic relationship is one factor shaping the conscious and unconscious sense of right and wrong of each participant. All dyadic relationships involve ambivalence on the part of each partner toward the other. Ambivalence is represented by positive and negative orientation. For purposes of model building, the assumption is first made that positive and negative orientations can exist in pure form, which is not possible in reality.

Positive orientation in the hypothetical pure form is defined again in id, ego, and superego terms. From the viewpoint of the id, it involves libidinal cathexis of the other person and gratification of instinctual drives. In less technical terms, each gratifies the other's needs for physical and psychological satisfaction. Positive orientation with regard to the ego involves cooperative behavior in each member of the dyad which redounds to the advantage of both. With regard to the superego, there is a shared value system and general moral approval of the behavior of each by the other. Regarding affect, both members of the dyad experience and acknowledge loving feelings toward the other, defined in the broadest sense of the term.

Negative orientation in its hypothetical pure form is defined from the id viewpoint as thwarting of libidinal drives of each other and the presence of conscious or unconscious destructive drives. From an ego standpoint, it implies interactions that impede the adaptation of one or both persons. On the superego level, there is harsh criticism and negative value judgment by each of the other and sometimes of the self. The predominant factor is anger, sometimes reaching hatred or rage. Self-depreciation and depression, however, may occur in addition to or in place of overt anger in one or both persons. Guilt over rage, including death wishes, is frequent and often severe. Another phenomenon that may occur is mutual projective identification. Each partner projects unacceptable attributes of the self on the other and also subtly induces responses in the other that allow partial confirmation of the projection.

Predominantly negatively oriented relationships can be stable over years because they frequently afford an opportunity for discharge of anger. Guilt is relieved by the punishment that each inflicts upon the other. Alternately, guilt can be diminished by periods of reconciliation, during which a partner tries to undo the real or fantasized injury done to the other. Another important reason for the stability of these relationships is that in practice they are not purely negative and the combination of positive and negative aspects underlies their tumultuous nature. It may also be the only type of relationship available to the participants because of their psychological makeup or because of lack of opportunity for more adaptive interactions.

Positive and Negative Orientation in Bereavement

Orientation is defined here as that existing prior to the death of the spouse. For example, a relationship that had a positive character over a long period of time may become increasingly negative during a serious illness. Furthermore, the postulation of a positive relationship does not exclude the presence of anger after the death as a response to the bereavement.

The following is the postulated situation when death interrupts hypothetically pure, positively oriented dyadic relationship: Reality testing leads to the conclusion that all aspects of the relationship have terminated. Introjection occurs, leading to identification with positive results, including the integration of loving feelings formerly experienced as coming from the other as well as coping skills and values into the survivor's psychic structure. Anger that results from the bereavement is acknowledged as normal and does not lead to introjection and depression. Guilt is minimal or absent. Reinvolvement eventually ensues in another dyadic relationship or in relationships involving several persons, which fulfill functions relative to instinctual drives, ego, and superego that were previously carried out within the former dyad.

The fact that a relationship was positively oriented prior to death does not assure an adaptive outcome. Other social and psychological factors are involved, such as suddenness of the death, degree of attachment, or availability of social supports. Whether or not these variables operate by way of intense and at times unconscious rage over the "abandonment" by death is a question we cannot yet answer.

When death interrupts a hypothetically pure, negatively oriented dyadic relationship, the outcome will vary as a function of the extent to which the survivor is able to consciously recognize and acknowledge the negative orientation, both in the external reality while the other was alive and in the anger and generally negative feelings of the survivor toward the deceased before and after the death. Such recognition is easier when the survivor acknowledges the relationship existed mainly for external reasons, such as financial necessity, and/or was ready to give up the relationship before the death or became ready to do so thereafter. A good outcome is likely when the anger at the deceased is neither denied nor repressed after the death. Guilt may be present in a tolerable amount for any real injury done to one or both partners, but it will not be unrealistic or excessive. There will be no fantasy that the deceased died as a result of the survivor's anger. Understanding what went wrong in the relationship will result in behavior that can be used in the future. Reinvolvement in new relationships that are more adaptive than the former dyad was may eventually ensue.

On the other hand, let us take a situation in which the survivor is unable to face the reality of either the negative character of the relationship or of rage toward the deceased. Let us assume that at the time of death the relationship, however unhappy, continued to meet important psychological needs and that the bereavement is painful. In the absence of awareness of the issues, pathogenic introjection will ensue in an attempt to deal with the loss. Attacks on the self will result, with depression and guilt as the corollary. The greater the felt loss and the less the conscious acknowledgment of the negative reality and the rage, the worse the outcome will be. The reaction ends when self-attacks have spent themselves, but residual self-depreciation and/or anger at the world may remain. Eventually, either prolonged withdrawal occurs or new negatively oriented relationships are established.

Ambivalence is a universal reality. From this point of view, the principle underlying the adaptive resolution of loss does not differ from that fostering adaptation in an ongoing relationship: the ability to *recognize and accept one's own (and by implication others') conflicting feelings about a person.* This ability develops originally in the mother–child relationship when the child is aware of both loving and hating feelings and impulses toward the mother. Klein referred to this stage as the depressive position,[46] and others have described it as the development of object constancy.[47] Failure to work these feelings through at this stage causes subsequent developmental problems. This is not an all-or-nothing matter, however. There can be partial resolution, but residual difficulties may be activated in the bereavement situation.

In bereavement, the task is to acknowledge as truthfully as possible the positive *and* negative aspects of the relationship and to accept that both have been terminated. If this occurs, the positive aspects can in a sense be preserved through introjection and identification; the negative ones do not result in introjection but are recognized as reality. There is clear differentiation between the self and the deceased. Eventually new and adaptive relationships are formed.

Response to Loss by Divorce

The above framework can lead us to an understanding of the key issues involved in divorce with the two very important modifications: there is a living ex-spouse and the orientation is normally weighted to the negative, whereas in bereavement, at least prior to the terminal illness, it was typically weighted to the positive side.

Because of the presence of a living spouse, divorce allows active interplay of intrapsychic factors in each spouse and allows interactions between the spouses. Whether or not resolution is adaptive must be determined by reference to each arena: intrapsychic and interpersonal.

Adaptive *intrapsychic* resolution is identical to the adaptive resolution of bereavement. Positive and negative aspects are acknowledged and surrendered. This means that eventually one comes to grips with both one's own and the former spouse's contribution to the failure of the marriage. Sadness, anger, and guilt cannot be totally escaped in most instances, but they are moderate and congruent with reality. Eventually there is readiness to invest in new and better relationships.

Adaptive *interpersonal* resolution involves both spouses recognizing that the relationship no longer meets their mutual needs. Each expects and accepts anger in the other as an appropriate response to the situation and this anger is expressed within limits without evoking blame. The relationship is redefined in accordance with the reality of the divorce. Adversary positions in regard to financial settlements often occur and are accepted, and each party protects its own interests without being punitive to the other. When applicable, coparenting relationships are worked out that do not serve as covert ways to maintain consciously terminated marital attachments. Each party is free to invest in new dyadic relationships without interference from the former spouse.

Maladaptive resolutions may also be viewed from an intrapsychic and interpersonal viewpoint. Relationships ending in divorce are often intensely negatively oriented. An unhappy marriage, however, can serve many needs: some satisfaction may coincide with the negative aspects, guilt may be relieved through being punished by the partner or through reconciliation and undoing, and projective identification may temporarily relieve intrapsychic tension. For any or all of these reasons, an unhappy marriage may be consciously or unconsciously preferred to no marriage by one or both partners. With such a marriage, after separation the same maladaptive intrapsychic resolution may ensue that occurs with bereavement under similar circumstances. One or both partners do not acknowledge and renounce the positive and negative aspects. In the physical absence of the partner, the negative aspects are introjected just as in bereavement, with resulting depression, guilt, and suicidal ideation. Anger may be expressed at the spouse, but this tends to take the form of criticism of specific acts or qualities, rather than acknowledgement of one's own angry feelings. The resulting internal state may be very painful.

The divorced person at this point usually has an option that the bereaved one does not have: the former spouse can be contacted in person, by phone, or through others. The result can be a reconciliation, either at the previous unhappy level or on a better one. Another possibility is that the former spouses renegotiate a new modus vivendi of lessened intensity. If this occurs, some of the pain may be relieved, but each partner's ability to relate to someone new may be impaired by the continued bond to the former spouse. A common yet relatively maladaptive occurrence is that the renewed contacts may temporarily assuage the pain of the loss but will result in renewed and probably increased negatively oriented interaction. At this point, readiness to acknowledge the reality of the end of the marriage may occur, and resolution will proceed along more adaptive lines.

In a significant number of couples, however, renewed contacts do not resolve the issue but lead to further conflict. A new contact may leave one or both partners bruised if rage increases but is not acknowledged and tolerated without excessive guilt, or if depreciation by one partner results in the other's loss of self-esteem. Separation occurs again and increases depression, which may again cause an attempt to resume contacts—a situation that can remain stormy for months and perhaps years. It is characterized by varying frequency and intensity of contact and by peaks of turmoil whenever events highlight the reality that the relationship is terminating, such as a new involvement for one partner. The situation may abate or continue indefinitely, in which case, an unhappy marriage is replaced by an unhappy divorce.

A Vicious Circle in Divorce

Only in the divorced is there a possible alternation of intrapsychic maladaptive resolution with introjection and depression, with resumption of an unhappy and potentially mutually destructive interaction. In bereavement the end of the relationship, no matter how painful, must sooner or later be acknowledged. The opportunity for vacillation between the pain of ending a relationship and the pain of continuing it constitutes a unique risk factor for the divorced. There exists a potential, for an indefinite time, of a combination of the most pathogenic aspects of an unhappy marriage with the most pathogenic aspects of bereavement.

We can now return to the question, Are there psychological factors that can contribute to the greater incidence in disturbance among the divorced than among the widowed? The answer is yes, based on the considerations just given. To the extent that divorce permits ongoing unhappy interaction with the former spouse, resolution may be deferred for significantly longer than is possible among the widowed. Whether or not differences in fact exist is not yet known. But if the differences prove to be real, a rationale exists to explain them. The vicious circle potential among the divorced still represents an important phenomenon from the standpoint of clinical understanding and as basis for research design.

Like all models, the above is necessarily oversimplified. Determinants of outcome are in fact many and complex. For instance, conscious recognition of negative orientation and anger is desirable, but much lies between conscious acknowledgement of the reality of one's own affect on one end of the continuum and introjection with suicidal ideation on the other. Various defenses of different degrees of adaptiveness can be made, such as channeling one's anger into the support of a socially important cause. Also, the establishment of a good new relationship can be a cause as well as an effect of adaptive resolution of divorce.

Granting these qualifications, however, the model will be useful to analyze factors in the divorce process. What role do such phenomena as ongoing contacts and emotional reliance on the spouse, reconciliation and renewed separations, hostility, and other aspects of interspouse relations have on the mental health of the divorcing? We shall address these topics in subsequent chapters, immediately following the introduction to the research design and the relationship of mental health status to demographic factors, socioeconomic factors, and time elapsed since various separation events.

REFERENCES

1. Gove WR: Sex, marital status and mortality. Am J Sociology, 79:45–67, 1973
2. Ilfeld FW: Psychological status of community residents among major demographic dimensions. Arch Gen Psychiatry 35:716–724, 1978

3. Mellinger GD, Bacter MB, Manheimer DI, et al: Psychic distress, life crises and use of psychotropic medication. Arch Gen Psychiatry 35:1048–1052, 1978

4. Bergler E: Divorce Won't Help. New York, Harper Bros, 1970

5. Briscoe CW, Smith JB: Depression in the bereaved and divorced. Relationship to primary depressive illness. A study of 128 subjects. Arch Gen Psychiatry 32:439–443, 1975

6. Parsons T: The Social System. Glencoe, Ill, Free Press, 1951

7. Kessler S: Building skills in divorce adjustment groups. J Divorce 1:210–216, 1978

8. Divorce: Part I, film produced by Kessler S, Whitely J. Distributed by American Personnel and Guidance Assoc, 1607 New Hampshire Avenue NW, Washington DC 20009

9. Carter H, Glick PC: Marriage and Divorce: A Social and Economic Study. Cambridge and London, Harvard University Press, 1976, p 440

10. Freud S: Draft G. Melancholia, in Strachey S (Ed): The Standard Edition of the Complete Psychological Works of Sigmund Freud, vol 1. London, Hogarth Press, 1966, pp 200–206

11. Shakespeare W: Macbeth, Act IV, scene 3, lines 208–229

12. Freud S: On transience, in Strachey S (Ed): The Standard Edition of the Complete Psychological Works of Sigmund Freud, vol 14. London, Hogarth Press, 1957, pp 305–307

13. Pollock GJ: Mourning and adaptation. Int J Psychoanal 42:341–361, 1961

14. Greenblatt M: The grieving spouse. Am J Psychiatry 135;41–47, 1978

15. Parkes CM: The first year of bereavement. Psychiatry 33:444–467, 1970

16. Parkes CM: Psycho-social transitions: A field for study. Soc Sci Med 5:101–115, 1971

17. Bowlby J: Attachment and Loss (vol 1). New York, Basic Books, 1969

18. Bowlby J: Making and breaking of affectional bonds. I: Aetiology and psychopathology in the light of attachment theory. Br J Psychiatry 130:201–10, 1977

19. Lindemann E: Symptomatology and management of acute grief. Am J Psychiatry 101:141–148, 1944

20. Fried M: Grieving for a lost home, in Duhl LJ (Ed): The Environment of the Metropolis. New York, Basic Books, 1962

21. Freud S: The interpretation of dreams: I, in Strachey S (Ed): The Standard Edition of the Complete Psychological Works of Sigmund Freud, vol 4. London, Hogarth Press, 1958, pp 1–338

22. Holmes TR, Rahe RH: The social readjustment rating scale. J Psychosom Res 11:213–218, 1967

23. Hartman H: Ego psychology and the problem of adaptation. Psychoanal Assoc Monograph, Series 1. New York, International Universities Press, 1958, pp 26–27

24. Parkes CM: Bereavement, Studies of Grief in Adult Life. New York, International Universities Press, 1972

25. Bowlby J, Parkes CM: Separation and loss, In Anthony EJ, Koupernik C (Eds): International Yearbook for Child Psychiatry and Allied Disci-

plines: The Child in his Family (vol 1). New York, Wiley, 1970, pp 197–216

26. Parkes CM: Bereavement and mental illness: I. A clinical study of bereaved psychiatric patients; II. A classification of bereavement reactions. Br J Med Psychol 38:1–26, 1965

27. Freud S: Mourning and melancholia, in Strachey S (Ed): The Standard Edition of the Complete Psychological Works of Sigmund Freud, vol 14. London, Hogarth Press, 1957, pp 237–259

28. Freud S: The ego and the id, in Strachey S (Ed): The Standard Edition of the Complete Psychological Works of Sigmund Freud, vol 19. London, Hogarth Press, 1961, pp 12–59

29. Parkes CM: Unexpected and untimely bereavement: A statistical study of young Boston widows and widowers, in Schoenberg B, Gerber I, Wiener A, et al (Eds): Bereavement. Its Psychosocial Aspects. New York and London, Columbia University Press, 1975, 119–138

30. Bohannon P: The six stations of divorce, in Bohannon P (Ed): Divorce and After. New York, Doubleday, 1970, pp 33–62

31. Fisher EO: Divorce: The New Freedom. New York, Harper and Row, 1974

32. Goode WJ: After Divorce. Glencoe, Ill, The Free Press, 1956, pp 184–185, 186

33. Wiseman RS: Crisis theory and the process of divorce. Soc Casework 56:205–212, 1975

34. Weiss RS: Marital Separation. New York, Basic Books, 1975

35. Hetherington EM, Cox M, Cox R: The aftermath of divorce. Read at the 54th annual meeting of the American Orthopsychiatric Association, New York, 1977

36. Chester R: Health and marriage breakdown: Experience of a sample of divorced women. Br J Prevent and Social Med 25:231–235, 1971

37. Hunt M, Hunt B: The Divorce Experience. New York, McGraw-Hill, 1977

38. Heimann MF: Suicide among police. Am J Psychiatry 134:1286–1290, 1977

39. Rose KD, Rosow I: Physicians who kill themselves. Arch Gen Psychiatry 29:800–805, 1973

40. Chiriboga PA, Cutler L: Stress responses among separating men and women. J Divorce 1:95–106, 1977

41. Brown CA, Feldberg R, Fox EM, et al: Divorce: Chance of a new lifetime. J Soc Issues 32:119–133, 1976

42. White SW, Asher SJ: Separation and divorce: A study of the male perspective, in Raschke V, Raschke H (Eds): Computer printouts on current research on marital separation and divorce (unpublished), Feb 1978

43. Jaffe DT, Kanter RM: Couple strains in communal households: A four-factor model of the separation process. J Soc Issues 32:169–191, 1976

44. Simon W, Lumry GK: Suicide of the spouse as a divorce substitute. Dis Nerv System 31:609–612, 1970

45. Glick IO, Weiss RS, Parkes CM: The First Year of Bereavement. New York, Wiley-Interscience, 1974
46. Klein M: Envy and Gratitude. A Study of Unconscious Sources. New York, Basic Books, 1957
47. Shapiro BR: The psychodynamics and developmental psychology of the borderline patient: A review of the literature. Am J Psychiatry 131:1312, 1978

5

The Research Study: Introduction, Demographic Characteristics, and Time Elapsed Since Separation

The next several chapters contain findings of a research project on the relationship of mental health status to various aspects of the marital separation and divorce process. This chapter introduces the research project. There will follow consideration of the relationship of mental health status to demographic and socioeconomic variables in a population undergoing marital dissolution. Lastly I will address the issue of the relationship of mental health level to time elapsed since various separation events.

THE RESEARCH STUDY

The original title of the study was "Relation of Suicide to Marital Separation and Divorce." Before it actually was implemented the study was broadened to include the relationship of mental health status to marital separation and divorce. The goal was to study in depth individuals undergoing various aspects of the dissolution process. The main focus was on transactions between these spouses and on psychological responses to these transactions. Information was also obtained on demographic variables, involvements with persons other than the spouse, and variables unrelated to separation/divorce that have been described in the literature as predictive of mental health status. One of the goals of the study was to consider the relative power of separation-related and non–separation-related variables in predicting levels of mental health.

Study Population

The study population was drawn from successive applicants to the Benjamin Rush Center, a crisis clinic associated with the Los Angeles Psychiatric Service, a nonprofit outpatient facility.* The decision to draw the study population from this source rather than from court records or from a community survey deserves comment. Clearly, a population drawn from the latter sources would allow for greater generalizability to the population of the separated and divorced. Court samples however, are limited to those who have already filed for a decree. Some of the most important events in the dissolution process occur prior to and immediately subsequent to the separation, when divorce often has not been filed for. As to community surveys, two overriding problems existed: First, the cost would have been prohibitive, as a very large area would need to have been surveyed to locate a sufficient number of recently separated individuals. At the same time, obtaining the in-depth psychological information necessary to shed light on some of the issues, including those of attachment and anger, would have had to have been done by trained mental health professionals making home visits, rather than by the type of interviewers normally used in social science surveys. The task would have been formidable and for practical reasons was not feasible at the time the study was undertaken.

The population of applicants to a crisis clinic also may be more representative, particularly of the recently separated and divorced, than might be immediately apparent. The Benjamin Rush Center identifies itself as a "Center for Problems of Living," in a deliberate attempt to avoid the stigma attached in the minds of some to a psychiatric service and to maximize utilization by a broad cross-section of the population. There are also indications that many of those separating utilize some form of helping facility and that the group using services resembles the group that does not. Chester[1] noted that 130 of 150 women who were petitioners in mental health suits reported adverse health effects as a result of their marital termination and two thirds had sought

---

*Since November 1, 1974, the Benjamin Rush Center has been part of the Didi Hirsch Community Mental Health Center.

medical help. More recently, Kitson and Sussman[2] reported that 61% of divorcing women and 41 percent of divorcing men in their study had consulted at least one professional in the year prior to interview. Only replication studies using other sources can definitely resolve this issue.

The sample used in this project consisted of consecutive applicants to the Benjamin Rush Center between July 1973 and March 1975 who were either separated or divorced at the time of their first interview or who stated that they were seriously considering marital separation or divorce. The goal was to continue data collection until there were at least 100 subjects who had experienced one of the following events within 13 months prior to admission to the study: separation from the spouse, filing for divorce, or obtaining a final decree of divorce. In addition, 50 subjects who were seriously discussing separation but were not actually separated and 50 more who had received a final decree 14 or more months prior to interview were desired for the study. The actual numbers in each subgroup for which data are available and the distribution by men and women are shown in Table 5-1.

Looking at the data another way, there were 55 separated persons who have not filed for divorce, 36 who have filed, and 85 who have received a final decree. It is interesting to compare the ratio of separated to divorced in the study sample to the ratio reported for the general population. Unfortunately, there is no generally accepted standard for classifying those who have filed for divorce into either the separated or divorced category. Self-report is usually the method used, and

Table 5-1
Study Sample

Seriously discussing separation or divorce (Sub 1: M = 23, F = 39)	**62**
Last event 1 to 13 months ago (Sub 2)	
Separated 1 to 13 months previous, not filed (M = 15, F = 32)	47
Filed 1 to 13 months ago, not final (M = 11, F = 17)	28
Final decree 1 to 13 months ago (M = 8, F = 23)	<u>31</u>
Total last event 1 to 13 months ago (M = 34, F = 72)	**106**
Last event 14 months or more previous (Sub 3)	
Separated 14 months or more ago, not filed (M = 3, F = 5)	8
Filed 14 months or more ago, not final (M = 1, F = 7)	8
Final decree 14 or more months ago (M = 18, F = 36)	<u>54</u>
Total last event 14 or more months ago (M = 22, F = 48)	**70**
Total (M = 79, F = 159)	**238**

it is frequently inconsistent. If filers are considered as separated, then the ratio of divorced to separated is less than 1:1. If, on the other hand, filers are considered as divorced, then the ratio becomes 2.2.

This general lack of clarity only makes comparisons with the general population of divorcing and divorced people more difficult. As noted in Chapter 3, the 1976 ratio of divorced to separated people nationally was 1.9. It was considerably higher in Los Angeles County in 1977 to 1978, at 3.1 for men and 4.5 for women. Assuming some ambiguity in regard to those who have filed for divorce only, it is probable that those who are separated and those who have filed but have not received a final decree are overrepresented in our sample. This becomes important when we consider how mental health changes during the separation/divorce process.

The data are analyzed separately for the three major subgroups: persons discussing separation but not separated (Sub 1), those having experienced the last separation event within the previous 13 months (Sub 2), and those for whom separation occurred more than 13 months previous (Sub 3). Differences between these groups were anticipated. The more detailed subcategories within the three broad ones were analyzed only occasionally.

The study population consisted of 79 men and 159 women. There were no significant differences as to sex between the marital dissolution categories ($X^2 = 1.74$; 4 df; NS).

Ages ranged from 18 to 67 years (SD = 11.0, $\bar{x} = 35.2$, and median = 32.3). Age distribution did not differ significantly for men ($\bar{x} = 36.2$) or for women ($\bar{x} = 34.7$). There was, however, a difference in ages between the dissolution groups, those whose last separation event occurred 14 or more months ago being older ($\bar{x} = 38.0$ years) than the other two groups ($F = 3.283$; 2 df; $p = .039$).*

The entire sample was white. Blacks were excluded because the divorce experience both may differ for blacks and because the population of the Rush Center treats insufficient blacks to adequately assess their experience.

Socioeconomic status was indicated by a two-factor index involving education and occupation. Five categories were employed, with 1 being the highest and 5 the lowest; 15.6 percent were in classes 1 and 2, 39.4 percent were in class 3, 35.5 percent were in class 4, and 9.5 percent were in class 5. About three fourths of the sample was composed

---

*Throughout this book, F is the F ratio statistic calculated in analysis of variance procedures.

of middle- and working-class people (those with white- and blue-collar occupations). There were no significant differences regarding social class by sex and by marital dissolution categories.

Current monthly family income was determined on the basis of information given at the clinic intake interview. Because the clinic fee is determined on the basis of ability to pay, there may be a tendency to decrease the amount of income indicated. Stated income ranged from none in 38 cases to $5000 per month in one case. The mean was $578 and the median was $500. (It should be kept in mind that those were 1973–1975 dollars.) The standard deviation was $542, indicating that a wide range existed. There was no significant difference in income by sex, though women averaged slightly less ($X^2 = 6.15$; 4 df; NS). There was, however, a relationship between income and dissolution status. When income was grouped into five categories, ranging from $0–249 to $1500 and more, and compared to the three dissolution categories, there was a significant difference ($X^2 = 25.82$; 8 df; $p = .001$). Inspection reveals that this difference is due to higher income levels among those discussing separation who are still married, indicating that persons with higher income are less likely to separate and/or that a drop in income characteristically accompanies marital separation. The mean income for those still married was $776 compared to $540 for those with a recent separation event and $461 for the long-term separated or divorced.

Subjects had been married for a relatively long period of time. The mean length of marriage at the time of interview was 7 years 5 months, and the median was 4½ years (SD = 7 years 3 months). The range was from 1 month to 38 years. There was no difference as to sex ($X^2 = 0.17$; 4 df; NS) or marital dissolution category ($X^2 = 8.79$; 8 df; NS).

The majority of the subjects were parents. Fifty had children from previous marriages and 129 had children from the present marriage. Only about a third did not have any children.

It is interesting to compare some of the characteristics of this sample with national statistics. Previously cited statistics show an age peak ranging from 25 to 34 years; 47 percent of my sample were in that group. Nationally, approximately 62.5 percent of the divorced are women; my sample has 67 percent. Women are overrepresented in the divorced population because men often remarry single women. In my sample, however, women are also overrepresented in the separated and filed groups but not in the divorced group. Thus women are represented disproportionately in the study. The national median between first marriage and divorce is 6.7 years for men and 7.3 years for women. The figures for remarriage are lower. Our figures are only roughly comparable, since we do not distinguish between first and subsequent marriages. However, our mean of approximately 7.5 years and median of 5.5 years are roughly of the same magnitude. Nationally, about 60 percent of those divorcing had children; in our sample, the figure is approximately 66 percent. For these basic demographic characteristics, then, our sample does not differ sharply from the national picture. The sample does, however, overrepresent the separated and those who have filed but have not received a final decree, compared to those whose divorce is final.

Method

Each participant was interviewed by a research assistant and either a senior psychiatric social worker or senior psychologist.* The clinically significant data were obtained in face-to-face interviews by the social worker or psychologist. Several instruments were designed for the study: (1) A marital-problems survey, questions about marital dissolution status, nature and frequency of recent spouse contacts, emotional reliance on spouse, aggression by and toward the spouse, alliances with friends and relatives, romantic involvements, and the occurrence of events increasing the likelihood of separation or reconciliation. (2) A separation-coping scale further dealt with wishes for and likelihood of reconciliation; the presence of sadness, anger, and guilt and its relationship to the separation; and the presence and intensity of memory and fantasy about the spouse. Also included in this instrument were questions relating to the capacity to test reality regarding separation and the clarity and consistency of communication between the spouses. (3) Other instruments assessed the existence and nature of the crisis and the presence and nature of new love-object relationships.

Eight measures of mental health were employed:

1. The somatic disturbance subscale of the Frank Discomfort Scale (SOM)[3]
2. The anxiety subscale of the Frank Discomfort Scale (ANX)[3]
3. The depression subscale of the Frank Discomfort Scale (DEP)[3]
4. The Brief Psychiatric Rating Scale (BPRS)[4]
5. The Social Dysfunction Rating Scale (SOC or SDRS)[5]

---

*Margaret Bonnefil, A.C.S.W. and Kenneth Wurtz, Ph.D. contributed greatly to the study in these roles.

6. Suicide Prevention Center Assessment of Suicide Potential[6], retrospective to the time of entry into the Benjamin Rush Center (SPC1) (usually between one day and one week before the research interview)
7. Suicide Prevention Center Assessment of Suicide Potential as measured at the time of research interview (SPC 2)
8. Suicide potential assessed by the mental health rater at the time of interview (ASP). The marginals for the total sample and for Sub 2 can be found in Appendix 1 at the end of this book.

The first three measures were directly reported by the respondent. They therefore have the advantage of not requiring an outside rater and not involving any possible rater bias. They reflect an individual's subjectively experienced level of well-being and do not include references to more serious psychiatric pathology. The Frank Discomfort Scale was specifically designed for use with outpatient populations.[3] The Brief Psychiatric Rating Scale includes indicators of more serious pathology as well as some of the symptomatology reflected in the Frank Discomfort Scale. It was included in this study to determine to what extent this widely used measure of psychiatric pathology would be sensitive to divorce-related phenomena. The Social Dysfunction Rating Scale primarily assesses functioning in interpersonal and social areas. Three measures of suicide potential were employed, in part because of the original focus of the study on suicide phenomena. Two of these used a scale that has been widely employed in suicide prevention centers as a practical measure of suicide risk. That scale, ranging from 1 to 9, was administered only when the person gave some clinical indication of suicide potential. If it was not administered, the score was automatically 0. Because several days often elapsed since the person entered the Rush Center, we anticipated that the suicide potential might have diminished as help was sought and offered. We therefore asked the respondent questions to assess suicide potential both at the moment of entry into the Center and at the time of the research interview. Lastly, we asked the mental health professional raters to indicate their views of the person's suicide potential on a scale of 1 through 4, ranging from no potential to severe potential.

Inter-rater reliability was assessed for 22 cases using the Spearman rho coefficient (p). The correlation was .96 for the Social Dysfunction Rating Scale, .87 for the Brief Psychiatric Rating Scale, and .90 for the Suicide Prevention Center Assessment of Suicide Potential.

A Pearson correlation matrix involving the eight outcome measures for the total study population showed highest correlations among the subscales of the Frank Discomfort Scale. The correlation between the somatic and anxiety subscale was $r = .727$; it was .567 between somatic and depression and .635 between anxiety and depression. There was also a high correlation ($r = .705$) between the Brief Psychiatric Rating Scale and the Social Dysfunction rating scale. The three suicidal measures also showed correlations ($r = .775$ to .821). There were thus three major subgroups: the three subscales of the Frank Discomfort Scale; the Brief Psychiatric Rating Scale and Social Dysfunction Rating Scale; and the three suicidal measures.

The correlations between these groups were lower than those within the groups. The Frank Discomfort subscales correlated with the Social Dysfunction Rating Scale at levels from $r = .277$ to .307 and with the Brief Psychiatric Rating Scales at levels from $r = .451$ to .476. The correlations of the Frank Discomfort subscales to the suicidal variables ranged from $r = .238$ to .335. The Social Dysfunction Rating Scale and the Brief Psychiatric Rating Scale were correlated with the suicidal variables at levels of $r = .352$ to .427.

When we look at the relationships between the three subgroups of outcome variables with each other, we find that while each is related to the other, the least relationship prevails between the Frank Discomfort Scales and the suicidal variables. The Brief Psychiatric Rating Scale occupies an intermediate position in that it shows moderate correlations with all other mental health variables ($r = .352$ to .476). The Social Dysfunction Rating Scale is also intermediate showing low to moderate relationships to the Frank Discomfort measures ($r = .277$ to .307) and slightly higher ones to the suicidal variables ($r = .390$ to .428).

These relationships are expected. The Brief Psychiatric Rating Scale reflects both subjective discomfort and more serious indicators of pathology, while the Social Dysfunction Rating Scale assesses social interaction and therefore associates with both discomfort and suicide potential. The only surprising finding was that the three indicators of subjective discomfort show a relatively low association with the indicators of suicide potential.

A note of caution needs to be introduced. The number of persons indicating any degree of suicide potential was relatively low. Of the entire sample population ($N = 231$), 75.3 percent were rated as non-suicidal at the time of entry. At time of interview, 83.2 percent were rated non-suicidal on the Suicide Prevention Center instrument,[6] and 80.7 percent were so judged by the raters. The high proportion of non-suicidal subjects resulted in a highly skewed distribution curve. Kendall's tau (τ) was used in all correlation analyses when significant levels were reported because of the extent of skewing. Nevertheless, the reader should keep in mind the relatively low proportion of suicidal individuals.*†

DEMOGRAPHIC AND SOCIOECONOMIC
CHARACTERISTICS AND MENTAL HEALTH

This section discusses the relationship of sex, age, socioeconomic status, income, and presence or absence of children to the mental health status of those involved in the marital dissolution process. In each instance we will review some general considerations based on the literature and proceed to findings from the research study.

Sex and Mental Health

PREVIOUS STUDIES

As Hunt and Hunt[7] pointed out, there has been a widespread belief that the typical divorce involves a hedonistic man who abandons his wife and children, marries or lives with a younger woman, and leads a self-indulgent, pleasurable life while his abandoned wife suffers greatly. The reality is far more complex. A number of recent studies have related sex to various measures of mental health or general satisfaction in the separated and divorced. The Hunts' study indicates that almost as many men as women in the early phase of separation report being unable to sleep, eat, or concentrate on their work and use alcohol, smoke heavily, and suffer from a sense of failure or worthlessness. Later on in the separation, the women's practical problems, especially if she has young children, often make life harder for her than for the man, but "at the outset, the emotional impact is much the same." Also more women than men are likely to feel good immediately after the separation.[7]

---

*While not so extreme in their distribution as the suicide indicators, other mental health measures also showed degrees of skewness and/or kurtosis, which called for the use of Kendall's tau as a correlation measure whenever significance levels were of interest.

†In subsequent chapters findings for Sub 2 men and women will be reported. However, there were not enough suicidal men in Sub 2 to analyze their suicide potential.

Although most workers agree that some differences do exist between men and women in regard to divorce, there is no consensus on what the differences are. Brown and Fox[8] stated that the question is not which gender does better or worse, overall, but what the combination of stresses and coping are for each. Such factors as economics, children, social relations, emotional separation, and reestablishment of identity must be considered separately for men and women.

Kitson[9] reported that women experience more subjective distress than men ($r = .13$, $p < .05$). However, the relationship becomes insignificant when controls are introduced for having sought mental health help, income, receiving help from the family, and having friends with whom one can talk over confidential matters as well as for how long ago the divorce was suggested. The association with sex is strengthened when controls are introduced for self-esteem and attachment.[9] Kitson and Raschke[10] concluded that the evidence thus far on whether males or females have more difficulty in adjusting to divorce is contradictory.

Chiriboga and associates[11,12] studied persons who had filed for divorce in San Francisco and Alameda counties. Using a trauma and relief index, they found that "men appear more vulnerable to stresses of separation."[11] The relationship of gender to outcome in their study differed, however, depending on the dependent variable employed. When self-report of happiness was the indicator, divorcing men reported themselves as significantly less happy; 31 percent of men and 16 percent of women indicated that they were "not too happy."[12] The authors did not feel that this difference reflects sex differences in the general population regardless of whether or not the marriage was intact, since surveys do not indicate differences between men and women as a whole in regard to self-report of happiness. On the other hand, when depression and "tension" were the criteria, women were significantly worse off than men. The authors concluded that "men and women simply react in different ways to separation,"[12] men being more likely to report enduring unhappiness while women experience more temporary depression and unrest.

Mellinger et al.[13] used an index of psychic distress and found that a higher proportion of women, regardless of marital status, experienced high levels of psychic distress (34 percent compared to 19 percent of men). Among the separated and divorced, the proportion indicating high levels of distress rises in both women and men to 49 percent and 28 percent respectively. The increase is somewhat higher for men than for women, though no test of statistical significance is reported.

STUDY FINDINGS

Findings for the group are summarized in Table 5-2. Women reported more distress on the somatic, anxiety, and depression subscores of the Frank Discomfort Scale than did men (*p* ranging from .000 to .003). There were, on the other hand, no significant differences between the sexes on the Brief Psychiatric Rating Scale, the Social Dysfunction Rating Scale, or on any of the three measures of suicide potential.

Table 5-2
Relationship of Sex to Mental Health Measures (All)

Mental Health Measure	Sex	Cases (No.)	Mean	SD	*t*	*df*
SOMA	M	79	1.381	0.408	-4.35^b	235
	F	158	1.645	0.457		
ANX	M	79	1.674	0.717	-2.98^a	235
	F	158	1.966	0.708		
DEP	M	79	2.350	0.817	-3.36^b	235
	F	158	2.729	0.821		
SOC	M	77	1.993	0.633	0.87	231
	F	156	1.922	0.570		
BPRS	M	77	1.682	0.419	0.21^c	124
	F	156	1.671	0.331		
SPC 1	M	75	0.684	1.523	-1.13	229
	F	156	0.932	1.577		
SPC 2	M	76	0.475	1.293	$-.68$	230
	F	156	0.598	1.287		
ASP	M	77	1.247	0.588	$-.70$	231
	F	156	1.308	0.649		

For explanation of mental health measures see Appendix 5-A.
$^a p \le .01$.
$^b p \le .001$.
$^c F$ test for homogeneity of variances indicates significant differences in variances of the two groups. Therefore, separate variance estimate has been provided and the *t* test consequently adjusted.

Table 5-3
Relationship of Sex to Mental Health Measures
(Married and Discussing Separation—Sub 1)

Mental Health Measure	Sex	Cases (No.)	Mean	SD	t	df
SOMA	M	23	1.303	0.178	-4.35^b	53
	F	39	1.671	0.476		
ANX	M	23	1.391	0.445	-3.26^a	60
	F	39	1.885	0.638		
DEP	M	23	1.957	0.630	-3.52^b	60
	F	39	2.675	0.851		
SOC	M	23	1.975	0.630	1.23	60
	F	39	1.799	0.487		
BPRS	M	23	1.628	0.446	-0.17^c	35
	F	39	1.646	0.306		
SPC 1	M	23	0.235	0.778	-1.19^c	60
	F	39	0.562	1.387		
SPC 2	M	23	0.00	1.00	1.80	60
	F	39	0.428	1.137		
ASP	M	23	1.131	0.344	-0.81^c	60
	F	39	1.231	0.627		

For explanation of mental health measures see Appendix 5-A.
$^a p \leqslant .01$.
$^b p \leqslant .001$.
$^c F$ test for homogeneity of variances indicates significant differences in variances of the two groups. Therefore, separate variance estimate has been provided and the t test consequently adjusted.

The further breakdown of sex differences pertaining to self-reported discomfort is of interest. Highly significant differences ($p = .000$ to .002) exist for all three subscales (SOM, ANX, and DEP) for those persons who were seriously discussing separation and divorce but who were not separated at the time of interview (Sub 1). These findings are reported in Table 5-3.

The situation changes when we look at Sub 2, the group who have experienced their last separation event less than 14 months before the

Table 5-4
Relationship of Sex to Mental Health Measures
(Separated or Divorced Within Previous 14 Months—Sub 2)

Mental Health Measure	Sex	Cases (No.)	Mean	SD	t	df
SOMA	M	34	1.423	0.526	-2.48^a	103
	F	71	1.680	0.481		
ANX	M	34	1.780	0.766	-1.54	103
	F	71	2.033	0.802		
DEP	M	34	2.618	0.766	-1.01	103
	F	71	2.794	0.869		
SOC	M	32	1.960	0.636	0.21	100
	F	70	1.933	0.558		
BPRS	M	32	1.729	0.399	0.95^b	48
	F	70	1.653	0.301		
SPC 1	M	32	0.834	1.699	-0.70	
	F	70	1.086	1.676		
SPC 2	M	32	0.594	1.444	-0.39	100
	F	70	0.710	1.361		
ASP	M	32	1.250	0.622	-0.38	100
	F	70	1.300	0.622		

For explanation of mental health measures see Appendix 5-A.
$^a p \leq .05$.
$^b F$ test for homogeneity of variances indicates significant differences in variances of the two groups. Therefore, separate variance estimate has been provided and the t test consequently adjusted.

interview. The details will be found in Table 5-4. Here, the only mental health indicator differing statistically between women and men is SOM ($\tau = -2.48$; 103 df; $p = .015$). The reason for the change is that distress in men tends to catch up with that of women once the separation has actually occurred.

When we turn to Sub 3, the group that experienced their last separation event more than 13 months prior to the interview, we find that there are no longer any significant differences between the sexes (Table 5-5). Only somatic distress approaches significance ($\tau = -1.73$; 68 df; $p = .088$). While distress levels remain slightly higher for women than

Table 5-5

Relationship of Sex to Mental Health Measures
(Separated or Divorced More than 14 months Previously—Sub 3)

Mental Health Measure	Sex	Cases (No.)	Mean	SD	t	df
SOMA	M	22	1.398	0.376	−1.73	68
	F	48	1.573	0.402		
ANX	M	22	1.807	0.809	−0.72	68
	F	48	1.932	0.610		
DEP	M	22	2.349	0.924	−1.61	68
	F	48	2.671	0.728		
SOC	M	22	2.060	0.656	0.32	67
	F	47	2.007	0.641		
BPRS	M	22	1.671	0.432	−0.44	67
	F	47	1.717	0.390		
SPC 1	M	20	0.960	0.805	−0.11	65
	F	47	1.010	1.556		
SPC 2	M	21	0.814	1.622	0.66	66
	F	47	0.571	1.302		
ASP	M	22	1.364	0.727	−0.10	67
	F	47	1.383	0.709		

For explanation of mental health measures see Appendix 5-A.

for men, two out of three suicide potential indicators are higher for men than for women though none of these differences are statistically significant.

We thus see that for women, disturbance is clearly higher prior to separation. For men, disturbance levels rise sharply after separation to the point where they are of the same intensity as in women. This phenomenon is corroborated by analysis of variance, comparing mental health measures for men in the groups Sub 1, Sub 2, and Sub 3. As seen in Table 5-6 the increase in disturbance for men after separation reaches statistical significance for depression and approaches significance for anxiety and SPC 2. Men tend to be more depressed, anxious, and suicidal after separation than men who discuss separation but are still married. No such findings exist for women, for whom a parallel analysis of variance shows no significant changes.

Table 5-6

Relationship of Depression, Anxiety, and Suicide Potential to Marital
Dissolution Status of Men

Analysis of Variance

	Source	df	SS	MS	f	p
DEP	Between	2	5.997	2.998	4.950	.0095
	Within	76	46.036	.606		
	Total	78	52.033			
ANX	Between	2	2.604	1.302	2.643	.0777
	Within	76	37.440	.493		
	Total	78	40.044			
SPC2	Between	2	8.058	4.029	2.508	.0884
	Within	73	117.28	1.607		
	Total	75	125.34			

Descriptive Statistics

		Sub 1	Sub 2	Sub 3	Total
DEP	Mean	1.957	2.618	2.349	2.350
	SD	.630	.766	.924	.817
	N	23	34	22	79
ANX	Mean	1.391	1.779	1.807	1.674
	SD	.445	.766	.809	.717
	N	23	34	22	79
SPC2	Mean	0.000	0.594	0.814	0.475
	SD	.000	1.444	1.622	1.293
	N	23	32	21	76

For explanation of mental health measures see Appendix 5-A.

CONCLUSIONS

These findings seem to corroborate that during separation there is
a tendency toward greater subjective distress among women. The existence of such distress, however, is most definite in persons whose future marital status is still unclear: they are discussing the possibility of
separation but they may or may not act on it. To some extent, the
gender differences in this subgroup may reflect Mellinger et al.'s[13] finding that married women—divorce discussions apart—show much higher psychic distress than do men. What is interesting is that in my study

the distress level rose more sharply after separation in men than it did in women, thus tending to reduce differences. If this finding is corrobo-·rated by future studies, certain explanations may be considered. One of these suggests that marriage provides more psychic support for men than for women and that they therefore have more to lose.[13] Another view might be that among the married, the traditional female role allows the wife to express emotions, including those of distress, more than the husband. The wife may be expressing feelings for both members of the couple. When the wife is no longer available, the husband must acknowledge his own distress.

My findings are compatible with the work of Kitson[9] and Chiriboga,[12] both of whom suggested that there is more overt distress among women. That the association reported by these authors is not strong may be explained by the increase in reported distress in men over time. My own data do not allow any conclusion regarding the view that men report more unhappiness, since questions in that area were not included in the study. As to whether men are more behaviorally disturbed, two of the mental health measures could be expected to shed some light on the question: the Brief Psychiatric Rating Scale and the Social Dysfunction Rating Scale. Scores for men and women on both of these measures were very similar for the group at all times. A differential along this axis was therefore not found.

My data support the tentative conclusion that the differences between psychological disturbances among divorcing men and women is a weak one. Those still married and discussing separation should be exempted from this conclusion. It is also possible that distress rises more sharply in men than in women after separation occurs. The clinician should be alert to the possibility that women will acknowledge and perhaps experience distress both before and after a marital separation, while men are more likely to be overtly disturbed after the event. It is also possible that suicide danger increases more sharply in men than in women following a marital separation.

Age

PREVIOUS STUDIES

Surveys have indicated that self-reported well-being or happiness tends to decline in the divorced with increasing age. Chiriboga[12] reported that those divorcing in later life tended to be less happy than younger persons. On the other hand, Raschke[14] found that post-divorce stress is less for older men than for younger men.

STUDY FINDINGS

My data suggest a trend similar to Chiriboga's. The association of age to the eight mental health measures was examined for the entire group, using Kendall's tau (τ) as the measure. Only one measure, rater-assessed suicide potential, increased with age ($\tau = .107$; $N = 233$; $p < .05$). When Sub 1, Sub 2, and Sub 3 were separately considered, there were no significant associations with age. For males, ASP increased with age at a level just missing significance ($\tau = .179$; $N = 77$; $p = .056$). For women, increasing age predicted higher scores (more impairment) on BPRS ($\tau = .136$; $N = 156$; $p < .05$).

CONCLUSIONS

The findings suggest that the generally accepted principle of a somewhat adverse effect of increasing age on mental health holds true for the separating and divorcing. The effect is quite weak, however, perhaps because many divorcing persons are in their thirties and the deleterious impact of aging may not be as great at that time in life as it is later on.

Socioeconomic Status

PREVIOUS STUDIES

Socioeconomic status is indicated by level of education, occupation, and in some studies by income. Chiriboga[12] found that education, work, and finances have an effect on the well-being of separating and divorcing persons. Raschke[14] notes that for divorcing males higher occupational status relates to lower stress and lower status relates to higher stress, but the association did not hold true when men and women were considered together. No association of stress was found with educational levels.

Pearlin and Johnson[15] used survey techniques to examine the relationship of marital status, life strain, and depression in 2300 persons from the Chicago area. Depression was related to marital status at a highly significant level. The widowed, divorced, and separated were more depressed than the married, and those separated were most depressed. Using statistical regression analysis, 69 percent of the variance of depression with marital status could be related to life stresses including economic hardship, social isolation, and number of children. Foremost of these in its impact on depression was economic hardship.

Similarly, Goode[16] pointed out that the highest trauma in his sample of women was among those who stated they would have been financially better off without divorce, while the lowest trauma was found among those who would be worse off if they had not divorced. Raschke[14] also reported that post-divorce stress is lower when a woman is economically independent of her husband. Kitson[9] reported that lower anticipated income in the coming year is related to distress in a group of persons who filed for divorce.

STUDY FINDINGS

The two-factor index of social position was used to measure socioeconomic status.[17] Weights were assigned to occupational groups according to their status, and weights arc also given to years of education completed. The resulting scores are divided into categories numbered from 1 (highest) to 5 (lowest). This measure was related to the mental health variables (Table 5-7). For the group as a whole, all outcome measures except for depression were significantly related to socioeconomic status using Kendall's tau ($p \leq .01$). The lower the socioeconomic status the greater the disturbance. It is of considerable interest that this association did not hold for any measures for Sub 1. For Sub 2, however, increased disturbance on all mental health measures except for two suicide variables were similarly associated with lower socioeconomic status using Kendall's tau ($p \leq .01$). Those separated or divorced for longer periods fell in the middle: measures indicating more social dysfunction and more suicide potential on all three suicide variables were significantly related to lower socioeconomic status ($p \leq .05$), while other variables did not so relate. Analysis separately by men and women showed that association for many of the mental health variables was present for both sexes. For men the strongest relationships prevailed in the non-suicide variables, while for women suicide variables were most strongly related.

Family income was self-reported. For the group as a whole, only the Social Dysfunction Rating Scale scores were associated with income levels. Persons with lower income showed poorer functioning ($\tau = -.121$; $N = 194$; $p < .05$). When the marital subgroups were examined, only the long-term separated showed a relationship of less income to more disturbance on the SDRS ($\tau = -.275$; $N = 56$; $p < .01$) and the BPRS ($\tau = -.198$; $N = 56$; $p < .05$). Income was also associated with SDRS for men ($\tau = -.185$; $N = 60$; $p < .05$) but not for

Table 5-7

Relationship of Socioeconomic Status to Mental Health Measures
(Kendall's tau)

Mental Health Measure	Total Sample	Sub 1	Sub 2	Sub 3	M	F
SOMA	.133[a]	−.073	.264[a]	.083	.208[b]	.094
	(231)	(60)	(102)	(69)	(77)	(154)
ANX	.164[a]	.007	.299[a]	.082	.291[a]	.090
	(231)	(60)	(102)	(69)	(77)	(154)
DEP	.068	−.099	.202[a]	.031	.205[b]	−.017
	(231)	(60)	(102)	(69)	(77)	(154)
SOC	.211[a]	.026	.322[a]	.189[b]	.279[a]	.177[a]
	(227)	(60)	(99)	(68)	(75)	(152)
BPRS	.153[a]	.091	.248[a]	.097	.224[b]	.105
	(227)	(60)	(99)	(68)	(75)	(152)
SPC1	.160[a]	.019	.155	.245[b]	.160	.160[b]
	(225)	(60)	(99)	(66)	(73)	(152)
SPC2	.187[a]	−.043	.236[a]	.240[b]	.179	.193[a]
	(227)	(60)	(99)	(68)	(75)	(152)
ASP	.179[a]	.113	.167	.224[b]	.155	.191[a]
	(227)	(60)	(99)	(68)	(75)	(152)

For explanations of mental health measures see Appendix 5-A.
Sample sizes are given in parentheses.
[a]$p \leq .01$.
[b]$p \leq .05$.

women ($\tau = -.085$; $N = 134$; NS). The relatively weak association of income with mental health may in part be due to the unreliability of income data obtained in a setting in which the establishing of fees depends on reported income.

CONCLUSIONS

The evidence strongly indicates that socioeconomic factors do matter, both among the general population and especially among the divorcing. In my study these differences do not appear relevant among those now married, although the marriage may be unhappy. Marriage may therefore exert a protective effect against the stresses of lower class status. On the other hand, those who have recently experienced separation events show the greatest association of poor mental health with lower socioeconomic status found among any subgroup. Those whose separation events occurred over 14 months ago, show a moderate association. One interpretation of these findings is that those who have most recently experienced the traumas of marital separation are most vulnerable when they do not have the protection of higher social status, whereas after a period of time those divorced achieve a new equilibrium with their environment and social status looms less large. Suicide potential, however, continues to be significantly associated with lower socioeconomic status in this group.

Presence or Absence of Children

PREVIOUS STUDIES

From a theoretical standpoint, there are conflicting expectations as to whether divorcing people with or without children may be expected to cope better with marital dissolution. Pearlin and Johnson[15] believed it is the number of children, rather than their presence or absence, that contributes to strain. The more children there are, the greater the likelihood of depression. On the other hand, the presence of children in the home is generally considered by suicidologists to lower the suicide risk.

In empirical studies, Hunt and Hunt[7] reported that separating persons with children are more likely to feel good immediately after separation than those without children; women who have custody of their children are more likely to feel good than their former husbands. Weiss,[18] on the other hand, reported that the presence of children in the home seems to reduce the proportion of women reporting themselves as happier and to increase the proportion of those who fear a breakdown. This finding occurs both in the separated/divorced and in the widowed, leading to the suggestion that being a single parent is stressful.[18]

STUDY FINDINGS

The only comparison made was between persons without children from either the current or a prior marriage and those with children. Using the *t* test, the only significant differences were observed for the

Table 5-8
Relationship of Presence or Absence of Children to Mental Health Measures
(All)

Mental Health Measure		Cases (No.)	Mean	SD	t	df
SOMA	Children	161	1.562	0.484	0.25	235
	No children	76	1.546	0.398		
ANX	Children	161	1.872	0.706	0.13	235
	No children	76	1.860	0.761		
DEP	Children	161	2.614	0.817	0.29	235
	No children	76	2.580	0.884		
SOC	Children	158	1.908	0.585	−1.42	231
	No children	75	2.025	0.600		
BPRS	Children	158	1.675	0.361	0.03	231
	No children	75	1.673	0.366		
SPC 1	Children	156	0.655	1.425	−2.61[a]	123[b]
	No children	75	1.260	1.750		
SPC 2	Children	157	0.407	1.135	−2.36[a]	115[b]
	No children	75	0.873	1.520		
ASP	Children	158	1.228	0.563	−1.93	117[b]
	No children	75	1.413	0.737		

For explanation of mental health measures see Appendix 5-A.
[a]$p \leq .05$.
[b]F test for homogeneity of variances indicates significant differences in variances of the two groups. Therefore, separate variance estimate has been provided and the t test consequently adjusted.

group as a whole (all) regarding suicide potential. Persons with children were significantly less suicidal ($p \leq .05$) than those without children on all three measures of suicide potential, thus confirming the prediction made in the literature (see Table 5-8).

Greater suicide potential was associated with absence of children on all suicide variables for the group as a whole, for Sub 2, and for women (Table 5-9). There was a non-significant tendency in the same direction for Sub 3. The only other measure that distinguished between the two groups was the SOC for the recently divorced, those with children showing less dysfunction ($\tau = .185$; $p < .05$) (Table 5-9). My

Table 5-9
Relationship of Presence or Absence of Children to Mental
Health Measures for Sub 2 (using Kendall's tau)

Mental Health Measure	Total Sample	Sub 2	F
SOMA	.013	.062	.017
	(237)	(105)	(158)
ANX	−.023	−.015	−.009
	(237)	(105)	(158)
DEP	−.013	.025	−.018
	(237)	(105)	(158)
SOC	.088	.185[b]	.106
	(233)	(102)	(156)
BPRS	−.002	.105	.019
	(233)	(102)	(156)
SPC 1	.185[a]	.198[b]	.225[a]
	(231)	(102)	(156)
SPC 2	.172[a]	.221[b]	.198[a]
	(232)	(102)	(156)
ASP	.130[b]	.210[b]	.167[b]
	(233)	(102)	(156)

For explanation of mental health measures see Appendix 5-A.
Sample sizes are given in parentheses.
[a] $p \leq .01$.
[b] $p \leq .05$.

data therefore confirm the existence of increased suicide risk for separated or divorced women who do not have children.

CONCLUSIONS

The negative effects on mental health of having children predicted by other researchers were not seen in our data. Such effects might have appeared, however, if the number of children, their ages, and the economic status of the family had been taken into account. Clearly, having children diminishes the tendency to be self-destructive, at least for women; whether it also increases the strain on the single parent under some circumstances remains unanswered.

MENTAL HEALTH AND TIME ELAPSED SINCE
SEPARATION-RELATED EVENTS

Is there a point in the separation process during which individuals are at greatest mental health risk? Does distress and associated symptomatic disturbance and disability reach a peak and then subside? This question is of considerable importance, from the standpoint of both the practitioner and the researcher.

Previous Reports

The modern phase of divorce research may be said to have begun with Goode,[16] who developed the trauma index discussed in Chapter 4. Its components were difficulty sleeping, poorer health, greater loneliness, low work efficiency, memory difficulties, increased smoking, and increased drinking. All of his respondents were interviewed after their final divorce decree and were asked to describe retrospectively whether they had experienced any of these disturbances during the divorce process and if so, when they felt the difficulty to have been greatest. The time periods studied were at the time of final decision to divorce, at the final separation, at the filing for the divorce, when the decree was granted, or at the time of interview. About 63 percent were high- or medium-trauma respondents.[16] Goode constructed a "curve of trouble"[16] to describe the peak incidence of difficulty. This curve rises from the point of the final decision to divorce to a high point at the final separation; it then tapers off gradually to the first filing and drops off somewhat to the point of final decree and drops further again to the point of the interview. The last drop is equivocal, Goode noted, due to the fact that in 25 percent of the cases the time interval between the final decree and the date of the interview was one to two months.

Chester,[1] also using retroactive inquiry, noted that most women reported feeling most upset at the time of actual separation; fewer indicated that the divorce decision represented the most difficult aspect; still fewer found the entering of the final decree the most stressful moment. However, Chester's own interpretation notwithstanding, his data indicate that 60 percent of the subjects reported that their feelings of upset were most intense before separation, while only 28 percent found the actual separation most difficult. Hunt and Hunt[7] stated that the length of leveling off of symptoms is variable, lasting one week to years, and that "most formerly married take two or more years to achieve genuine emotional stability."[7] Weiss[18] felt that there is an 8-

month to 1-year period during which initial disorganization and depression is followed by an attempt to regain one's footing. A subsequent phase involves periods of recovery interspersed with vulnerability to regression, which can shatter the attained equilibrium. This latter period ends after two to four years, when Weiss believes that a "stable and resilient new identity pattern is established."[18]

Chiriboga[11] used a scale based on that of Goode, adding items that converted it to a trauma and relief scale. He also modified the time periods to add the time prior to the decision to divorce, and he added an item indicating that distress was equal at all times. Summarizing his findings and those of Goode,[16] Weiss,[18] and Hetherington,[19] Chiriboga concluded that the evidence seems to imply at least two peaks and troughs associated with divorce. The first may correspond roughly to the period of separation and the second may involve long-term adaptation to the role and status of the divorced person. Ilfeld[20] stated that separated respondents "are the most distressed group; however, level of distress drops considerably for those who have passed through separation and are divorced." He compared the separated and divorced as a group, without consideration of the length of separation.

Study Findings

On the basis of Goode's observations and of crisis theory, I hypothesized that those who had recently undergone a separation experience (Sub 2) would be more impaired in terms of mental health measures than those who had undergone such an experience at some time in the past (Sub 3). We also studied how those discussing separation but who were not separated (Sub 1) would relate to the other two groups. For purposes of analysis, Sub 2 was studied as a whole and was also broken down into three subgroups: those that had been separated less than 14 months but had not filed for divorce; those that had filed less than 14 months ago but had not received a final decree; and those who had received a final decree less than 14 months previously. To test the hypothesis, analysis of variance was performed.

The results were the same whether three or five subgroups were used. Of the eight mental health measures, depression was significant at $p = .05$ and anxiety approached significance ($p = .069$). The details of the analysis of variance for depression are found in Table 5-10. Intensity of depression peaks in the recently separated group, drops after filing of the divorce suit, drops further after the final decree, and shows a slight rise thereafter. It should be noted here that the statistical

Table 5-10

Relationship of Marital Dissolution Status to Depression

Analysis of Variance

Source	df	Sum of Squares	Mean Square	F Ratio	F Prob
Between Groups	4	7.030	1.757	2.575	.039[a]
Within Groups	232	158.351	0.683		
Total	236	165.380			

Means and Standard Deviations

Group	Cases (No.)	$\bar{X}$	SD
Seriously discussing separation (Sub 1)	62	2.409	0.846
Recently separated (Sub 2)	46	2.866	0.842
Recently filed (Sub 2)	28	2.798	0.825
Recently received final decree (Sub 2)	31	2.491	0.815
Long-term separated/divorced (Sub 3)	70	2.574	0.803

[a]$p \leq .05$.

results reported above only refer to tests performed regarding overall differences among the various groups. The particular pattern of differences was not analyzed for significance.

The results suggest that since only depression changed significantly, the crisis-rich period around the separation events is not as unequivocally associated with greater mental health impairment compared to the long-term separated and divorced as was expected.

The fact that all of our subjects were applicants to a crisis clinic must be kept in mind. It is likely that individuals early in the separation/divorce process are overrepresented in the study population. If this is true, the most logical explanation is that they were more likely to see themselves as being in crisis. To definitively distinguish between the degree of disturbance in the recently separated/divorced versus the long-term separated/divorced, one would need to know the degree of disturbance of the entire population—a very difficult endeavor. It is likely that the recently separated/divorced are even more disturbed relative to their long-term counterparts than can be determined through the present study.

Yet, even given this consideration, the fact that among applicants to a crisis clinic, degree of disturbance does not differ as sharply between the recently and long-term separated/divorced as was hypothesized is of interest. To understand this finding better, some other analyses of the data were made. The questions underlying the further studies are: Taking those among the separated/divorced who are sufficiently troubled to seek help, can we distinguish a pattern in degree of disturbance over time? How would it relate to studies in the general population, such as the "curve of trouble" of Goode?[16]

If there is a gradual improvement in functioning as time goes on, one would expect lower levels of impairment (lower scores) on the mental health measures. For that reason the number of months that elapsed between date of separation and date of interview were related to the mental health variables. The time elapsed ranged from one month to several years. For men there was no change over time. Women, however, showed diminished depression as the number of months since separation increased ($\tau = -.211$; $N = 114$; $p \leq .01$) and less anxiety ($\tau = -.154$; $N = 114$; p < .05). Somatic symptoms approached significance ($\tau = -.122$; $N = 114$; $p = .066$). When only Sub 2 was studied, the pattern was similar, with anxiety, depression, and BPRS. Improvement occurred as time since separation lengthened.

There are some complicated findings, however. This analysis was of all persons in the study, regardless of whether or not they had gone on to file for and to receive their final decrees. I then looked at only those who were separated and had not filed. Data were available for 50 subjects in the study—32 who were separated one or two months at the time of interview and 18 who were separated three or more months. Surprisingly, there was a tendency for the latter group to score *higher* on all measures except depression. The difference was statistically significant only for the SDRS ($\tau = -3.13$; 45 *df*; $p \leq .01$) and approached significance for BPRS ($\tau = -1.91$; 45 *df*; $p = .062$) and SPC 1 ($\tau = -1.72$; 45 *df*; $p = .092$) (Table 5-11). While the small samples, particularly in the three-or-more month group, suggest caution, the findings are of interest and suggest that the separated who do not file may get worse as time goes on.

There is another set of findings that run counter to the optimistic generalization that things get better over time for all separated and di-

Table 5-11

Relationship of Length of Separation to Mental Health Measures in
Separated Persons Who Have Not Filed for Divorce

Mental Health Measure	Length of Separation	Cases (No.)	X̄	SD	t	df
SOMA	1–2 mo	32	1.533	0.515	−1.50	48
	3 or more mo	18	1.761	0.515		
ANX	1–2 mo	32	1.992	0.846	−0.32	48
	3 or more mo	18	2.069	0.780		
DEP	1–2 mo	32	2.859	0.835	−0.11	48
	3 or more mo	18	2.833	0.739		
SOC	1–2 mo	30	1.866	0.605	−3.13[a]	45
	3 or more mo	17	2.462	0.667		
BPRS	1–2 mo	30	1.658	0.299	−1.91	45
	3 or more mo	17	1.863	0.433		
SPC 1	1–2 mo	30	0.713	1.640	−1.72	45
	3 or more mo	17	1.677	2.158		
SPC 2	1–2 mo	30	0.597	1.410	−1.47	45
	3 or more mo	17	1.306	1.871		
ASP	1–2 mo	30	1.233	0.568	−1.62	45
	3 or more mo	17	1.588	0.939		

For explanation of mental health measures see Appendix 5-A.
[a]$p \leq .01$.

vorced. These are from analysis of Sub 3 regardless of whether or not
they divorced. Whether they also improved as the date of separation
receded into the past was considered. They did not. On the contrary,
all correlations except somatic suggest that there is more disturbance
as time goes on. The difference is significant for SPC 2 ($\tau = 0.186$; $N =
94$; $p \leq .05$) and ASP ($\tau = 0.162$; $N = 95$; $p = .05$) and approaches
significance for BPRS ($\tau = 0.117$, $N = 95$; $p = .10$).

What happens when we look at the data using the standard categories of separated, filed for divorce, and final decree, regardless of the
length of time elapsed since each event? Does this approach help us
resolve the question of what happens to the divorcing over time? Only
to a degree. Using analysis of variance, we find that only on the depression variable did the groups differ ($F = 3.24$; $df = 2.168$; $p = .042$).
The group that had received the final decree was less depressed than
the separated and those who have filed. There was a similar difference

for anxiety that was not statistically significant, and there were no trends in either direction on other measures.

Conclusions

These findings, along with the work of others, raise some questions on the "curve of trouble" of Goode. There is indeed some evidence that, broadly speaking, disturbance on some mental health measures peaks during the separation period and diminishes thereafter. The finding that the separated as a group are more disturbed than the divorced thus will probably prove to be accurate.

These data and the data of others indicate that the course of mental health during the separation and divorce process is more complex than it first appears. The implication from my data is that at least among those in sufficient trouble to seek help, the groups contributing most to the generalization of high disturbance in the period following upon the separation followed by improvement appear to be women, persons proceeding fairly rapidly after separation with filing, and persons who have recently become divorced. On the other hand, the generalization may not hold for men, for those who are separated for longer periods without filing, and for persons remaining divorced over an extended period. It may well be that those reporting continued gradual improvement after the divorce was obtained may have based their conclusions on those persons who remarried; in recent years they may also have included persons who shared stable dyadic relationships without marriage. Others may remain at the same levels of mental health or possibly get worse.

The rather small group that waits for more than two months after separation before filing for divorce is of special interest. They may be wavering between reconciliation and separation, which our theoretical model would expect us to lead to impaired functioning.

The failure of the long-term separated (whether divorced or not) to continue to improve over time may be due to the chronic strains of divorce, which for reasons different from those of the crises of the separation period may adversely affect mental health. For those who remarry, mental health may again begin to improve. Since the present study did not include remarried individuals, this must remain speculation. We are making inferences about processes over time from data on different individuals who are at various points in the process. This limitation makes longitudinal study essential. Such studies are quite costly, however, and until they are done the above considerations may provide useful data.

The clinician must be alert to the possibility of increased disturbance in all individuals undergoing marital separation and divorce.
Time may, but will not always, be a healer.

SUMMARY

In this chapter the research study has been introduced. The goal of
the study is to relate mental health levels to various aspects of the
process of marital separation and divorce. The study population is
drawn from successive applicants at the Benjamin Rush Center, a crisis
clinic associated with a community mental health center in Los
Angeles, California. A case is made for the possibility that in spite of
the fact that this is a population of help-seekers, there may be some
generalizability of the findings to the population at large. Methodology
included the use of well-trained clinicians as raters who administered
instruments indicative of various aspects of the separation process.
Mental health status was measured by eight variables. Three of these
are subscales of the Frank Discomfort Scale. Two others are the Brief
Psychiatric Rating Scale and the Social Discomfort Rating Scale.
Lastly, there were three measures of suicide potential.

Demographic and socioeconomic characteristics of the separating/
divorcing are related to mental health. Somewhat greater distress during the separation process occurs for women than for men. This differential is clearest among persons who are discussing divorce but are not
yet separated. Once separation occurs, disturbance tends to rise more
rapidly among men than among women, thus tending to reduce differences between them.

There is a weak trend toward greater disturbance with increasing
age, but this factor is not important, probably due to the effect that the
divorcing group as a whole is relatively young.

There is strong evidence that socioeconomic factors do matter
among the general population and among the divorcing in particular. In
data the differences did not appear to be relevant among those now
married and discussing divorce but became clear among those who had
recently experienced separation. Lower socioeconomic status appears
to increase vulnerability to the divorce process.

The presence of children tends to decrease suicide potential but
does not otherwise seem to affect the mental health functioning of the
separating/divorcing.

The relationship of time to mental health in the separating/divorc-
ing is examined. In general, there is a tendency for discomfort to dimin-

ish over time. The data suggest, however, that experience over time may differ for various subgroups. Those proceeding from separating to filing to final decree tend to improve over time but those who do not file and those who are separated 14 months or more (whether or not they file) do not tend to improve further and may even worsen. These findings are tentative and longitudinal studies are needed for more conclusive data.

REFERENCES

1. Chester R: Health and marriage breakdown: Experience of a sample of divorced women. Br J Prevent Soc Med 25:231–235, 1971
2. Kitson G, Sussman MB: The impact of divorce on adults. Conciliation Courts Rev 15:20–24, 1977
3. Parloff MB, Kleman HC, Frank JD: Comfort, effectiveness and self-awareness as criteria of improvement in psychotherapy. Am J Psychiatry 111:343–351, 1954
4. Overall JE, Gorham DR: The Brief Psychiatric Rating Scale. Psychological Rep 10:799–812, 1962
5. Linn M, Sailthorpe WB, Williams B, et al: A social dysfunction rating scale. J Psychiatr Res 6:299–306, 1969
6. Farberow NL, Heilig SM, Litman RE: Techniques in crisis intervention. A training manual. Los Angeles Suicide Prevention Center, Inc., 1968
7. Hunt M, Hunt B: The Divorce Experience. New York, McGraw-Hill, 1977
8. Brown P, Fox H: Sex differences in divorce, in Gomberg E, Frank V (Eds): Gender and Disordered Behavior: Sex Differences in Psychopathology. New York, Brunner-Mazel, 1979, pp 101–123
9. Kitson GC: Attachment to the spouse in divorce: A scale and its application. Journal of Marriage and the Family, May 1982, pp 379–393
10. Kitson GC, Raschke HJ: Divorce research: What we know and what we need to know. J Divorce 4(3):1–38, 1981
11. Chiriboga PA, Cutler L: Stress responses among separating men and women. J Divorce 1:95–106, 1977
12. Chiriboga PA, Roberts J, Stein JA: Psychological well being during marital separation. J Divorce 2:21–36, 1978
13. Mellinger GD, Bacter MB, Manheimer DI, et al: Psychic distress, life crises and use of psychotropic medication. Arch Gen Psychiatry 35:1048–1052, 1978
14. Raschke JJ: Social and psychological factors in voluntary post-marital dissolution adjustment. DAI (Dissertation Abstract Index), 1975, p 5549A
15. Pearlin LI, Johnson JS: Marital status, life strains and depression. Am Sociol Rev 42:704–715, 1977

16. Goode WJ: After Divorce. Glencoe, Ill, The Free Press, 1956.
17. Myers JK, Bean LL: A Decade Later. A Follow-up of Social Class and Mental Illness. New York, Wiley, 1968, pp 235–237
18. Weiss RS: A preliminary examination of potential contribution of quality of life data to an understanding of single parenting. Boston, Laboratory of Community Psychiatry, 1976
19. Hetherington EM, Cox M, Cox R: The aftermath of divorce. Read at the 5th Annual meeting of the American Orthopsychiatric Association, New York, 1977
20. Ilfeld PW: Psychological status of community residents among major demographic dimensions. Arch Gen Psychiatry 35:716–724, 1978

APPENDIX 5-A: ABBREVIATIONS

Respondents

Group as a whole: **All**

Persons seriously discussing separation but not separated: **Sub 1**

Persons who experienced their last separation-related (last of separation, filing, final decree) event 1 to 13 months previous to the interview: **Sub 2**

Persons who experienced their last separation-related event 14 months or longer previous to the interview: **Sub 3**

Measures of Mental Health (Higher Scores Indicate Greater Disturbance)

Somatic Subscale of the Frank Discomfort Scale: **SOMA**

Anxiety Subscale of the Frank Discomfort Scale: **ANX**

Depression Subscale of the Frank Discomfort Scale: **DEP**

Brief Psychiatric Rating Scale: **BPRS**

Social Dysfunction Rating Scale: **SDRS, SFRS,** or **SOC**

Suicide Prevention Center Assessment of Suicide Potential at time of entry to Rush Center: **SPC 1**

Suicide Prevention Center Assessment of Suicide Potential at time of research interview: **SPC 2**

Assessment of Suicide Potential by clinical rater at time of research interview: **ASP**

APPENDIX 5-B

The study's three subgroups divided by men and women provide six groups for analysis. There are eight indicators of mental health. For each independent variable there are thus 6 × 8, or 48, possible measures of association, not including further breakdowns of the population subgroups, which has been undertaken in some instances. The following chart indicates *all* potential measures of association for any one independent variable.

	All	Sub 1	Sub 2	Sub 3	Men	Women
SOMA						
ANX						
DEP						
BPRS						
SDRS						
SPC 1						
SPC 2						
ASP						

A cluster of independent variables is frequently used to make a particular point. On the other hand, there are times when conclusions are drawn based on a large number of individual analyses and the relationships between them. It quickly can be seen that there is risk of becoming inundated by figures and tables. I am aware that some readers wish to know the specific aspects of the statistical analyses, while others are more interested in general conclusions and clinical implications. The text will allow the reader who is not familiar with research methodology and statistics to follow the broad argument. Only essential data are presented in the text.

6

The Continuing Tie Between Spouses

There is general agreement that continuing ties between spouses are an important element of the divorce process. According to Weiss,[1] "separation is an incident in the relation between the spouses, rather than the ending of the relationship." He added that "the postmarital relationship is unique among relationships (and is one of) extraordinary ambivalence."[1] Hunt and Hunt stated that "divorce puts a formal end to marriage but often does not and cannot wholly end the relationship."[2] Most of the newly divorced remain connected to a degree, "some by only a single strand, a few by a surprising entanglement of them—for months, for years, or even for most of their lives."[2]

Adaptive resolution of the divorce process involves giving up the spouse as a marital partner and working through the resulting grief. The relationship between the spouses either ends or is sharply redefined, as may occur when the interaction becomes limited to parenting. For this reason the extent and nature of the post-separation and divorce relationship between (former) spouses are important. This chapter deals with the amount of contact and the extent of emotional and everyday reliance on the spouse at two points in time: before the first serious discussion of separation and in the two weeks prior to the research interview. Subsequent chapters will deal with other facets of the continuing interspouse relationship.

Although there is general agreement that a continuing tie exists between separated spouses, there is no such unanimity on the nature of the tie. Hunt and Hunt stated that divorced people may be bound to each other by one or more of several ties: "love, hate, money, co-parenthood, dependence, moral obligation, or habit."[2] Two of these ties are, at least on the surface, based on situations not in the control of the former spouses: money and co-parenthood. The former has often been imposed by court order; the latter is presumably governed by the need to jointly resolve child-rearing issues. Psychological factors play a great role in determining whether the communication in both areas is relatively neutral and limited to the issues at hand or whether it pro-vides an opportunity for the manifestation of other forces, such as a wish to cling to the relationship or to avenge oneself. In this sense, we can set aside realistically determined interaction and look at the under-lying motivation. Several theoretical frameworks have been put for-ward to explain this motivation, including attachment theory, psy-choanalytic theory, and sociological and economic explanations.

Attachment theory is based in good part on Bowlby's concept that a primary instinct of attachment of the child to the mother is fundamen-tal to attachment throughout life.[3,4] Separation anxiety, as well as pain and anger, are associated with the dissolution of attachment. A number of current writers, notably Weiss,[1] have used Bowlby's concept in con-sidering responses to divorce. Weiss saw the ties between marital part-ners as analogous to the child's early tie to the mother.[1] He defined pre-separation attachment in terms of "a bonding that gives rise to feelings of at-homeness and ease when the other is present, or, if not actually present, is felt to be accessible." He defined post-separation attach-ment as the spouses' wish to be in touch with each other.

Levinger and Moles[5] questioned Weiss' emphasis on the remaining attachment between separated and divorced spouses, pointing out that Weiss used an urban middle-class sample and wondering if his general-izations extend beyond the population of men and women living in iso-lated households.[5] They also asked to what extent the emotional impact noted by Weiss is a function of the newness of the separation or of the kinds of people who sought out his seminars.[5] Recently, some workers have proposed to define and measure attachment to the spouse in sepa-rated or divorced individuals (see Chapter 9).

Attachment theory is an important framework for understanding relationships, and some observations can be most parsimoniously un-derstood in its terms. However, it falls short of being a comprehensive explanation of the continuing tie between marital spouses. One limita-tion is that attachment theory still has its most important implications in the area of *de*tachment. Among the original stimuli for Bowlby's work were Robertson's observations[6] of young children who were separated from their mothers and exhibited distress. Overall, the theory tells us more about what happens when a tie is broken than when it is not.

Attachment theory views attachment in terms of a non-specific need for an important person's (originally the mother's) love and presence. This description is an oversimplification. Even in the child the motivation to be in the parents' presence is more complex than this, and in the adult the tie between the spouses certainly is more than the expression of an inborn instinctual pattern.

The psychoanalytic theory allows us to investigate what drives are expressed in relation to others. Basically, libidinal (broadly, loving) and aggressive drives are involved. Libidinal drives involve need-satisfaction, whereas aggressive drives are associated with anger and may have the goal of injuring or destroying. Anna Freud[7] pointed out that in children aggressive drives and fantasies play an important role in school phobia as a motivation of the child not to separate from the parents: "In (the parents') absence, the hostile side of the ambivalence assumes frightening proportions, and the ambivalently loved figures of the parents are clung to so as to save them from the child's own death wishes, aggressive fantasies, etc." In adults as well, including those divorcing, the wishes to gratify needs and/or to be reassured that one's anger has not been deadly may be motives for a continuing tie. We can add to this the wish for revenge, a more direct expression of the aggressive drive, which can contribute to a powerful bond.

From a sociological standpoint, the marital role may be preferable to the single role. This may be particularly true for the woman whose social status is higher as a wife, such as in the case of a woman who is married to a high-status professional or executive and who does not have a career of her own. In broader terms, the assumption of a new role in society is difficult, and one may seek out the spouse to avoid it.

From an economic standpoint divorce commonly represents a hardship for one or both spouses. Resumption of the marital tie, at least for a while, can prevent that hardship.

The continuing ties between separated or divorced couples are clearly complex. How does an empirical study address these issues? First, there must be awareness that a series of studies involving various designs and populations will be needed before definitive statements can be made. Second, variables must be quantifiable and measurable.

CONTACTS BETWEEN SEPARATED AND DIVORCED COUPLES

Previous Studies

Goode pointed out that there is "no specification of appropriate role behavior between the spouses."[8] For the women in his study the husband was "a continuing, living person whom the wife may see on his visits to the children, whom (she) may even continue to date for a while. What he does, seems to affect what she does."[8] Goode developed a "contact index" based on whether the respondent (the wife) dated her former husband, whether she found out about him (with or without seeing him), whether she saw him, and whether she would avoid seeing him. Goode constructed five "latent contact" classes. The percentage of the respondents falling into each group is shown in Table 6-1. Goode's respondents had been divorced 2 to 26 months, and women who had remarried were also included. Goode stated that his index measured intensity rather than frequency of contact.

Goode also related the contact index to whether the predominant attitude of respondent to former husband was positive or negative. Among those not remarried at point of interview, the percentage of positive attitudes was highest for high-contact respondents and diminished as contact intensity diminished, while negative and indifferent attitudes increased as contact decreased. However, 17 percent of the high-contact (not remarried) individuals had negative attitudes toward the former spouse. According to Goode, "Contact alone may create greater *antagonism* or maintain an attachment."[8] As Anna Freud noted, it can often do both simultaneously, and high contact may be the result as well as the cause of antagonism.

Sexual contact with the (former) spouse, particularly its frequency and whether its presence or absence affects mental health, is of special

Table 6-1
Respondents in Each Latent Contact Class
($N = 440$)

High contact	10%
Medium-high contact	21%
Medium contact	41%
Medium-low contact	19%
Low contact	9%

interest. Weiss[1] believed that many separated couples maintain a sporadic sexual relationship for a few weeks or months after the separation. They may have sexual relations with each other despite a generally hostile relationship. He quoted one member of his "Seminars for the Separated" as stating, "I come to see the children and later we fight and go to bed."[1] Bohannon[9] indicated that several "ceremonial bouts" of sexual intercourse may occur right before divorce. He reported that some judges have refused to grant a divorce because they cannot condone "litigation by day and copulation by night."[9] Bohannon also told of a man who murdered his about-to-be-ex-wife after sexual intercourse.

To date there have been few quantitative studies regarding the occurrence and frequency of sexual relations between separated and divorced spouses. Burke and Grant "estimated" on the basis of workshops they conducted that 30 percent of persons experienced sex with their former spouse during and after divorce.[10] However, Goldsmith found that of 129 divorced spouses of mother-custody families, none acknowledged having had sexual intercourse with their former spouse in the past several months.[11]

Present Study

My approach to studying contacts between former spouses owes much to Goode's concept of a contact index, but unlike Goode I separated quantity and quality of contacts. It seemed preferable to first look at what is most readily measurable—whether the spouses were in contact, in what manner, and how often. A separate set of questions was asked regarding their emotional and everyday involvement with each other.

The following questions in the marital problems survey pertained to the types of contact with the former spouse: speaking in person; speaking on the telephone; writing; receiving written communication; finding out something about him or her; seeing spouse without speaking; any other form of contact. In each instance, the time period in question was the two weeks prior to the interview. Supplementary questions were also asked regarding each separate type of contact, including how recently the contact had occurred. In addition, questions were asked about how consistent respondents were in making arrangements about contacting one another, seeing children, etc. Observation of separating or divorcing couples has led to the conclusion that failure to be clear about such arrangements occurs commonly.

As mentioned in Chapter 5, the study population was divided into three subgroups: those seriously discussing separation (Sub 1), those who experienced their last separation-related event (last of separation, filing, final decree) less than 14 months earlier (Sub 2), and those who experienced the last such event 14 months or longer earlier (Sub 3). Data for all men and all women were also analyzed separately, regardless of their subgroups. When there were sufficient numbers, men and women within the Sub 2 group were analyzed. Data on the issue of contacts were not relevant for Sub 1, since, living under the same roof, they were presumably in daily contact.

EXTENT OF CONTACT

Table 6-2 lists the number of contacts with the former spouse. Separate analysis by men and women regardless of dissolution status revealed no difference in the number of contacts. The recently separated remained in contact with their former spouses by a ratio of almost 11 to 1. After filing for divorce, the ratio of those in contact to those not was 3 to 1, and over half of those who received their final decree within the past 14 months still remained in touch. Close to half continued to maintain contact 14 months or more since the last separation event. As expected, the number of contacts diminished as the time after the separation increased.

These findings confirm the expectation that the bond between former marital partners is tenacious. Although the presence of children is important, it does not account for the extent of the bond: there was no difference between couples with and without children in the amount of contact for the recently separated and recently filed. For the recently divorced and long-term separated/divorced, persons with children

Table 6-2

Contacts with Spouse in the Two Weeks prior to Interview

	Separated less than 14 Mo before Interview	Filed for Divorce less than 14 Mo before Interview	Final Decree less than 14 Mo before Interview	Last Separation Event 14 or more Mo before Interview
In contact	43	21	17	31
Not in contact[a]	4	7	14	39

[a]Those who did not respond to the contact questions were designated as not in contact.

were in contact significantly more often than those without children. However, even among couples without children whose divorce or last separation occurred 14 or more months earlier, about a third had been in contact with their former spouse in the two weeks prior to interview.

SPECIFIC CHARACTERISTICS OF THE CONTACT

For Sub 2, types of contact are shown in Table 6-3. The most common form of contact was the telephone: 65.1 percent. (The percentage may be slightly higher, since those for whom this information was not available were counted as not being in touch.) Next most common was in-person contact, acknowledged by 51 persons (48.1 percent). Contrary to expectation, the most common source of information about the spouse was not children but friends followed by relatives and others; children were the least common source. Of those with in-person speaking contact, 47.1 percent were in contact on the day prior to interview, and 82 percent were in contact within three days of interview. In regard to phone contact, 46.4 percent were in touch on the day prior to interview and 66.7 percent were in touch within the previous three days. For Sub 3, the most common form of contact was again the telephone.

To evaluate sexual contact, data obtained from the question "How often did you rely on your (former) spouse for sexual satisfaction in the last two weeks?" were used. The answers ranged from "not at all" to "all the time." Only persons who had been in contact in the last two weeks were asked the question. Sixty-five of 85 persons in Sub 2 who had been in contact answered the question; 49 respondents (75 percent) denied any sexual contact, six (9.2 percent) stated that it occurred rarely or occasionally, three (4.6 percent) said frequently, and only one person said always.

Table 6-3
Contact with Former Spouse in the Two Weeks prior to Interview

Type of Contact with Spouse	Sub 2 (N=106)	Sub 3 (N=68)
Spoke in person	48.1%	22.1%
Telephone	65.1%	33.8%
Wrote	14.2%	4.4%
Received correspondence	11.3%	2.9%
Found out information	29.2%	14.7%
Saw without speaking	3.8%	1.5%

CONSISTENCY OF ARRANGEMENTS

To explore the question of how consistent arrangements were between separating spouses, respondents were asked how often they said one thing and did another on a series of topics: spouse contacts, custody of children, arrangements to see children, and property settlement. Answers were on a five-point scale ranging from "almost never" to "almost always." Over half of the respondents claimed never to say one thing and do another on any matter. The percentages were 52.6 regarding spouse contacts, 87.5 regarding custody of children, 91.1 regarding arrangements with children, and 76.2 regarding property settlement. Meaningful responses were found only regarding spouse contacts, and these are therefore considered in greater detail.

There were significant differences between the marital separation categories for the group as a whole ($N = 156$). The question was asked of all respondents, including those still living together, and was answered by those who were or had recently been in contact. Those who never said one thing but did another increased from 28.6 percent of those still living with their spouse to 63.3 percent of the long-term separated/divorced. ($X^2 = 38.25$; 16 df; $p = .0014$). Similarly, there was a difference between subgroups of Sub 2. Divorced persons were less likely to be inconsistent in arranging for spouse contacts than those in earlier stages ($X^2 = 16.06$; 8 df; $p = .042$). There were no significant differences between men and women. In Sub 2 ($N = 84$), 60.7 percent said they almost never said one thing but did another, 9.5 percent did so very infrequently, 9.5 percent sometimes, 16.7 percent very frequently, and 3.6 percent almost always. Slightly over one third of Sub 2 respondents thus acknowledged at least occasional inconsistency regarding spouse contacts, and about a fifth acknowledged its frequent occurrence.

RELATIONSHIP BETWEEN CONTACTS AND
MENTAL HEALTH MEASURES

The hypothesis in this area was that the more frequent the contacts between spouses in Sub 2, the greater the disturbance as indicated by selected mental health measures. The rationale for this hypothesis was that contact between spouses undergoing separation or divorce is likely to be associated with frustration of emotional needs and with expression of mutual hostility resulting in loss of self-esteem and/or guilt, in turn resulting in measurable changes in indicators of emotional well-being.

The originally designated contact measures to test the hypothesis were (1) the sum of all contacts of all kinds over the past two weeks; (2) the number of such contacts in the past 72 hours; and (3) the presence or absence of sexual relations in the past two weeks. The total number of persons in Sub 2 ($N = 106$) were divided as follows: no contacts, 24 persons; 1 to 5 contacts, 35; 6 to 10 contacts, 23; 11 to 15 contacts, 15; and 16 to 20 contacts, 9. The number of contacts was related to mental health measures using Kendall's tau. Significance at $p = .05$ was considered to confirm the hypothesis. A one-tailed test of significance was used for Sub 2 because predictions were made for that group. For all other analyses, a two-tailed test was employed.

The association of the sum of the contacts to mental health measures was determined both with and without the no-contact group. When those who had no contact were included, there were no significant associations for Sub 2 group. For Sub 3 ($N = 67$), suicide potential at entry was in the opposite of the predicted direction: those with more contact were less suicidal ($\tau = -.212$; $p < .05$).

The picture was somewhat different when those with no contact were excluded. For Sub 2 women ($N = 58$), the correlation of more contact with greater depression was significant ($\tau = .192$; $p < .05$). There were no significant associations for Sub 2 men or for Sub 3.

The relationship between the number of contacts in the last 72 hours with the former spouse and mental health variables could not be directly addressed since there was no breakdown as to the number of contacts in this time period. To approximate a test of the hypothesis, those who had contact of any sort in the last 72 hours were compared with those who did not, using Kendall's tau. In Sub 2, 62 persons had contact in the last 72 hours, 36 did not, and information was not available for 8. No differences were observed.

As to the association of sexual relations with the spouse to mental health measures, the SDRS was significantly related in the opposite of the expected direction for Sub 2 ($\tau = -.202$; $N = 65$; $p < .05$). There were no significant associations in Sub 3.

The findings on the relationship of contacts with the former spouse to mental health measures result in no clear-cut confirmation of the hypothesis. When those with no contacts are included, there is an association of greater depression with more contacts in Sub 2 women. On the other hand, there is a suggestion that continued contact is associated with *better* functioning. If those with no contact are included, such an association is found between the number of contacts and SPC 1 for Sub 3. Similarly, in Sub 2 relying on the spouse for sexual satisfaction was associated with lower scores (better functioning) on the SDRS.

In future studies, the problem of contacts may be approached by breaking down respondents into three groups: those with no contact, those with infrequent contact, and those with frequent contact. It is possible that a U-shaped curve may emerge, with dysfunction highest among those with no contact and with frequent contact, and lower distress among those with few contacts. For now, however, we cannot confirm any strong association between contacts as such and mental health. For more light on this issue we therefore turn to other aspects of the interspouse relationship.

RELATIONSHIP BETWEEN CONSISTENCY OF INTERACTION AND MENTAL HEALTH MEASURES

It was considered possible that inconsistency in various facets of interaction between the spouses is related to difficulty in separating. Inconsistency was also seen as an indicator of the inability to deal with the separation cognitively. Mainly for the latter reason, an association with various mental health measures was possible. No formal predictions were made, however, and therefore a two-tailed test of significance was used in the analysis of this item. The extent to which the respondent said one thing and did another in relation to spouse contacts was related to mental health measures. There were no significant findings for Sub 1 or Sub 3, except for BPRS ($\tau = .349$; $p < .05$; $N =$

Table 6-4

Relationship Between Consistency of Interaction with Spouse and Mental Health Measures (Sub 2)[a]

Mental Health Measure	Men ($N = 29$)	Women ($N = 55$)	Total ($N = 84$)
SOMA	.302[c]	.282[b]	.276[b]
ANX	.350[c]	.207	.257[b]
DEP	.183	.202	.202[c]
SOC	.123	.314[b]	.256[b]
BPRS	.174	.320[b]	.246[d]
SPC 1	.076	.027	.039
SPC 2	.094	.099	.104
ASP	.101	.048	.070

For explanation of mental health measures see Appendix 5-A.
[a]Measured by Kendall's tau.
[b]$p = .01$
[c]$p = .05$

30). Table 6-4 shows the relationship of mental health measures to Sub 2 as a whole and to men and women in that group.

It appears clear that *inconsistency regarding contacts with the (former) spouse is related to all mental health measures for sub 2 group with the exception of the suicidal group.* Except for somatic discomfort and anxiety, this relationship appears to be stronger for women than for men. This finding suggests that the cognitive confusion associated with the marital separation is definitely related to dysfunction. A cause-and-effect relationship cannot be stipulated. It is likely that the relation is reciprocal. Inconsistency is in part a result of poor functioning, but the consequent uncertainty can further impair coping.

EMOTIONAL RELIANCE

Emotional reliance is defined in this study as the number of times an individual has relied on the spouse for such forms of emotional satisfaction as feeling loved, feeling taken care of, etc. This reliance is assessed before separation was discussed and in the two weeks prior to interview.

Previous Studies

There are no empirical studies that deal specifically with these aspects of emotional reliance. The literature does deal with positive and negative *feelings*, but the concept of reliance is different in that it describes an interaction between two people. Fisher[12] mentioned dependence, which is a similar concept to that of reliance. He suggested that how people feel after divorce depends on the extent to which they are locked in by intensive dependence so that "divorce is psychic death."

Present Study

Areas of reliance on the spouse are companionship, feeling loved, feeling successful, feeling like a good person, feeling taken care of, feeling understood, and receiving sexual satisfaction. The last has already been considered in the section on contacts.

EXTENT OF EMOTIONAL RELIANCE

Emotional reliance was assessed by (1) responses to the questions regarding extent of reliance in each of the above seven areas using a five-point scale including "not at all," "rarely," "sometimes," "most of the time," and "always"; (2) the mean score of the responses to these seven items; (3) the respondent's answer to the question, "Overall, how much did you rely on the spouse?" as rated on the same five-point scale; and (4) the rater's assessment of how great the respondent's overall reliance was on a five-point scale ranging from "minimal or non-existent" to "extremely great."

Before first serious discussion of separation. Information on emotional reliance prior to the first serious discussion of separation was retroactively assessed for 232 of 238 subjects; the remainder indicated that they relied on the spouse either rarely or never. This group reported relying heavily on the spouse before the first serious discussion of separation (Table 6-5). In all areas, over half indicated that they turned to the spouse at least some of the time. The overall reliance rating both by the respondents and by the raters is higher than the average of the individual items, indicating that in the minds of both respondent and rater the areas of greatest reliance are weighted more heavily than the others. There were no statistically significant differences for men and women. For this analysis Sub 1, Sub 2, and Sub 3 were compared. Statistically significant differences were found for feeling loved ($X^2 = 18.26$; 8 *df; p* = .02) and for receiving sexual satisfaction ($X^2 = 17.52$; 8 *df; p* = .03). Sub 3 reported less reliance before the separation discussion than did Sub 1 or Sub 2. This may well be retrospective falsification—the longer ago the separation discussion

Table 6-5
Reliance on Spouse prior to First Serious Discussion of Separation for All Groups ($N = 232$)

Area	%
Companionship	86.3
Feeling loved	84.5
Sexual satisfaction	76.3
Feeling taken care of	73.2
Feeling understood	67.2
Feeling like a good person	61.2
Feeling successful	50.8
Overall emotional reliance (respondent)	81.9
Overall emotional reliance (rater)[a]	79.8

[a]Inter-rater reliability was assessed in 22 cases. The Spearman rho was .39, *p* = .02.

Table 6-6
Reliance on Spouse prior to First Serious Discussion of
Separation (Sub 2, $N = 102$)

Area	%
Companionship	91.2
Feeling loved	88.3
Sexual satisfaction	77.4
Feeling taken care of	71.7
Feeling understood	70.3
Feeling like a good person	69.6
Feeling successful	57.8
Overall emotional reliance (respondent)	81.4
Overall emotional reliance (rater)	83.3

occurred, the more the memory of relying on the spouse for love or
sexual gratification may have faded or been repressed.

Sub 2 is especially interesting. Data on pre–separation-discussion
emotional reliance variables for this group are given in Table 6-6. Percentages includes respondents who relied on the spouse sometimes,
most of the time, or always. The order in which these appear is the
same as for the group as a whole. The percentages in each case are
slightly higher, probably because they were brought down for the total
sample by the retrospective lowering of estimates on the part of Sub 3.

The two weeks prior to interview. Because our main interest is in
Sub 2 (the recently separated/divorced), figures for the group as a
whole and for other subgroups will not be detailed. Briefly, as expected, there are sharp differences in the amount of reliance in the two
weeks prior to the interview between the groups. Sub 1 had the heavi-
est reliance, followed by Sub 2, with Sub 3 reporting the least emotional reliance. In all but one instance, these differences are statistically
significant ($p = .001$ to $p = .01$). The one exception is "feeling like a
good person," for which the difference only approaches significance ($p = .08$). There were no statistically significant differences between men
and women. Information was asked of the recently separated/divorced
only when the respondent had been in contact with the spouse in the
two weeks prior to interview and was therefore in a position to experience emotional reliance. Percentages include reliance on the spouse
sometimes, most of the time, or always (Table 6-7). There are some
interesting points to be noted here. First, naturally there was a sharp

Table 6-7

Reliance on Spouse in the Two Weeks prior to Interview (Sub 2)

Area	N	%
Feeling understood	72	33.3
Companionship	67	25.4
Feeling taken care of	71	25.3
Feeling like a good person	73	23.3
Feeling loved	72	22.3
Sexual satisfaction	65	15.3
Feeling successful	70	10.0
Overall emotional reliance (respondent)	71	23.9
Overall emotional reliance (rater)	102	27.4

decrease in the number of persons relying on the spouse compared to the pre-separation discussion in all areas. The diminution may even be greater than indicated, since those not in contact and thus presumably not having any emotional reliance were excluded from the two-week assessment. The decrease is not equal in all areas however, and the order of importance of the items is quite sharply changed. Feeling understood now leads the list, and feeling loved and feeling sexual satisfaction have dropped to near the bottom. This suggests that, at least insofar as respondents are willing to admit, turning to an estranged or former spouse to feel understood is maintained longer than other forms of reliance, particularly feeling loved and receiving sexual gratification.

Most important is the difference between overall emotional reliance as indicated by the respondent and as assessed by the raters.* The difference is greater than it appears, since individuals not in contact were included by the raters and were rated as having zero reliance. The total number was therefore 102. Had only the 71 who reported their self-assessment of overall reliance in the last two weeks been included, the raters would have assessed 39.4 percent as having a reliance of moderate or greater proportions. It is likely that we can place more confidence in the raters' assessment, since it is generally accepted that separated respondents tend to play down continued reliance on the (former) spouse.[1] Goode[8] also stated that an unmeasurable amount of "bias toward indifference" exists among divorced persons. Slightly

---

*This finding must be viewed with some caution because the inter-rater reliability is relatively low. On 22 cases on which it was assessed, Spearman rho = .29, p = .05.

more than 10 percent of Sub 3 still had moderate or greater overall reliance on the (former) spouse, according to the raters, and over one-fourth had at least limited reliance in the previous two weeks.

RELATIONSHIP TO MENTAL HEALTH MEASURES

Several hypotheses regarding the relationship of emotional reliance to mental health measures were proposed.

Before the first serious discussion of separation. The hypothesis was that in the recently separated/divorced, the greater the emotional reliance on the spouse before the first serious discussion of separation,* the more disturbance will be observed in mental health measures.† The rationale underlying this hypothesis was as follows: Emotional reliance before the first serious discussion of separation was viewed as a baseline, characterizing the period when the marriage was still more or less functional. Strictly speaking, the period to be considered should have been the time before the marriage was in difficulty, since difficulty may exist before any discussion of separation takes place. For practical purposes, however, such a point is hard to define. Furthermore, the answers to the questions themselves indicate that the kind of reliance reported before the first separation discussion could reasonably be expected in a marriage that fulfills many of the respondent's emotional needs. If that is the case, then the extent to which these needs are met should parallel the extent to which a loss has occurred as a result of the separation. The greater the loss, the greater the pain and the greater other indices of psychological malfunctioning are expected to be. In simpler terms: The greater the emotional reliance before the first serious discussion of separation, the more meaningful the marital tie; the more meaningful the marital tie, the greater the expected psychological dislocation after separation.

To test this hypothesis, mental health measures at the time of interview were related to the following three measures of pre-separation-discussion emotional reliance: (1) overall reliance as reported by the respondent, (2) overall reliance as reported by the rater, and (3) average score on the seven individual reliance items. The possible scores on each of the reliance variables were 1, never relied on spouse; 2,

---

*As originally formulated, the period before separation was to be studied. Before the study actually began, the period was changed to pre-separation discussion.

†As originally formulated, the dependent variable was suicide potential. Before the study began, this was revised to include other mental health measures.

rarely relied on spouse; 3, relied on spouse some of the time; 4, relied on spouse most of the time; and 5, relied on spouse always.

The correlation between the numerical score on the emotional reliance variable and the numerical score on the mental health measures was assessed using Kendall's tau. Significance at the .05 level with a one-tailed test was considered to confirm the hypothesis.

As Table 6-8 indicates, the hypothesis is confirmed for Sub 2 as a whole for depression in relation to all three measures indicating reliance on the spouse before the first serious discussion of separation. Somatic discomfort, anxiety, and the Brief Psychiatric Rating Scale had associations that were significant at the .05 level for rater-rated emotional reliance. The data for pre–separation-discussion emotional reliance were also analyzed separately for men and women in Sub 2 using the same variables. For men there were no significant associations with any of three measures used. On the other hand, there were a number of significant associations for women. These are summarized in Table 6-9. There was a significant association for women between the three independent variables and somatic discomfort, anxiety, depression, and the BPRS.

In summary, these data support the hypothesis regarding subjective discomfort and rated psychiatric disturbance for both the group as a whole and for women, but not for men. The reasons for the difference between the sexes is not clear. It is possible that terms describing emotional reliance are less meaningful for men than for women, and that therefore the loss of such reliance, as men define it, is less significant. We shall see that men do show increased disturbance in relation to pre–separation-discussion everyday (as distinct from emotional) reliance. Perhaps men can consciously relate more to questions of practical reliance than of emotional dependence.

Males and females were also analyzed regardless of dissolution status, using the same group of variables.* Thus respondents discussing separation and the long-term separated/divorced (Sub 3) were included along with Sub 2. Men ($N = 76$) again showed no associations in the expected direction. In fact, anxiety was associated in the opposite direction, achieving significance on one independent variable, and approaching significance on another. This finding is difficult to interpret.

Women, regardless of dissolution status, showed associations of independent variables with somatic discomfort, anxiety, and depres-

---

*Predictions were made only for Sub 2; therefore, a one-tailed test was employed for that group. For all other analyses, including respondents regardless of separation status and Sub 3, a two-tailed test was used.

Table 6-8

Relationship Between Emotional Reliance on Spouse prior to
First Serious Discussion of Separation and Mental Health Measures
(Sub 2, N= 102)[a]

Mental Health Measure	Overall Emotional Reliance (Self-Rated)	Overall Emotional Reliance (Rater-Rated)	Average of Individual Reliance Items
SOMA	.104	.152[c]	.043
ANX	.109	.205[b]	.070
DEP	.177[b]	.176[b]	.151[c]
SOC	.038	.059	.059
BPRS	.111	.126[c]	.098
SPC 1	.046	−.013	−.093
SPC 2	.078	.073	−.039
ASP	.124	.056	−.073

For explanation of mental health measures see Appendix 5-A.
[a]Measured by Kendall's tau.
[b]$p \leq .01$
[c]$p \leq .05$

Table 6-9

Relationship Between Emotional Reliance on Spouse prior to
First Serious Discussion of Separation and Mental Health Measures
(Sub 2 Women, $N = 70$)[a]

Mental Health Measure	Overall Emotional Reliance (Self-Rated)	Overall Emotional Reliance (Rater-Rated)	Average of Individual Reliance Items
SOMA	.193[c]	.177[c]	.202[b]
ANX	.189[c]	.256[b]	.202[b]
DEP	.270[b]	.231[b]	.262[b]
SOC	.047	.067	.034
BPRS	.201[c]	.198[c]	.172[c]
SPC 1	.001	−.036	−.173
SPC 2	.097	.112	−.042
ASP	.096	.090	−.102

For explanation of mental health measures see Appendix 5-A.
[a]Measured by Kendall's tau.
[b]$p \leq .01$
[c]$p \leq .05$

sion, which achieve or approximate significant relationships with rater-rated pre-separation reliance. This is probably the most sensitive measure. Of special interest are the findings for this group in relation to the suicidal variables. Rater-rated pre–separation-discussion reliance is significantly associated with suicidal ideation for two of three measures, and self-rated reliance is significantly associated for one of the three measures. Since there are no significant associations of the suicidal measures to pre–separation-discussion reliance in Sub 2 women, the explanation seems to lie in the findings for Sub 3. There was not a sufficient number to analyze separately by men and women. Taking the group as a whole ($N = 68$), there is a significant association between two of three suicidal variables and rater-rated reliance. On the other hand, Sub 3 no longer showed significant associations with other mental health variables. These findings are not conclusive, but they suggest that the short-term effects of loss of emotional reliance are psychological discomfort (somatic, anxiety, depression) and psychiatric disturbance (BPRS), whereas a longer-term effect may be increased suicide potential, particularly in women.

The two weeks prior to interview. The hypothesis was that in the recently separated/divorced, the greater the emotional reliance on the spouse in the two weeks prior to interview, the more disturbance will be observed in the mental health measures. This hypothesis requires a comment. It is reasonably self-evident why one would expect that pre–separation-discussion reliance would relate to post-separation mental health, but no such simple expectation exists as to continued degree of reliance. It was my expectation that relying on an individual from whom one is separated involves frequent frustrations as well as inner conflict. This is because one needs an individual for whom one may have a great deal of anger. The hypothesis was tested in a parallel manner to that involving pre–separation-discussion reliance, substituting only the last two weeks for the earlier time period: (1) overall reliance in the last two weeks as reported by the respondent; (2) overall reliance in the last two weeks as reported by the rater; and (3) average score on the seven individual reliance items.

The results are shown in Table 6-10. Only individuals who were in contact with the spouse were asked to rate their emotional reliance on the spouse in the last two weeks. However, the raters assessed everyone, assigning a "no reliance" rating to those not in contact. Therefore, the number of respondents differs between the columns. It should be noted that the raters were blind to the hypotheses.

The relationship between self-reported overall emotional reliance

Table 6-10

Relationship Between Emotional Reliance on Spouse in the Two Weeks prior to Interview and Mental Health Measures (Sub 2)[a]

Mental Health Measure	Overall Emotional Reliance (Self-Rated) ($N = 71$)	Overall Emotional Reliance (Rater-Rated) ($N = 102$)	Average of Individual Reliance Items ($N = 64$)
SOMA	−.150	.088	.063
ANX	−.074	.169[b]	.159[b]
DEP	−.069	.159[b]	.118
SOC	−.169[b]	.067	.039
BPRS	−.140	.119	.032
SPC 1	−.209[b]	−.007	−.007
SPC 2	−.211[b]	.122	−.034
ASP	−.253[b]	.120	−.136

For explanation of mental health measures see Appendix 5-A.
[a]Measured by Kendall's tau.
[b]$p \le .05$

on the spouse in the previous two weeks and mental health measures was in the opposite direction of that predicted. The correlations were negative in every instance; the association was statistically significant for four measures including all three suicidal variables. A *different* picture emerged, however, when rater-rated current emotional reliance on the spouse was examined. Now two associations were significant in the predicted direction. The third reliance measure, the average of the individual items, was significant in the expected direction for anxiety. Emotional reliance in the two weeks prior to interview was analyzed separately for Sub 2 males and females. In men, there were no significant associations regarding any of the three indicators of current emotional reliance with mental health measures. The total number of cases, however, was very small ($N = 25$, 32, and 21 respectively).

In women, *self*-reported overall emotional reliance is associated in the direction opposite of that expected for ASP ($\tau = -.293$; $N = 46$; $p < .05$). A different picture exists, however, when *rater*-rated rather than self-rated current reliance is considered. Here there are significant associations in the predicted direction for somatic discomfort ($\tau = .205$; $N = 70$; $p < .05$), anxiety ($\tau = .258$; $N = 70$; $p < .01$), depression ($\tau = .208$; $N = 70$; $p < .05$), and the BPRS ($\tau = .247$; $N = 70$; $p =$

.01). On the third indicator of reliance (the average of the items), there were no significant findings.

There is a clear discrepancy between self-assessed current reliance and rater-assessed current reliance concerning mental health measures. In the former, the association tends to be opposite to the predicted direction. In the latter, the hypothesis is confirmed that subjective dysfunction (somatic discomfort, anxiety, depression) and greater psychiatric disturbance (BPRS), are seen in women but not in men.

In interpreting these findings, rater-rated reliance is more meaningful than self-rated reliance. Many separated and divorced individuals do not acknowledge current reliance on a former spouse. Furthermore, it is possible that the reliance most likely to be associated with psychological dysfunction is that which is present but not acknowledged. If this interpretation is employed, we can cautiously infer confirmation of the hypothesis for Sub 2 as a whole and for women, but not men, within that group.

Another group of study respondents was used to analyze current emotional reliance. For men, regardless of dissolution status ($N = 79$), the associations regarding anxiety were opposite to the predicted direction and were significant in relation to rater-rated reliance. For women, regardless of dissolution status, the results parallel those for Sub 2 women. Self-rated current reliance tended to relate in the opposite of the expected direction to mental health indicators (SPC 1: $\tau = -.145$; $N = 102$; $p = .10$). However, in relation to rater-rated current reliance, depression was associated in the predicted direction ($\tau = .127$; $N = 156$; $p < .05$). There was no consistent association of current reliance with mental health indicators in the long-term separated or divorced.

The differences between genders in regard to current rater-rated reliance are interesting. It is possible that men are indeed more gratified by continuing to rely on an estranged spouse than women are. A phenomenon similar to the finding that marriage has a more protective effect on men than on women may be in effect for couples who continue to rely on each other after separation. It is also possible that the raters understated the emotional reliance of those men for whom separation is associated with dysfunction. Men may be more able than women to hide their reliance on their former spouse and may be particularly prone to deny reliance because the resulting unmet needs may be incompatible with a masculine self-image.

These findings provide some support for the hypothesis that continued reliance on a spouse is associated with psychological disturbance. The findings runs contrary to some assumptions held by the public and mental health professionals that separated spouses may still be a valuable resource for one another. More often than not, continued reliance may not be associated with better levels of mental health, particularly in women, and in the recently separated or divorced, the opposite may be true. Attempts to turn to former spouse in an effort to avoid working through the loss and associated grief are likely to reactivate earlier conflicts, thereby aggravating the emotional suffering they were intended to allay. It is important to keep in mind that there will undoubtedly be individual cases where current reliance on the former spouse is associated with higher levels of mental health.

It will be noted that I have referred throughout to association and not to causality. The findings as such allow no inference as to causality; the theoretical framework presented in an earlier chapter suggests a reciprocal relationship: suffering, manifested by measurable mental health disturbance, increases emotional reliance on a (former) spouse, and that reliance in turn may increase suffering and manifestations of disturbance, as indicated on mental health measures.

EVERYDAY RELIANCE

Everyday reliance was defined as the extent of reliance on the spouse for various aspects of everyday functioning: doing household chores, transportation, taking care of children, managing financial matters, dealing with the church, dealing with the school, dealing with medical care, dealing with legal matters, visiting friends, going to the movies, involvement in social groups, and work. I am not aware of any prior studies of this subject in separated or divorcing individuals. The variables were assessed by asking whether any of the items occurred never, rarely, some of the time, most of the time, or always. Everyday reliance was assessed as reported before the first serious discussions of separation and in the two weeks prior to interview. Relationship at both points of time to mental health measures was also assessed.

EXTENT OF EVERYDAY RELIANCE

Results will be reported for Sub 2.

Before the first serious discussion of separation. Table 6-11 shows the percentage of respondents who relied on the spouse for the named activities some of the time, most of the time, or always.

As expected, there was a good deal of everyday reliance on the spouse before the first serious discussion of separation. The reliance was in accordance with common sex role assignments. Men relied on

Table 6-11
Everyday Reliance on Spouse prior to First Serious Discussion of
Separation (Sub 2)

Area of Reliance	Sex	N	Never/ Rarely	Some of Time	Most of the Time/ Always
Doing household	M	34	11.8	20.6	67.6
chores	F	72	68.1	27.8	4.2
Transportation	M	34	91.2	2.9	5.9
	F	72	62.5	15.3	22.2
Taking care of children	M	23	0.0	26.1	73.9
	F	40	55.0	35.0	10.0
Managing financial	M	34	35.3	26.5	38.2
matters	F	72	41.7	19.4	38.9
Dealing with the church	M	16	62.5	12.5	25.0
	F	39	87.2	10.3	2.6
Dealing with school	M	25	36.0	20.0	44.0
	F	48	77.1	14.6	8.3
Dealing with medical	M	33	33.3	18.2	48.5
care	F	71	47.9	21.1	31.0
Dealing with legal	M	30	63.3	23.3	13.3
matters	F	60	40.0	18.3	41.7
Visiting friends	M	34	32.4	35.3	32.4
	F	72	27.8	37.5	34.7
Going to movies	M	33	15.2	30.3	54.5
	F	70	25.7	17.1	57.1
Involvement in social	M	31	32.3	35.5	32.3
groups	F	62	48.4	8.1	43.5
Respondent's work	M	32	68.8	18.8	12.5
	F	65	75.4	15.4	9.2

women for taking care of children and for doing household chores, and
for dealing with the school, and to some extent with medical matters.
Women tended to rely on men for dealing with legal matters. Men and
women relied on the spouse in roughly similar numbers for managing
financial matters, visiting friends and going to the movies. There was
little reliance of men or women on the spouse in the areas of transportation, dealing with the church, or work.

The responses of 103 respondents in Sub 2 to questions about the
extent of financial dependence on the spouse before the first serious
discussion of separation indicate that financial support was fairly even-

ly divided between respondent and former spouse. Slightly less than
two-fifths (38.8 percent) indicated that they provided the only or main
financial support; 27.2 percent stated that both contributed equally;
and 34 percent said that the spouse was only or mainly responsible for
providing financial support before the separation discussion.

The two weeks prior to interview. Everyday dependence on the
spouse was sharply diminished, as Table 6-12 indicates. The relatively
high continued reliance on the spouse for care of children reflects responses of non-custodial parents, mainly men. The other categories

Table 6-12
Everyday Reliance on Spouse in the Two Weeks prior to Interview (Sub 2)

Area of Reliance	Sex	N	Never/ Rarely	Some of Time	Most of the Time/ Always
Doing household	M	9	44.4	22.2	33.3
chores	F	30	93.3	0.0	6.7
Transportation	M	20	100.0	0.0	0.0
	F	40	90.0	5.0	5.0
Taking care of children	M	20	15.0	15.0	70.0
	F	27	55.6	18.5	25.9
Managing financial	M	21	76.2	0.0	23.8
matters	F	49	85.7	2.0	12.2
Dealing with the church	M	14	85.7	0.0	14.3
	F	23	95.7	4.3	0.0
Dealing with school	M	19	63.2	0.0	36.8
	F	28	75.0	7.1	17.9
Dealing with medical	M	23	69.6	4.3	26.1
care	F	40	72.5	7.5	20.0
Dealing with legal	M	21	61.9	28.6	9.5
matters	F	36	75.0	8.3	16.7
Visiting friends	M	22	86.4	4.5	9.1
	F	44	97.7	2.3	0.0
Going to movies	M	19	89.5	5.3	5.3
	F	38	86.8	7.9	5.3
Involvement in social	M	20	100.0	0.0	0.0
groups	F	37	97.3	2.7	0.0
Respondent's work	M	20	95.0	5.0	0.0
	F	40	92.5	7.5	0.0

Table 6-13
Everyday Reliance on Spouse in Two Weeks Prior to Interview when
Reliance (Existed) prior to First Serious Discussion of Separation (Sub 2)

Area of Reliance	N	Never/ Rarely	Some of Time	Most of the Time/ Always
Taking care of children	19(M)	10.5	15.8	73.7
	12(F)	33.3	33.3	33.3
Managing financial matters	16(M)	68.8	0.0	31.3
	28(F)	85.7	3.6	10.7
Dealing with the school	14(M)	50.0	0.0	50.0
	6(F)	66.7	16.7	16.7
Dealing with medical care	16(M)	56.3	6.3	37.5
	26(F)	57.7	11.5	30.8
Dealing with legal matters	6(M)	33.3	50.0	16.7
	21(F)	71.4	9.5	19.0

with more than very small amounts of continued reliance were dealing with medical care, legal matters, schools, and finances.

Table 6-13 shows the distribution of current everyday reliance for respondents whose reliance before the separation discussion relied some of the time, most of the time, or always. (Only those categories for which nine or more respondents indicated current reliance other than never/rarely was included in the table.)

RELATIONSHIP BETWEEN EVERYDAY RELIANCE
AND MENTAL HEALTH MEASURES

We next turn to two hypotheses. The first states that the higher the amount of pre–separation-discussion everyday reliance among the recently separated or divorced, the greater the disturbance as indicated on mental health measures at time of interview. This is based on an expectation that the more the prior dependence, the greater the loss; the greater the loss, the more the disturbance.

Before first serious discussion of separation. The hypothesis was tested by assigning values of 1 (never) to 5 (always) to applicable everyday reliance variables and relating the average of the scores on these variables to mental health measures using Kendall's tau. The results show that for Sub 2 (the recently separated/divorced) as a whole, there were no significant associations. When the relationship of individual areas of reliance to mental health measures was considered, greater reliance in three areas was associated with *less* somatic disturbance: Doing household chores ($\tau = -.193$; $N = 105$; $p < .01$), taking care of children ($\tau = -.207$; $N = 62$; $p < .05$), and dealing with the school ($\tau = -.250$; $N = 73$; $p < .01$). On the other hand, greater reliance was associated with *more* somatic disturbance in dealing with legal matters ($\tau = .156$; $N = 73$; $p < .01$) and in going to movies ($\tau = .156$; $N = 102$; $p < .05$). Greater reliance in dealing with legal matters was also associated with more anxiety ($\tau = .142$; $N = 90$; $p < .05$).

When Sub 2 was divided by gender and the same analysis carried out, there were significant associations of greater pre–separation-discussion everyday reliance for men with anxiety ($\tau = .287$; $N = 34$; $p < .05$), and depression ($\tau = .372$; $N = 34$; $p < .01$). Analysis of individual items indicated that in men greater reliance in the following areas was associated with increased anxiety: dealing with medical care ($\tau = .367$; $N = 33$; $p < .01$) and work ($\tau = .280$; $N = 32$; $p < .05$). Greater reliance in the following areas was associated with more depression in men: dealing with medical care ($\tau = .321$; $N = 33$; $p < .01$) and going to the movies ($\tau = .244$; $N = 33$; $p < .05$). There were too few suicidal men to make associations with suicidal variables meaningful. For women there was no association with mental health measures.

Regarding emotional reliance, women, not men, showed a relation to pre-separation discussion levels. When everyday reliance is at issue, only men related current distress to pre–separation-discussion reliance. Women respond to loss of emotional dependence, men respond to loss of everyday dependence. These findings apply only to the recently separated/divorced. Analysis by men and women in the total sample resulted in no significant associations of pre–separation-discussion everyday reliance and mental health status.

The second hypothesis stated that the greater the dependence on the spouse for financial support, the greater the emotional disturbance at time of interview. The greater the dependence on the spouse before the separation, the greater the likely loss of financial resources and therefore the greater the disturbance. The hypothesis was tested by assigning increasing numerical scores to the extent to which self or spouse was responsible for financial support before the first serious discussion of separation. This variable was related to the score on mental health measures using analysis of variance involving three groups: support by self only or mainly; mutual support; and support by spouse mainly or only.

The hypothesis was not supported for the recently separated/divorced ($N = 99$). Sub 3 ($N = 67$), however, showed significant associations in the expected direction when tested by analysis of variance for somatic discomfort ($F = 5.76$; 2 df; $p = .005$); and for anxiety ($F = 3.51$; 2 df; $p = .04$). In both cases the greater the degree of prior spouse support, the greater the symptoms.

The two weeks prior to interview.   A hypothesis relating everyday reliance in the last two weeks to score on mental health measures predicted that the greater the everyday reliance in the last two weeks, the greater the emotional disturbance would be. To test this hypothesis, a score ranging from 1 (never relied on the spouse) to 5 (always relied on the spouse) was assigned for each variable. The average scores for each of the applicable measures was then related to the score on mental health measures by means of Kendall's tau. Only individuals who were in contact with the spouse were considered. The results are shown in Table 6-14. The hypothesis was confirmed regarding somatic discomfort and the BPRS. Reliance on the spouse in the following individual areas was associated with greater somatic disturbance: managing financial matters ($\tau = .237$; $N = 69$; $p = .01$) and dealing with legal matters ($\tau = .219$; $N = 57$; $p < .05$). More disturbance on the BPRS was associated with reliance in the areas of managing financial matters ($\tau = .232$; $N = 68$; $p < .05$) and legal matters ($\tau = .186$; $N = 55$; $p < .05$).

Gender analysis within Sub 2 indicates that for men, although the small number suggest caution, somatic discomfort ($\tau = .271$; $N = 28$; $p < .05$) and depression ($\tau = .312$; $N = 28$; $p < .05$) were related to current everyday reliance in the expected direction. Reliance on the spouse was associated with greater somatic disturbance in Sub 2 men in the areas of managing financial matters ($\tau = .560$; $N = 21$; $p < .01$) and legal matters ($\tau = .356$; $N = 21$; $p < .05$). More depression was associated with more reliance on the spouse in regard to managing financial matters ($\tau = .372$; $N = 21$; $p < .05$). For women, however, while somatic discomfort is related in the expected direction ($\tau = .270$; $N = 51$; $p < .01$), two of the three suicidal variables are significantly associated in the opposite direction (SPC 2: $\tau = -.243$; $N = 51$; $p < .05$; ASP: $\tau = -.359$; $N = 51$; $p < .01$). Overall, the results suggest but do not clearly establish confirmation of the hypothesis for men in Sub 2 in particular. For Sub 2 women, increased suicide potential is related to less, rather than more, current everyday reliance on the spouse. Men in Subs 2 and 3 combined in contact with the spouse showed a significant association in the expected direction with somatic discomfort ($\tau = .237$; $N = 60$; $p = .01$). Females in Subs 2 and 3 in contact with the former spouse ($N = 111$) showed an association in the predicted direc-

Table 6-14
Relationship Between Everyday Reliance on
Spouse in Two Weeks prior to Interview and
Mental Health Measures (Sub 2, $N = 79$)[a]

Mental Health Measures	τ
SOMA	.155[b]
ANX	.120
DEP	.123
SDRS	.080
BPRS	.151[b]
SPC 1	−.035
SPC 2	−.089
ASP	−.106

For explanation of mental health measures see
Appendix 5-A.
[a]Measured by Kendall's tau.
[b]$p \leq .05$

tion for somatic discomfort ($\tau = .154$; $N = 111$; $p < .05$). For Sub 3
there is an association of greater current reliance with more disturbance regarding social dysfunction ($\tau = .374$; $N = 29$; $p = .01$) and two
suicidal variables (SPC 1: $\tau = .380$; $N = 28$; p < .05; ASP: $\tau = .380$; $N = 29$; $p < .05$).

Men and women may respond differently to current reliance on an
estranged or former spouse. Sub 2 men do not appear to be obviously
distressed by continued emotional reliance, at least insofar as such reliance is recognizable by themselves or by raters. In fact, such emotional reliance may improve their functioning. On the other hand, men
seem to deal poorly with everyday reliance on the spouse. Women appear to be troubled by emotional reliance, but not to the same extent by
continued everyday reliance. In fact, Sub 2 women appeared to be less
suicidal if they continued some everyday reliance.

Men may view what they define as continued emotional reliance
on an estranged or former wife as acceptable and even protective, but
do not see everyday reliance in the same light. Reliance in the area of
finances and legal matters is specifically associated with disturbance.
These are the areas in which post-divorce conflict commonly occurs.
Women may find continued emotional reliance on the spouse particularly unacceptable. They are not as troubled by everyday reliance and
may find it protective. The socialization of women to expect practical
dependence on men may make such dependence more ego-syntonic.

SUMMARY

This chapter suggested that attachment theory, while important, does not fully explain the continuing tie between spouses. The nature and frequency of contacts between the spouses; emotional reliance prior to the first serious discussion of separation and in the two weeks before the interview; and everyday reliance, prior to the first serious discussion of separation and in the two weeks prior to interview specifically delineate the continuing tie. Among those recently separated and who have not filed for divorce, those who had some form of contact in the two weeks prior to research interview outnumbered those who did not by 11 to 1. The ratio decreased with time but close to half of all respondents and about one-third of childless persons continued some contact after 14 or more months elapsed since the last separation event. No clear-cut confirmation of the hypothesis that contacts per se would be associated with dysfunction, on the grounds that in the context of separation and loss they would be more painful than not, emerged. It is possible that distress may be related to contacts by a U-shaped curve, with greatest distress in those who had no contact or frequent contact, and lower distress in those having infrequent contact.

Before the first serious discussion of separation, from half to four-fifths of the respondents reported relying on the spouse in one or more defined areas of emotional reliance. In the last two weeks before interview, the percentage was much lower, ranging from 10 to 33 percent, depending on the type of reliance. The professional raters estimated emotional reliance higher than the respondents themselves did; individuals undergoing marital separation are presumably reluctant to acknowledge continued emotional dependence.

It was predicted that the level of emotional dependence before the first serious discussion of separation would vary directly with mental health functioning at interview in the recently separated/divorced, because the greater the prior reliance, the greater the loss. That hypothesis was generally supported in regard to the three component scales of the Frank Discomfort Scale (somatic discomfort, anxiety, and depression) and the Brief Psychiatric Rating Scale. Significant associations were found for the group as a whole, and for women when analyzed separately, but not for men.

It was further predicted that the level of current residual emotional dependence would be associated with increased disturbance on the mental health measures, because continued reliance on an estranged or former spouse would be painful and disturbing. Regarding self-assessed current reliance, the hypothesis was not sustained, but was confirmed when rater-rated current emotional reliance was considered. Since rater-rated reliance is probably more valid due to the respondent's probable reluctance to acknowledge emotional reliance, confirmation can be cautiously inferred.

High levels of everyday reliance occurred before the first serious discussion of separation, and much lower levels in the last two weeks. Child care was rated the highest, no doubt due to the frequency of custody by one parent.

A hypothesis was proposed that the greater pre-separation everyday dependence, the greater current dysfunction. There was suggestive confirmation for the recently separated or divorced as a whole, with confirmation present for men but not for women. The prediction that financial reliance before the separation discussion would be associated with high levels of disturbance was not borne out.

Increased disturbance was associated with current everyday reliance for the recently separated and divorced as a whole, particularly for men. Gender analysis suggests that for men everyday reliance both before the separation discussion and in the last two weeks is most clearly associated with disturbance on the outcome variables, whereas emotional reliance shows either no relationship or some association in the opposite direction. Just the reverse seems true for women. When current reliance is assessed by the raters, women respond adversely to high levels of emotional reliance both before the separation discussion and in the last two weeks, but less or not at all to everyday reliance.

The possible adverse effects of continued reliance of estranged spouses on each other run somewhat counter to the conventional wisdom, and provides some support for the theoretical framework proposed in Chapter 4.

REFERENCES

1. Weiss RS: Marital Separation. New York, Basic Books, 1975
2. Hunt M, Hunt B: The Divorce Experience. New York, McGraw-Hill, 1977
3. Bowlby J: Attachment and Loss (vol. 1). New York, Basic Books, 1969
4. Bowlby J: Making and breaking of affectional bonds: I. Aetiology and psychopathology in the light of attachment theory. Br J Psychiatry 130:201–210, 1977
5. Levinger G, Moles O: In conclusion: Threads in the fabric. J Soc Issues 32(1):193–207, 1976

6. Robertson J: A two-year-old goes to hospital (film). London, Tavistock Child Development Research Unit. Distributed by New York University Film Library, 1952

7. Freud A: Normality and Psychopathology in Childhood. New York, International Universities Press, 1965

8. Goode WJ: After Divorce. Glencoe, Ill, The Free Press, 1956

9. Bohannon P: The six stations of divorce, in Bohannan P (Ed): Divorce and After. New York, Doubleday, 1970

10. Burke MA, Grant JB, quoted in Marriage and Divorce Today 7(43), 1982

11. Goldsmith J: Relationships between former spouses: Descriptive findings. J Divorce 4(2):1–20, 1980

12. Fisher EO: Divorce: The New Freedom. New York, Harper and Row, 1974

7

Aspects of the Separation Process

This chapter deals with the separation process. Separation is neither a single event nor one that moves inexorably in a single direction. Rather, the ending of a marriage occurs slowly, with wishes to reconcile and save the relationship alternating with movement towards separation and divorce. The process of ending a marriage has been compared to the course of a terminal illness: there is the diagnosis, with its ensuing shock; then treatment brings about remission and renewed hope, only to be followed by relapses, perhaps alternating with new remissions until the ultimately fatal outcome. Of course, just as some seriously ill patients recover, some marriages are "cured," i.e., more or less lasting reconciliation occurs.

This chapter will emphasize the separation rather than the divorce because the psychologically crucial aspect of the separation/divorce process is the physical separation, not the legal divorce. Three aspects of the separation process will be discussed: (1) which partner initiates the separation; (2) vacillation in the decision to separate; and (3) reconciliation issues, which include intensity of these wishes, beliefs about the spouse's attitude to reconciliation, and the likelihood of reconciliation.

INITIATING THE SEPARATION

The question of which marital partner initiates the separation is an important one. It is too simple to expect that only the partner who did not want the separation is adversely affected, while the initiator, who gets his or her wish, is pleased with the outcome. The intricacies of marital bonding are such that this simplistic statement is unacceptable. It is an important empirical question whether there is an association between which partner initiates the separation and the spouse's mental health.

Previous Studies

Given the complex interaction between separating spouses, it is not surprising that investigators have found no simple answer to the question as to who initiated a separation or divorce. Goode[1] asked divorced women which partner had instigated the divorce; 62.1 percent reported that they themselves, 24.7 said the husband, and 13.2 percent reported mutual intent.[1] Goode, however, went a step further. He suggested without citing specific evidence that it is the husband more often than the wife who wants to escape from the marriage and "adopts strategy to force the wife to ask for a divorce."[1] In any event, he found that there was a relationship between who the reported instigator was and the trauma index mentioned previously. Women who stated that their husband suggested the divorce had the highest trauma index, followed by those reporting self-initiation, and those who said that the decision was mutual showed the least trauma.[1] There is some question as to the implications of Goode's findings in light of his view that husbands instigate divorce more frequently than his respondents indicated.

Hunt and Hunt[2] also referred to the difficulty in obtaining clear answers to the question of who wanted a divorce. They noted that although only 20 percent of the respondents in their study said that both spouses wanted the divorce, Brown (cited in Hunt and Hunt) estimated that a mutual wish for divorce occurs in over half of the concerned couples. Hunt and Hunt did not take information about instigation at face value and came to a conclusion opposed to Goode's view that husbands initiate divorce more often than wives. Hunt and Hunt stated that even though men more often move out, "the woman is more often the one who wants the separation."[2] The woman was the "discarder" in "about half" of their cases, in "about a third" the man, and in "about a fifth" the decision was mutual. Although they did not specifically refer to Goode's contrary view, Hunt and Hunt suggested that the tendency for women to seek divorce more often than men is a recent development. From their point of view, their conclusions that wives are more frequent instigators and Goode's earlier conclusion that husbands are more frequent instigators could both be valid.

Weiss suggested that there is a difference between the response of the instigator and that of the spouse on whom the separation is imposed. Weiss believed that the latter feels more hurt and anger,[3] while the spouse who takes the lead in the separation, having less reason to be angry, may attempt to establish friendly post-marital relations.[3] However, Weiss has also suggested that the difference between instigator and other is more in the kind than in the intensity of distress, and that separation distress appears in both groups. The person who is left may feel a traumatic rejection, but the instigator tends to feel guilty.[3]

Present Study

Both Goode[1] and Weiss[3] have pointed out that there is no easy way to produce meaningful information on the issues of whether one of the spouses wanted the separation more than the other, who that spouse was, and whether the decision was mutual.

Hunt and Hunt believe that there is an increase in female-instigated divorces.[2] There is evidence that women with more income and education are likely to leave unhappy marriages more readily than those not so fortunate. With more women achieving higher social and economic status, the number of such initiators may well increase. In addition, some women may see divorces as "the chance of a new lifetime."[4] At the same time, however, there is a bias in both men and women toward identifying women as instigators of separation and divorce. Goode's view is that men salve their consciences and try to absolve themselves of blame in the eyes of others by attributing the decision to separate to their wives.[1] Men, particularly in states that have adversary proceedings, may also feel that they will obtain a better financial settlement if the wife is the initiator. At the same time, both men and women may see designating the women as the initiator as protective of her position, which historically has been held to be more vulnerable in that it implies that the husband is at fault.

There is a serious methodological issue regarding the determination of who is "really" the initiator. Ideally, the matter should be addressed by means of a detailed interview focused on the subject of initiation and attuned to the conscious and unconscious reluctance, to confront this issue head on. The present study tries to deal with the issue by asking four questions and then concentrating on the one most likely to yield valid responses. The questions were: Who first seriously suggested separation? Who initiated the current separation? Who first brought up a divorce? Who filed for divorce? Replies are first described for men and women combined (Table 7-1).

The responses to the two questions related to separation are shown in Table 7-1. Over half of those questioned stated that they themselves initiated the last separation. At first it would seem that

Table 7-1

Replies to Questions about Separation for Men
and Women Combined (Sub 2)

Initiator	First Seriously Suggested Separation (N = 100)	Initiated Current Separation (N = 100)
Self	56%	56%
Spouse	42%	35%
Mutual	2%	9%

among those whose decision is not mutual, there should be an equal number reporting self- and spouse-instigation. Women, however, were the reported initiator more often than men, and the majority of our respondents were women. Further, there are probably a number of instances in which both husband and wife both state—as a matter of pride—that they were the initiator. Between the first discussion of separation and the initiation of the current separation, there is an increase in the "mutual" category, indicating that at least consciously, some of the respondents whose spouses initially brought up separation came to accept the idea over time.

The picture changes somewhat when the question of initiation of divorce is considered. Not all persons in Sub 2, it will be recalled, had considered or filed for divorce. The responses to the two questions related to instigation of divorce are shown in Table 7-2. Self-initiated divorce was reported slightly less frequently than self-initiated separation, and the spouse was reported as filing for divorce more often.

The question, Who initiated the last separation? is the least likely to be subject to distortion for two reasons: it refers to a relatively re-

Table 7-2

Replies to Questions about Instigation of Divorce
for Men and Women Combined (Sub 2)

Initiator	First Brought up Subject of Divorce (N = 84)	First Filed for Divorce (N = 84)
Self	51.2%	46.0%
Spouse	42.8%	54.0%
Mutual	5.9%	NA

cent event and it focuses on that specific occurrence. Who first brought up the issue of separation and divorce may be less clearly remembered. The matter of who filed, while it is the least ambiguous, may be invalid because women more often file.

Theoretically, the category of mutual agreement is of interest since, as Goode found,[1] this group is the least disturbed. However, there were too few cases in this category in the present study to warrant further analysis.

Self- and spouse-initiated separation was compared, by means of cross-tabulation, for 156 respondents in Sub 2 and Sub 3 (long-term separated/divorced). There were no statistically significant differences between individuals who had recently separated, recently filed, recently been divorced, or experienced the last of these events 14 or more months earlier ($X^2 = 3.71$; 3 df; $p > .05$, NS). There were, however, significant differences between men and women (Table 7-3). Men reported that the last separation was spouse-initiated significantly more often than did women. Combining the statements of our male and female respondents, we find that men initiated the last separation in 53 (21 + 32) cases (34.0 percent) and women in 103 (75 + 28) cases (66.0 percent). Both Goode[1] and Hunt and Hunt[2] found—many years apart—that about two thirds of all separated initiators are wives. If the mutual group is omitted, Goode's percentage of wife-initiated divorce was 71.5. Hunt's and Hunt's report, when adjusted in the same manner, found wife-initiated divorce to be 60 percent. It is possible that women overestimate the extent to which they initiate a separation and that men underestimate their own role. Further work remains to be done in this area. Nevertheless, the results suggest that both men and women say that women initiate separation and divorce considerably more often.

When considering only Sub 2 ($N = 91$), the way men and women see the separation is no longer statistically significant (Table 7-4). The

Table 7-3
Replies to Question of Which Partner
Initiated Separation (Subs 2 and 3)

Initiator	M	F	Total
Self	21	75	96
Spouse	28	32	60
Total	49	107	156

X^2 (corrected) = 9.41; 1 df; $p \leq .01$

Table 7-4
Replies to Question of Who Initiated
Current Separation (Sub 2)

Initiator	M	F	Total
Self	14	42	56
Spouse	15	20	35
Total	29	62	91

X^2 (corrected) = 2.39; 1 df; $p \leq .12$, NS.

finding that there are no statistically significant differences is probably due to the smaller number of cases. However, the preponderance of reported woman-initiated separations may be a distortion. Such distortion is less likely when the separation has recently occurred and defenses have not yet changed this recollection.

RELATIONSHIP BETWEEN SEPARATION AND MENTAL HEALTH MEASURES

Hypotheses. The following hypotheses were formulated prior to the beginning of the study: (1) If the spouse is perceived by the respondent as being the one who most wanted the separation or divorce, the respondent is likely to be rated as more disturbed by the chosen mental health measures; (2) A respondent who indicated that the decision to obtain a separation was mutual will be less disturbed than an individual who wanted the separation or whose spouse wanted the separation. The criterion for the first hypothesis was the relationship between the response to the question, Who initiated the current separation? and mental health measures. It was not possible to test the second hypothesis because there were too few cases in the "mutual" category.

Results. The results (Table 7-5) indicate that there are associations between the respondents' mental health and who the respondent identified as the initiator of the current separation. In all analyses, only those reporting that the respondent or the spouse initiated the separation were included. Spouse initiation is significantly related to increases in depression, social dysfunction, BPRS, and suicide potential. When Sub 2 men and women are considered separately (Table 7-6), there are no statistically significant associations for males, but on all but two suicidal variables, women whose spouses initiated the last separation were significantly more disturbed than women who initiated

Table 7-5
Relation Between Reported Self- or Spouse-Initiated
Current Separation and Mental Health Measures
(Sub 2)[a]

Mental Health Measure	τ	Number
SOMA	.074	90
ANX	.086	90
DEP	.216[b]	90
SOC	.172[c]	87
BPRS	.250[b]	87
SPC 1	.073	87
SPC 2	.195[c]	87
ASP	−.011	87

For explanation of mental health measures see Appendix
5-A.
[a]Initiator: Self = 1; Spouse = 2
[b]$p \leq .01$
[c]$p \leq .05$

the last separation themselves. It remains to be seen whether the difference in findings for men and women in this area will remain true when greater numbers of men are available for study.

The association between who initiated separation and mental health measures was also analyzed for Sub 3. Surprisingly, all coefficients except ASP were in the opposite direction from that observed in Sub 2. Those who said that they instigated the last separation now reported more distress than the individuals who identified the spouse as the initiator. Only one measure, SOMA, showed a significant relationship ($\tau = -.232$, $p < .05$; $N = 65$). Pending further studies, we cannot dismiss these indications as spurious.

These findings suggest that among the recently separated/divorced, those who say the spouse initiated the last separation are more depressed, socially dysfunctional, and psychiatrically disturbed than those who say they initiated the separation themselves. This finding is much more clearly true of women than it is of men. The question whether the "rejected" are also more suicidal is not clearly answered by these findings. Common sense and clinical observation would suggest that this is so, but only one of three suicidal indicators was significant for the group as a whole.

Table 7-6

Relationship Between Reported Self- or Spouse-Initiated
Last Separation and Mental Health Measures (Sub 2)[a,b]

Mental Health	Males		Females	
Measure	τ	N	τ	N
SOMA	.039	29	.182[c]	61
ANX	−.052	29	.199[c]	61
DEP	.178	29	.276[d]	61
SOC	.099	27	.225[c]	60
BPRS	.120	27	.309[d]	60
SPC 1[f]	—	—	.113[e]	60
SPC 2[f]	—	—	.204	60
ASP[f]	—	—	−0.29	60

For explanation of mental health measures see Appendix 5-A.
[a]Initiator: Self = 1; Spouse = 2
[b]Measured using Kendall's tau
[c]$p \leq .05$
[d]$p \leq .01$
[e]$p \leq .051$
[f]There were not enough suicidal males to warrant computation
of correlations.

The finding that those who said that their spouse initiated the separation are more disturbed may imply that the spouse initiation causes the disturbance. While such an explanation is plausible, it is theoretically possible that mentally healthy persons rationalize a rejection better and convince themselves that they, not the spouse, wanted the separation. The finding that there is no longer an association between who initiated separation and mental health measures in Sub 3, and that one measure is associated in the opposite direction, is puzzling. One possible explanation is that people may with time become better able to rationalize the separation as their own doing, even though they may not have seen the situation this way before.

VACILLATION REGARDING THE DECISION TO SEPARATE

Marital separation is as a rule anything but the result of a single irreversible decision. This differentiates loss of a partner by separation, which is potentially reversible, from loss of a partner by death. As mentioned, the possibility to interact with a living partner may be, for some, one of the reasons for greater disturbance among the separated and divorced than among the widowed.

One result of the continued presence of the marital partner is the option to change one's mind regarding separation. This aspect of the separation process will be addressed by considering whether separated individuals report that since they originally decided to separate, they and their spouse decided not to carry it out and, if so, how many times such a change of mind occurred. This study is not concerned with people who at the time of interview were reconciled; for them vacillation may or may not have the same impact on mental health. We are at this time only interested in people who at the time of the study had not decided to reconcile.

Previous Studies

Goode examined what he called the stability of the decision to divorce.[1] His focus was divorce, not separation. He found that 67 percent never reconsidered; 12 percent did so rarely; 12 percent reconsidered several times, and 9 percent did so frequently. He found that the more frequent the decision not to divorce, the higher was the trauma index.[1]

Hunt and Hunt and Weiss stated that reconciliation is frequently attempted and is not uncommonly maintained,[2,3] but they did not supply figures on the frequency of vacillation. Since Goode, no study other than the present one addresses the question of vacillation in quantitative terms. Weiss stated that "the on again off again relationship is too painful to be sustained."[3] Hunt and Hunt stated that the bulk of reconciliations occur soon after the breakup.[2] Thereafter, most separated couples will go on to divorce.

Present Study

Unlike the difficulties in formulating questions designed to ascertain who the "true" instigator is, the question of vacillation is a relatively straightforward one. The major research decision is whether to be concerned with vacillation regarding the decision to separate or regarding the decision to divorce. The decision to separate is psychologically more meaningful, and therefore questions were asked in regard to this area.

In our population, vacillation in the decision to separate was con-

Table 7-7

Percentage of Vacillation in the Decision to Separate

Number of Times Decided Not to Carry Out Separation	Sub 1 (N = 61)	Sub 2 (N = 100)	Sub 3 (N = 68)	Sub 4 (N = 229)
0	13.1	30.0	41.2	28.8
1	13.1	11.0	14.7	12.7
2	21.3	12.0	4.4	12.2
3	8.2	12.0	7.4	9.6
4–6	11.5	12.0	7.4	10.5
7–9	3.3	2.0	1.5	2.2
10 or more	29.5	21.0	23.5	24.0

siderably more frequent than Goode found in regard to the decision to divorce, as Table 7-7 indicates. The responses are to the question, "Since your first serious discussion of separation, how often did you and your spouse decide not to carry it out?" Results are given for Sub 1, Sub 2, and Sub 3. In the whole group, less than 30 percent indicated that they and their spouse had never reconsidered their decision to separate. It is interesting to note that the number who said they never reconsidered the decision to separate declined with time since the first actual serious discussion. The largest proportion who said they had never reconsidered the decision to separate was in Sub 3 (41.2 percent), followed by Sub 2 (30.0 percent). The smallest proportion was Sub 1 (13.1 percent). This is probably due to the fact that reconciliations most often occur early in the separation process.[2] (Follow-up information [Table 7-8] was obtained for the majority of subjects after the series of crisis intervention interviews was completed, which was in most instances four to six weeks after the first research interview. It is anticipated that data based on these respondents will be separately published at a later time.) It is also possible that the more time that elapses since the separation crisis, the more vacillations may be forgotten.

One explanation for the differences between the frequency of vacillation found in this study and the much lower number Goode reported is that this study included people earlier in the separation process, some of whom will reconcile. Goode studied only those who had irrevocably terminated their marriages. There may also be a difference between vacillation regarding divorce and that regarding separation. Finally, the difference may be due to the time that has elapsed since the Goode study, differences in the sample, or other methodologic varia-

Table 7-8

Follow-Up Information Obtained Approximately Four to Six Weeks after First Research Interview

Status at Follow-Up	Status at First Research Interview					
	Discussing Separation (Sub 1)	Recently Separated, not Filed (Sub 2)[a]	Recently Filed (Sub 2)[a]	Recently Divorced (Sub 2)[a]	Long-Term Separated/Divorced (Sub 3)	Total
Discussing separation	14	0	0	0	0	14
Recently separated, not filed	8	21	0	0	0	29
Recently filed	6	5	20	0	0	31
Recently divorced	0	0	2	21	0	23
Long-term separated/divorced	0	0	0	1	50	51
Reconciled	20	12	0	1	0	33
Unavailable for follow-up	14	9	6	8	20	57
Total	62	47	28	31	70	238

[a] Within 13 months before first research interview.

153

tions. In the present study, it is clear that vacillation *is the rule, not the exception* and that about one quarter of all the subgroups change their minds ten or more times.

The question, How often did a change of mind occur in the two weeks prior to interview? was introduced, anticipating that recent vacillation might be especially disturbing. There were only few vacillations, however, in the prior two weeks. For the group as a whole ($N = 173$), 75.4 percent reported no recent vacillation. Only 3.5 percent reported ten or more changes of mind in this time period. Only those still in Sub 1 had any significant number of vacillations in the previous two weeks: 49.2 percent ($N = 61$) reported one or more changes of mind. In Sub 2, only 14.5 percent reported any vacillation, and there were no reported vacillations in Sub 3. These data confirm that frequent changes of mind occur early in the separation process.

RELATIONSHIP BETWEEN VACILLATION AND MENTAL HEALTH MEASURES

Hypothesis. The hypothesis was that the greater the degree of vacillation in the decision of the respondent to divorce in the recently separated/divorced, the greater the rated mental health disturbance. Prior to the beginning of data collection, the reference to divorce was replaced with separation. The original criteria related responses to the frequency of vacillation since the first decision to divorce (subsequently, to separate) and to vacillation in the previous two weeks. There was an insufficient number of cases to test the hypothesis regarding the previous two weeks. The tests of the hypothesis to be described are therefore based on vacillation since the first serious discussion of separation. The respondents were asked, "Since your first serious discussion of separation, how often did you or your spouse decide not to carry it out?" The range of scores was from 0 to 6, with 6 referring to six or more changes of mind.

Results. As Table 7-9 indicates, there were a number of significant associations with mental health measures for the recently separated/divorced (Sub 2) as a whole and particularly for women within that group. All but the SDRS, BPRS, and one of three suicidal indications were significant for women. None did so for men, however. Even though the sample was small, inspection suggests that the absence of a relationship might have been found even if the group of men had been larger. It is of interest that while men and women differed in their response to vacillation, they did not differ significantly in the number of separations they experienced ($X^2 = 8.23$; 6 *df;* $p = .22$, NS).

Table 7-9
Relationship Between Vacillation and Mental Health
Measures (Sub 2)[a]

Mental Health Measure	M ($N = 31$)	F ($N = 69$)	Total ($N = 100$)
SOMA	$-.069$	$.191^b$	$.090$
ANX	$.098$	$.192^b$	$.158^b$
DEP	$.007$	$.165^b$	$.116^c$
SOC	$-.063$	$.017$	$.008$
BPRS	$.047$	$.143$	$.097$
SPC 1[d]	—	$.201^b$	$.165^b$
SPC 2[d]	—	$.177^b$	$.169^b$
ASP[d]	—	$.114$	$.093$

For explanation of mental health measures see Appendix 5-A.
[a]Measured by Kendall's tau, two-tailed test.
[b]$p \leq .05$
[c]$p \leq .10$
[d]There were not enough suicidal males to warrant computation of correlations.

While no predictions were made for any subgroup other than Sub 2 (the recently separated/divorced), the findings regarding other subgroups are of interest. In Sub 1 ($N = 61$), correlations were in general of greater magnitude than was true of those already separated. Four correlations were significant (using in this case a two-tailed test, since no hypotheses were formulated). Three were significant at the $p \leq .01$ level: anxiety ($\tau = .273$), social dysfunction ($\tau = .257$), and BPRS ($\tau = .247$); and one at the $p \leq .05$ level: SPC 1 ($\tau = .222$). Sub 1 also had the greatest actual incidence of vacillation. On the other hand, and not surprisingly, there were no significant associations of this variable with mental health measures in Sub 3 (long-term separated/divorced).

The findings indicate that there is a consistent inverse association of vacillation with mental health levels as measured by our instruments. Persons considering separation and the recently separated/divorced tend to be more symptomatic in relation to vacillation in terms of somatic symptoms, anxiety and depression, and also tend to appear more psychiatrically disturbed and suicidal. Again, we are noting association, not etiology. It may be that the vacillation is painful and disturbing or that the disturbance is designed to motivate the partner to reverse the separation—and it is sometimes effective in doing so. While this is not a major factor, there may be some reciprocal association between vacillation in marital separation and mental health status.

It is not clear why the findings are strikingly different for men and women. On a number of variables men do not respond by changes in mental health whereas women do. This cannot be attributed to men as a group being less disturbed because the general level of disturbance in men after separation (but not before) is approximately the same as that in women. Perhaps men tend to take more of an all-or-nothing posture toward marital separation: the distress is there once it has occurred and the to-and-fro movement may affect them less than women.

RECONCILIATION ISSUES

To say that whether or not a separated spouse wants to reconcile is likely to be significantly related to the respondent's mental health is almost to state the obvious. Yet in scientific investigation, even the apparently obvious needs to be empirically demonstrated. In addition, there are some questions to which there are no readily available answers, such as the incidence and intensity of reconciliation wishes and the extent to which persons undergoing separation or divorce adequately reality test the likelihood of separation.

Previous Studies

To some extent, studies of vacillation previously quoted have a bearing on the desire to reconcile, since vacillation is clearly one result of such a wish. Hunt and Hunt reported that 55 percent of the men and 44 percent of the women had thought about reconciliation[2] and about two thirds of the men and slightly fewer of the women had actually suggested it to their spouses. Weiss said that most separated couples give at least a passing thought to reconciliation.[3] Insofar as writers discuss divorce, they deal with the incidence of actual reconciliation, and perhaps with its chances of success, but only rarely do they address the incidence of wishes for reconciliation in a separated or divorced population.

Present Study

The questions of reconciliation in this present study originally stemmed from an interest in the issue of reality testing. Reality testing is often thought of as an indication of ego strength or adequacy in coping. To address the extent to which there were distorted perceptions in regard to the probability that reconciliation would in fact occur, the interviewers and respondent were asked to indicate the likelihood of reconciliation. It was assumed that the raters would be more objective than the respondents and thus closer to the reality. The difference between the two ratings was therefore considered to be the reality testing score.

A number of other questions were also of interest: What was the respondent's attitude toward reconciliation? What was the affect, whether or not a reconciliation is wanted? What did the respondent believe the spouse's attitude toward reconciliation to be?

All items in this series were recorded by the clinician-interviewers. In several instances the degree of inference was low and the clinician, for practical purposes, simply recorded the answer to the question. (Exceptions will be noted.) The inter-rater reliability using the Spearman rank correlation coefficient ranged from .82 to .91 ($p \leq .001$, $N = 22$). The one exception was the item rating intensity of affect about reconciliation, for which inter-rater reliability was $p = .07$.

• The first question in the series was, "What is the respondent's attitude toward reconciliation?" Answers were recorded on a five-point scale, ranging from "definitely does not want" to "definitely wants." The responses for Sub 2 ($N = 102$) were: definitely does not want (42); probably does not want (8); uncertain (28); probably wants (3); definitely wants (21). It is of interest that 24 persons definitely or probably wanted to reconcile, compared to 35 persons who said that the spouse instituted the last separation (Table 7-4). Therefore, some of these persons had either come to agree with the spouse in wanting the separation or were now uncertain.

There is a trend toward more reconciliation wishes in men. Over a third of the men (34.4 percent) but only one fifth (18.6 percent) of the women probably or definitely wanted a reconciliation. When the data are run without grouping, X^2 is significant (9.49, 4 df; $p = .05$), but 3 of 10 cells have expected frequencies of less than 5. When the data are grouped by combining those that definitely and probably wanted a reconciliation with those that definitely and probably did not want a reconciliation, X^2 is no longer significant (3.60, 2 df; NS); Pearson's R = $-.179$, $p = .036$ (men = 1; women = 2).

The earlier one is in the separation process, the greater the likelihood one wants to reconcile. For those not yet separated (Sub 1), 59.7 percent either probably or definitely wished for reconciliation. Among the long-term separated/divorced (Sub 3), 10.3 percent wanted reconciliation ($X^2 = 102.73$, 16 df; $p = .0001$).

• We next turn to the rater's statement as to the respondent's affection about reconciliation. On this point the clinicians made a judgment.

They rated the affect on a five point scale, ranging from "no affect" to "extremely strong affect." The significance of these findings is limited by the fact that the interrater reliability was not significant. The amount of affect did not depend upon whether or not one wished to reconcile. The responses for Sub 2 ($N = 102$) were: no affect, 17; mild affect, 16; moderate affect, 38; very strong affect, 23; extremely strong affect, 8.

Reconciliation is not a matter of indifference. Over two thirds of the group had at least moderate affect on the subject.

How is the intensity of affect related to wishes for reconciliation? In general, those wishing reconciliation had stronger affect ($\tau = .479$; $p = .001$; $N = 102$). While highly significant, the correlation is far below 1.0. When examining the relationship further by means of cross-tabulation, we find that all of the 24 persons who probably or definitely want reconciliation had moderate or stronger affect about it. The largest proportion of those with very strong and extremely strong affect wanted to reconcile. Among the 50 people who did not want to reconcile, almost half had moderate or stronger affect on the matter. Among those uncertain, 75 percent had moderate or stronger affect; this group may include many of the vacillators. Thus, a number of respondents indicated considerable affect on the subject, whether or not they wanted to reconcile.

Unlike the situation regarding wishes for reconciliation, there is no significant difference between men and women in Sub 2 on the dimension of the intensity of affect regarding reconciliation ($X^2 = 2.22$; 4 df; $p = .69$, NS). There is, of course, a highly significant difference if all groups including Sub 1, Sub 2, and Sub 3 are compared. Intensity of affect is very high early on and diminishes sharply over time ($X^2 = 69.78$; 16 df; $p = .0001$). It is noteworthy, however, that even among the long-term separated/divorced (Sub 3), 36.8 percent still had either moderate or strong affect on the subject of reconciliation.

• We next turn to the question, What does the respondent believe the spouse's attitude toward reconciliation is? Using the same categories as those regarding the respondent's own attitude, the results for Sub 2 ($N = 101$) were: spouse definitely does not want reconciliation (36); spouse probably does not want reconciliation (12); uncertain (17); spouse probably wants reconciliation (17); spouse definitely wants reconciliation (19).

Slightly less than half (47.5 percent) said the spouse probably or definitely did not want to reconcile; 35.6 percent believed the spouse did want to reconcile, and 16.8 percent were uncertain. Respondents stated that the spouse wanted reconciliation somewhat more often than the respondent did, probably in keeping with the greater frequency of designating oneself as the initiator.

There is no difference between men and women on this variable in Sub 2 ($X^2 = 1.48$; 4 df; $p = .83$, NS). There is, again as expected, a highly significant decline from Sub 1 to Sub 2 to Sub 3 in the number who state that the spouse wanted to reconcile ($X^2 = 100.46$; 16 df; $p = .0001$). A small but notable minority of the Sub 3 group (16.2 percent; $N = 68$) believe the spouse probably or definitely wanted to reconcile.

• The answers to whether the respondent believed a reconciliation would occur were rated on a five-point scale. For Sub 2 ($N = 100$) they were: reconciliation will definitely not occur (49); reconciliation will probably not occur (26); could go either way (26); reconciliation is probably going to occur (1); reconciliation is definitely going to occur (0).

The currently separated expected their status to remain unchanged; 75.0 percent did not anticipate a reconciliation.

There was no difference between men and women in Sub 2 on this point ($X^2 = 2.75$; 3 df; $p = .43$, NS). As expected, there was a highly significant difference when Sub 1, Sub 2, and Sub 3 were compared ($X^2 = 132.75$; 16 df; $p = .0001$). Of the Sub 3 group ($N = 62$), six (8.8 percent) still thought a reconciliation could go either way.

• The clinicians independently rated the likelihood of reconciliation. Their ratings for Sub 2 ($N = 102$) were: reconciliation will definitely not occur (45); reconciliation will probably not occur (29); could go either way (18); reconciliation is probably going to occur (10); reconciliation is definitely going to occur (0). The clinicians, in general, tended to see greater likelihood of reconciliation than the respondents did. Separated individuals are likely to under-report the residual attachment and thus the likelihood of reconciliation, especially if they consciously do not want it or are ambivalent about it. There was no difference between men and women in Sub 2 on this variable ($X^2 = 6.03$; 3 df; $p = .11$, NS). As expected, there was a highly significant difference between Sub 1, Sub 2, and Sub 3 ($X^2 = 128.24$; 16 df; $p = .0001$). In Sub 3 ($N = 68$), the clinicians thought that in only three cases might reconciliation take place.

• It seems reasonable that persons whose expectations about reconciliation dovetail with their wishes will do better than those who expect an outcome unlike the one they desire. To test this possibility, a score was derived from the difference between the respondent's own attitude toward reconciliation and the score on the measure of the respondent's expectation of whether reconciliation will occur. The latter was subtracted from the former. Thus, a person who definitely wants reconciliation (score of 5) but who believes that reconciliation is probably not going to occur (score of 2) will have a score of $(5 - 2 = 3)$ on this variable. A negative score indicates that reconciliation is relatively likely compared to the respondent's wishes. Scores potentially can range from -4 to $+4$. The results for Sub 2 ($N = 102$) were -1 (4); 0 (57); $+1$ (16); $+2$ (14); $+3$ (7); $+4$ (4).

Over half (57) the respondents indicated that their expectations of the outcome exactly matched their wishes. Only 4 expected a greater than desired probability for reconciliation. There were 41 persons who thought that reconciliation was less probable than they wished. There was no difference between men and women in Sub 2 ($X^2 = 6.67$; 5 df; $p = .25$, NS). There was, again, a highly significant difference between Sub 1, Sub 2, and Sub 3 ($X^2 = 49.31$; 20 df; $p = .0003$). The farther people are in the separation process, the greater the concordance between their wishes and their expectations. For Sub 1 ($N = 62$), only 40.3 percent had a difference score of 0 (perfect agreement between wish and expectation). On the other hand, in Sub 3 ($N = 68$), almost twice as many (77.9 percent) had a 0 score.

• The final comparison, the reality testing score, indicates the difference between the likelihood of reconciliation as seen by the respondent and by the interviewing clinician. The score was obtained by subtracting the score indicating the rater's estimate of the likelihood of reconciliation on a score of 1 to 5, from the respondent's estimate of this same likelihood, also scored 1 to 5. Thus, if the respondent thought that reconciliation was probably not going to occur (2) and the clinician indicated that it probably was going to occur (4), the difference score would be $(2 - 4 = -2)$. Conversely, if the respondent thought that reconciliation was probably going to occur (4) but the rater believed that it probably was not going to occur (2), the difference would be $(4 - 2 = 2)$. The results for Sub 2 ($N = 102$) were: -2 (5); -1 (22); 0 (57); $+1$ (16); $+2$ (2). There was no difference between men and women in Sub 2 on this variable ($X^2 = 3.79$; 4 df; $p = .44$, NS). There was a highly significant difference when Sub 1, Sub 2, and Sub 3 were compared ($X^2 = 57.50$; 16 df; $p = .0001$). As expected, consensus between respondent and rater increases over time. In Sub 1 ($N = 62$), there was agreement between respondent and rater in only a third of the cases; in Sub 3 there was agreement in 85.3 percent of the respondents.

In summary, we found that the majority of respondents in Sub 2 (recently separated/divorced) did not want reconciliation to occur; expressed moderate to strong affect on the subject; did not believe that their spouse wanted reconciliation nor that it would occur. However, close to half of the group showed a discrepancy between their wishes for reconciliation and their expectation that it would occur; and an equal number differed in their assessment of the likelihood of reconciliation from that of the clinical interviewers.

RELATIONSHIP BETWEEN RECONCILIATION AND MENTAL HEALTH MEASURES: ISSUES FOR STUDY

There were no formal hypotheses for this aspect of the study. The one specific question that was raised prior to the start of data collection had to do with reality testing, measured as the discrepancy between the respondents' estimate of the likelihood of reconciliation and the clinical raters' perception of the same issue. The question was raised whether failure to test reality would be associated with impairment on the mental health measures. For the other variables, the question of association with mental health measures was raised after the data were collected; it was of interest to see whether the other reconciliation-related variables would have a bearing on the mental health of the respondents. This subsection deals with the association of the reconciliation-related variables presented in the last subsection with mental health measures, using Kendall's tau as a measure of this association. Because no predictions were made, a two-tailed test was used. Emphasis will again be on the recently separated/divorced group (Sub 2), but some findings involving the other dissolution categories (Sub 1, Sub 3) will also be mentioned.

RESULTS

• There were a number of significant associations of respondents' attitude to reconciliation, as Table 7-10 indicates. Discomfort appears to be generally associated with wishes for reconciliation. Psychiatric disturbance, as measured by the Brief Psychiatric Rating Scale (BPRS), is also associated with reconciliation wishes for women particularly, and for the group as a whole. For Sub 1 (those discussing separation but not separated), all of the correlations are negative and two discomfort variables are significant (SOMA: $\tau = -.259$; $p \leq .01$; ANX: $\tau = -.204$; $p \leq .05$; $N = 62$). This finding suggests that among persons considering separation, there may be greater discomfort if one of the spouses does not want reconciliation. Wishing a marital state different from that in which one lives can increase discomfort. It is harder to explain the significant negative correlation for somatic dis-

Table 7-10

Relationship Between Attitude about Reconciliation and
Mental Health Measures (Sub 2)[a]

Mental Health Measure	M ($N = 32$)	F ($N = 70$)	Total ($N = 102$)
SOMA	.239	.200[c]	.160[c]
ANX	.269	.204[c]	.213[b]
DEP	.335[c]	.298[b]	.284[b]
SOC	.135	.078	.093
BPRS	.166	.263[b]	.227[b]
SPC 1[d]	—	−.007	.063
SPC 2[d]	—	.083	.137
ASP[d]	—	.037	.109

For explanation of mental health measures see Appendix 5-A.
[a]Measured by Kendall's tau, two-tailed test.
[b]$p \leq .01$
[c]$p \leq .05$
[d]There were not enough suicidal males to warrant computation of correlations.

comfort in Sub 3 (long-term separated/divorced) (SOMA: $\tau = -.240$; $p \leq .05$, $N = 68$). The other discomfort variables and the suicidal variables also correlate negatively and SPC 2 would approach significance with a one-tailed test ($\tau = -.156$; $p = .08$). This finding must be cautiously interpreted, since 75 percent of this group had a score of 1 (definitely did not want reconciliation). Future studies are needed to see if this finding is spurious or if there is some tendency for the longer-term separated and divorced to be disturbed by separation while still desiring it, while those who cling to the hope of reconciliation may do better.

• There are very strong observed associations between intensity of affect about reconciliation and mental health measures. For Sub 2 ($N = 102$), the variable was directly associated with all mental health measures at $p \leq .01$, except for SPC 2 ($p = .014$) and for SOC ($p = .06$). The association is interesting clinically, particularly since it does include two suicidal variables. It suggests that clinicians need to be alert to intensity of reconciliation wishes in separated couples when assessing suicide potential. However, methodologically, the mental health measures assess, to a significant extent, disturbance of affect. Agreement, then, between intensity of affect about anything and these measures is to some extent tautological. There was also inadequate reliability between the raters on this measure, so this finding should be treated with caution.

• One would not anticipate any association between mental health measures and respondent's belief regarding spouse's attitude to reconciliation. It might be important to know whether the spouse's wishes correspond with one's own but in themselves they are not likely to matter. In fact, no association was found.

• One would not anticipate any strong association between mental health measures and respondent-assessed likelihood of reconciliation. Respondents who wish a reconciliation and who anticipate it would have different responses from those who do not wish it. No significant associations were found.

• There is no conclusive association of clinician-rated likelihood of reconciliation and mental health. There is a significant association with suicide potential at entry (SPC 1) for Sub 2 as a whole ($\tau = .185; p \leqslant .05$), but this appears to be an isolated finding and is difficult to interpret.

• The greater the discrepancy score (the difference between the score describing the respondents' attitude to reconciliation and the score indicating their expectation of reconciliation), the greater the difference between wish for and expectation of reconciliation. When the discrepancy score is related to mental health measures there are a number of significant associations. The results are given in Table 7-11. These findings parallel those for attitude toward reconciliation alone; however, the correlations tend to be higher. All three measures of suicide potential achieve or approach significance for the group as a whole, and all would have been significant had the association been predicted and a one-tailed test used. Neither Sub 1 nor Sub 3 shows any significant relations to mental health indicators on this variable.

• Reality testing was assessed in relation to reconciliation. The score of the likelihood of reconciliation as seen by the clinical rater is subtracted from the corresponding score of the respondent. Positive values indicate that the individual thought reconciliation more likely than the rater; negative scores indicate the opposite. Relationship to mental health measures can be measured in two ways. The first involves the raw difference score, including negative and positive values. When these are related to mental health measures for Sub 2 as a whole, the only significant relationship is with two suicidal variables. The correlation is negative (SPC 2: $\tau = -.202; p \leqslant .05$; ASP: $\tau = -.175; p \leqslant .056$; $N = 102$. This indicates that persons who thought reconciliation was less likely than the clinical raters, were more suicidal than those whose estimates coincided with that of the clinicians or those who thought

Table 7-11

Discrepancy Between Wish for and Expectation of
Reconciliation as Related to Mental Health Measures
(Sub 2)[a]

Mental Health Measure	M (N = 32)	F (N = 70)	Total (N = 102)
SOMA	257	.227[c]	.199[b]
ANX	.240	.187	.194[c]
DEP	.368[b]	.350[b]	.328[b]
SOC	.159	.107	.119
BPRS	.215	.287[b]	.261[b]
SPC 1[d]	—	.075	.148
SPC 2[d]	—	.121	.174
ASP[d]	—	.138	.186[c]

For explanation of mental health measures see Appendix 5-A.
[a]Measured by Kendall's tau, two-tailed test.
[b]$p \leq .01$
[c]$p \leq .05$
[d]There were not enough suicidal males to warrant computation of correlations.

that reconciliation was more likely than the raters did. This finding is not conclusive, but it suggests that some individuals may re-enter marital situations even though denying that likelihood and that these persons may present an increased suicidal risk. Perhaps this phenomenon, if confirmed, is related to vacillation, which we have found to be associated with suicide potential. The other way of looking at this variable is in terms of its absolute value, i.e., making negative values positive. This method compares persons whose judgments agree with those of the clinicians with those for whom this is not true. Looking at the variable in this manner, there are no significant associations for men ($N = 32$) in Sub 2. For women in particular, and for Sub 2 as a whole, all but two mental health variables are significantly associated with poor reality testing. The results are shown on Table 7-12.

Lack of objectivity about the prospect of reconciliation is associated with indicators of discomfort, psychiatric and social maladjustment, and increased suicide potential in recently separated or divorced women. The size of the correlation coefficients for men suggests that failure to reach significance may be a function of the small size of the sample, in this instance, rather than being due to a fundamental differ-

Table 7-12

Relationship Between Reality Testing and Mental Health Measures (Sub 2)[a]

Mental Health Measure	M (N = 32)	F (N = 70)	Total (N = 102)
SOMA	.107	.205[c]	.139[c]
ANX	.200	.178	.173[c]
DEP	.158	.221[c]	.193[b]
SOC	−.096	.194[c]	.097
BPRS	.003	.237[c]	.146[c]
SPC 1[d]	—	.152	.135[b]
SPC 2[d]	—	.283[c]	.265[b]
ASP[d]	—	.248[c]	.247[b]

For explanation of mental health measures see Appendix 5-A.
[a]Measured by Kendall's tau, two-tailed test.
[b]$p \leqslant .01$
[c]$p \leqslant .05$
[d]There were not enough suicidal males to warrant computation of correlations.

ence between the sexes. Poor reality testing in separating or divorcing couples can be associated with greater suicide risk.

What we have learned about the association of reconciliation attitudes with mental health measures, including indicators of suicide potential, is not startling, but it is interesting. Those recently separated or divorced who still wish to reconcile are more disturbed as indicated by self-report and clinical rating than those who do not. Increased disturbance is also associated with the divergence between wishes and expectations regarding reconciliation. Suicide potential and other measures of disturbance are also increased, particularly in women, if reality testing as to the separation is faulty, especially if the person believes reconciliation to be more likely than it is in the opinion of a more objective clinician-rater.

COMMENT

The interaction between separating spouses is a highly emotionally charged one. One aspect of this process is the appearance of cognitive impairment. From the viewpoint of ego psychology we can observe regression to more primitive functioning and a reappearance of conflict in areas in which, using Hartman's terminology, there previously existed secondary autonomy.[5] Cognitive impairment is manifested in the frequently observed confusion as to who initiates the separation and who wants it at the present time. Even more clearly, the disturbance in both thinking and action is indicated by the frequency of vacillation in regard to the decision to separate and the relationship of that vacillation to disturbance, including suicide potential. Further, failure to adequately test the reality of the likelihood of reconciliation is quite common. The most frequent distortion consists of believing that reconciliation is less likely than a more objective observer views it to be. We have found that impairment of reality testing is associated with measures of discomfort, psychiatric disturbance, and suicide potential.

These give some support to the notion that the psychological and psychiatric risks in marital separation and divorce may not rest mainly with the fact of the separation as such. Rather, they may, to a significant degree, be related to psychological regression associated with an ongoing and disturbed pattern of interaction between the spouses.

SUMMARY

This chapter has dealt with three aspects of the separation process. The first involved the difficulty in determining who initiated the separation. The majority of persons in our sample indicated that they themselves are the initiators; and further, both men and women said that women were more likely to instigate the dissolution. These statements should not always be taken at face value. It is possible that women and men may have different reasons for designating the woman as the initiator more frequently than may "truly" be the case. Regardless of the difficulty in defining the true initiator, those who said they were the initiator tended to be less disturbed than those who said the spouse instigated the separation or divorce.

The next section dealt with vacillation regarding the decision to separate. Almost three-quarters of all participants in the study had changed their mind one or more times after they and their spouses had initially decided to separate. This is a surprisingly high percentage. About one-quarter of all of the subgroups reported changing their mind six or more times. The most frequent vacillations occur early in the separation process. Vacillation was associated with disturbances on the mental health measures, including suicidal measures in women, but not necessarily in men.

Third, there was a review of issues relative to reconciliation demonstrating, as expected, that those recently separated or divorced who want to reconcile and do not expect to do so, show increased evidence of disturbance. Of perhaps greater interest was the finding that poor reality testing regarding the likelihood of reconciliation was associated with disturbance on most mental health measures, including suicide potential, particularly in women.

The material presented in this chapter is compatible with the view that a significant portion of the disturbance in separating couples is due not only to the fact of the separation, but to psychological regression associated with being involved in disturbing and disturbed interactions between the separating spouses.

REFERENCES

1. Goode WJ: After Divorce. Glencoe, Ill, The Free Press, 1956
2. Hunt M, Hunt B: The Divorce Experience. New York, McGraw-Hill, 1977
3. Weiss RS: Marital Separation. New York, Basic Books, 1975
4. Brown CA, Feldberg R, Fox EM, et al: Divorce: Chance of a new lifetime. J Soc Issues 32:119–133, 1976
5. Hartman H: Ego psychology and the problem of adaptation. J Am Psychoanal Assoc Monograph, Series 1. New York, International Universities Press, 1958

8

Inter-Spouse Hostility and Mental Health*

Divorce and hostility are not pleasant subjects. Perhaps for this reason, interpersonal hostility between separating spouses has not been a frequent subject in the divorce literature. There is, in fact, a tendency among some to openly or subtly decry the presence of such hostility and place a premium on allegedly friendly divorce, often "for the sake of the children." Fisher, referring to the separating couple, said, "Burning with feelings of anger and distrust, they are often told to be friendly and achieve an 'amicable divorce' . . . I believe there is no such thing as an amicable divorce."[1]

Inter-spouse hostility among separating and divorcing couples is an important subject that merits investigation. Parenthetically, this subject is also significant to a study of intact marriages, but that is beyond the scope of this work.

PREVIOUS STUDIES

Goode found an association with emotional trauma in his female respondents who reported wishes to punish the husband at the time of divorce.[2] Further, he found that two or more years after the divorce 24 percent of the women had a negative attitude yet a high frequency of

---

*Adapted in part from a presentation to the American Orthopsychiatric Association Annual Meeting, 1979.

contact.[2] These are the people who go from an unhappy marriage to an unhappy divorce. Goode believed that antagonism is initially due to what the former husband has done to the wife; in most cases the husband was the initiator, in fact, if not always in law. This is later replaced by milder antagonism, which develops when the wife gets a "new standard" as she meets other men. Goode also found that women who report much affect, either positive or negative, toward the ex-husband are less likely to remarry than those who are indifferent.

Fisher stated that the first feelings toward the ex-spouse are "violent hostility and hatred, then guilt and feeling sorry for the spouse and finally, if you can make it, indifference."[1] Hunt and Hunt used a quote from the classics to make their point: "Odi et amo," Catullus wrote to his faithless lover Clodia, "I hate and I love . . . I am in torment."[3] Few separated people, they wrote, realize to what extent "every tug against the web of entanglement reawakens yearning and inflames anger at having been robbed."[3] For most newly separated persons, they believe, anger is the predominant feeling. Among the divorced as well as the separated, anger is still more common and more enduring than positive feelings.

Weiss noted that many separated people may try to avoid expressions of anger, yet "murderous fantasies do not seem especially rare."[4] He wrote of a post-marital mixture of affection and hostility. He noted that "least happy are those whose spouse acts as an enemy" and that "there is not really much a husband and wife can do in defense against a malevolent spouse."[4] He also noted that accusations and disparagements by the spouse are likely to remain vivid for months after the actual break and are related to self-condemnation. In Hetherington's study, two months after the divorce, 66 percent of the exchanges between spouses involved conflict about finances, support, visitation, child rearing, and intimate relations with others. With time, both conflict and attachment decreased, though anger and resentment were more sustained in women than in men.[5] Simon and Lumry, writing of "suicide as a divorce substitute," noted that of a group of 31 former patients in a Veterans Hospital and 9 spouses, all of whom committed suicide, 60 percent experienced serious marital discord, and two murdered their wives before committing suicide.[6] In a related work, Brown et al.[7] and Vaughn and Leff[8] have shown that the expressed hostility of relatives is associated with relapse of psychiatric patients independently of other social and clinical factors. In addition, Bowlby, Parkes, and Pollock recognized anger as an important and universal element of the response to loss.[9,10,11]

PRESENT STUDY

General Considerations

For this study, a list of verbal and physical behaviors was designed de novo, essentially on a common sense basis. The items were as specific as possible. The end was to gain objectivity. Most subtle and non-verbal forms of hostility were excluded, a point to which I will return in the Discussion. At the present stage of knowledge about the separation/divorce process the method employed will advance our understanding.

Five categories of behavior, each containing from two to four items, were addressed in this study. The categories were (1) everyday verbal expressions of hostility; (2) specific separation-related verbal expressions of hostility; (3) death-related expressions of hostility; (4) physical expressions of hostility; and (5) overall measures of hostility (see Table 8-1).

Table 8-1
Indicators of Hostile Inter-Spouse Behavior

Category	Item
Everyday verbal expression of hostility	Putting down the spouse with words* Teasing spouse* Making spouse feel everything he or she does is wrong*
Specific separation/divorce-related verbal expressions of hostility	Turning the children against spouse Using financial and custody matters against spouse
Death-related expressions of hostility	Telling spouse to drop dead* Saying one wishes spouse were dead* Serious wishing spouse dead (whether expressed or not) Encouraging suicide of spouse
Physical expression of hostility	Physically attacking spouse Trying to kill spouse
Overall measures of hostility	Summary index Rater's rating of overall hostility

*Included in summary index of hostility.

Respondents were asked whether they expressed each variant of hostility toward their spouse; and whether they had experienced the spouse expressing these types of hostility toward them. The statements respondents made about their own hostility can be considered more valid than those about their spouse since we can anticipate a distorted picture when seen through the eyes of the adversary.

It is important, nevertheless, to consider a spouse's frankly subjective report about experienced hostility from the former partner. Whether there is objective "truth" in the report, the fact that one experiences a spouse in a particular way may have important correlations with the reporting spouse's mental health.

The following procedure was followed regarding each of the eleven hostility behaviors. Respondents were asked if, in their opinion, hostile behavior had ever occurred in the relationship. If the answer was no, no further questions relating to this item were asked. If the answer was yes, the respondent was asked whether the behavior occurred before or after the first serious discussion of separation or both. If it occurred after the separation discussion, the respondent was also asked whether it occurred in the two weeks prior to interview. This question was only asked of persons who were in some form of contact with the former spouse. All questions were asked in regard to self-expressed hostility and hostility experienced from the spouse.

Results

EVERYDAY VERBAL EXPRESSION OF HOSTILITY

The three items asked were whether the respondent ever "put the spouse down with words"; whether the spouse was made to feel that everything he or she did was wrong; and whether the spouse was teased. The same questions were asked regarding whether the respondent experienced these behaviors expressed by the spouse toward them. The results are shown in Table 8-2. Verbal insults in either direction are virtually universally acknowledged: 91 of 102 respondents said that they at some time "put the spouse down" and that the reverse was also true. We can assume that the few who denied this behavior were deceiving themselves. The next most frequent behavior is making the spouse feel that anything he or she does is wrong. About half of the respondents state they had at some time done so and about two thirds attributed this expression to their former spouse. A somewhat smaller number stated that teasing occurred; about two fifths did this themselves; about half said the spouses did.

Table 8-2
Number of Respondents Reporting Everyday Expressions of Hostility (Sub 2)

Type of Behavior	At Any Time		Before Separation Discussion		Since Separation Discussion		Last Two Weeks[a]	
	To Spouse	From Spouse	To Spouse	From Spouse	To Spouse	From Spouse	To Spouse	From Spouse
Put down with words (N = 102)	91	91	83	84	82	79	28 of 64 (43.8)	40 of 63 (63.5)
Made to feel wrong (N = 101)	47	66	39	58	35	49	14 of 32 (43.8)	21 of 38 (55.3)
Teased (N = 101)	38	49	33	44	22	35	6 of 17 (35.3)	11 of 26 (42.3)

[a]Figures in parentheses refer to the percentage of those in whom the behavior occurred in the last two weeks as a proportion of all those in whom it could have occurred, i.e., those in contact in the last two weeks and in whom the behavior has occurred at some time since the separation discussion.

Respondents typically attributed more hostile behaviors to the spouse than they acknowledged having engaged in themselves. The difference, however, is not as great as one might expect, in light of the general tendency to blame the adversary more than oneself. For verbal putdown, there are practically no differences between hostility directed to the spouse except regarding the last two weeks; for making or being made to feel wrong, and for teasing and being teased, the respondents acknowledged engaging in the hostile behavior about 70 percent as often as they say the spouse did.

The only statistically significant sex difference occurred regarding teasing: 54.8 percent of the men but only 30.0 percent of the women stated that they did so at any time (corrected $X^2 = 4.64$; 1 df; $p < .05$).

Verbal expressions of hostility were common between separated/divorced spouses and occurred somewhat less frequently after the separation discussion than before; perhaps they are characteristic of what one might expect in an ongoing marital interaction, rather than in a situation of impending or actual separation.

SPECIFIC SEPARATION/DIVORCE-RELATED VERBAL HOSTILITY

We next turn to specific separation/divorce related verbal expressions of hostility (Table 8-3). The use of financial or custody matters to express anger could not, by definition, occur before separation. Turning the children against the spouse can and does occur at any time. It was included here because it was anticipated that such behavior is used or at least acknowledged after a separation is seriously considered. We found that this was indeed the case. About two-fifths of the respondents stated they have used financial or custody matters to express anger since the separation, while three fifths said their spouse did or is doing so. Only very few people acknowledged turning the children against the spouse; a somewhat larger, but still relatively small, number attributed this to the spouse. As anticipated, the behavior was more common after the separation discussion. There are no statistically significant sex differences in this area.

DEATH-RELATED HOSTILITY BEHAVIORS

Death-related hostility behavior is important because of the expectation that, under certain circumstances, suicide or homicide may ensue in marital dissolution crises. The items involved proceed from the relatively innocuous one of telling the spouse to "drop dead," to the wish, expressed or not, that the spouse should die, to the statement that one wishes the spouse dead and finally to the open encouragement

Table 8-3
Number of Respondents Reporting Specific Separation/Divorce-Related Verbal Expressions of Hostility (Sub 2)

Type of Behavior	At Any Time		Before Separation Discussion		Since Separation Discussion		Last Two Weeks[a]	
	To Spouse	From Spouse	To Spouse	From Spouse	To Spouse	From Spouse	To Spouse	From Spouse
Used financial or custody matters in divorce to express anger ($N = 102$)	NA	NA	NA	NA	40	60	17 of 33 (51.5)	27 of 50 (54.0)
Turned children against spouse	6 of 58	17 of 61	2	7	6	12	1 of 5 (20.0)	5 of 14 (35.7)

[a]Figures in parentheses refer to the percentage of those in whom the behavior occurred in the last two weeks as a proportion of all those in whom it could have occurred, i.e., those in contact in the last two weeks and in whom the behavior has occurred at some time since the separation discussion.

Table 8-4
Number of Respondents Reporting Death-Related Verbal Expressions of Hostility (Sub 2)

Type of Behavior	At Any Time		Before Separation Discussion		Since Separation Discussion		Last Two Weeks[a]	
	To Spouse	From Spouse	To Spouse	From Spouse	To Spouse	From Spouse	To Spouse	From Spouse
Told spouse to "drop dead" (N = 102)	32	33	25	22	25	27	5 of 20 (25.0)	9 of 23 (39.1)
Seriously wished spouse dead (yes and maybe combined) (N = 102)	31	27	10	16	27	24	11 of 26 (42.3)	11 of 20 (55.0)
Spouse says wished other dead (N = 102)	13	15	8	5	11	12	3 of 11 (27.3)	0 of 0
Encouraged suicide of spouse (N = 102)	4	6	1	4	3	3	0	1

[a]Figures in parentheses refer to the percentage of those in whom the behavior occurred in the last two weeks as a proportion of all those in whom it could have occurred, i.e., those in contact in the last two weeks and in whom the behavior has occurred at some time since the separation discussion.

175

of the spouse's suicide. These behaviors are progressive regarding their potential danger. The findings are shown in Table 8-4. About a third of the respondents indicated that telling the spouse to drop dead and seriously wishing the spouse dead have occurred at some time. In general, these more serious items tended to occur more frequently after the separation discussion. Death-related hostility behaviors are persistent: In about half the cases in which serious death wishes in either direction had been present since the separation discussions and when the spouses were in touch, they did, in fact, occur in the two weeks before the interview. Further, the previously observed differences between behavior acknowledged by the respondent and that attributed to the spouse, practically disappeared. Death-oriented rage was reported in the respondent as often as in the former spouse.

One item statistically differentiates between men and women: self-reported telling the spouse to "drop dead." Of the women, 38.6 percent but of the men only 15.6 percent said they had ever done so (corrected $X^2 = 4.36$; 1 df; $p < .05$; $N = 102$).

PHYSICAL EXPRESSION OF HOSTILITY

There are two items in this category: physically attacking the spouse and trying to kill the spouse. The results are shown in Table 8-5.

The matter of physical attack is of special interest, particularly in the present era, when there is much emphasis on the problem of family violence. A surprisingly high percentage (44 percent) of the respondents indicated that they had physically attacked the spouse and a somewhat greater number (55 percent) reported having been physically attacked. Physical fighting occurred more frequently before the separation discussion, although between one quarter and one third still continued physically fighting thereafter. This pattern often continued as long as there was contact. About one third of the respondents who stated they were ever physically attacked and who were in contact with their former spouses in the two weeks before interview reported an attack during that time; four of nine who had ever attacked their spouse and who were in contact within the last two weeks attacked the spouse during those two weeks.

Almost double the percentage of women (65.7 percent) reported being physically attacked at any time than did men (34.4 percent, corrected $X^2 = 7.52$; 1 df; $p < .01$; $N = 102$). There were however, no statistically significant differences by sex regarding reported physical attack at any other time period.

The picture is different when it comes to acknowledged physical attacks on the spouse by respondent. The number of women reporting

Table 8-5
Number of Respondents Reporting Physical Expressions of Hostility (Sub 2)

Type of Behavior	At Any Time		Before Separation Discussion		Since Separation Discussion		Last Two Weeks[a]	
	To Spouse	From Spouse	To Spouse	From Spouse	To Spouse	From Spouse	To Spouse	From Spouse
Physical attack ($N = 102$)	44 of 97	57	30	42	24	35	4 of 9 (44.4)	7 of 23 (30.4)
Try to kill spouse ($N = 102$)	3	12	2	5	2	10	0 of 0	2 (NA)

[a]Figures in parentheses refer to the percentage of those in whom the behavior occurred in the last two weeks as a proportion of all those in whom it could have occurred, i.e., those in contact in the last two weeks and in whom the behavior has occurred at some time since the separation discussion.

that they ever physically attacked their spouse was somewhat larger than that of men (48.5 percent versus 35.5 percent $N = 99$), but the differences do not reach significance at $p = .05$. Women reported that they attacked the former spouse significantly more often than men said they had after the separation discussion (66.2 percent compared to 18.2 percent, corrected $X^2 = 5.99$; 1 df; $p = .01$; $N = 44$). Before the separation discussion, the trend is in the reverse direction, though it does not reach significance at $p = .05$. While it is difficult to come to specific conclusions about gender-related patterns in physical attack, it is clear that in our sample interspouse violence among separating and divorcing couples is a two-way street.

The most serious result of the separation/divorce process is suicide or homicide. Of 102 respondents in the Sub 2 group, 12 (11.8 percent) believed that the spouse at one time—mainly after the separation discussion—tried to kill them. Only three respondents acknowledged trying to kill their spouse. When the answer of all subjects, regardless of separation status, are considered ($N = 233$), the number of percentage increases: 14 persons (5 men and 9 women) or 6 percent said they tried to kill their spouse at one time. These numbers are not large enough to be statistically significant, but the relatively high number who attributed homicidal potential to themselves and the much higher number who attributed it to the spouse are of considerable importance and concern to anyone working with the separating/divorcing population.

OVERALL MEASURES OF HOSTILITY

Overall measures of hostility include the summary index of hostility and an overall assessment of hostility by the professional raters. The *summary index* is the total of the three everyday verbal hostility items (put down with words, made to feel wrong, teased) and the two explicit verbal death-related items (told to drop dead; says wishes spouse dead).

As Table 8-6 shows, the hostility index is somewhat higher before the separation discussion than after the separation discussion. The index is lower in the last two weeks, but this may in part be due to the fact that a two week period is usually shorter than the entire period before or since the separation discussion. The lower figure for the past two weeks probably also reflects some gradual diminution of hostility over time after the separation discussion as a new equilibrium was slowly established. Table 8-6 also indicates that respondents saw hostility from the spouse as greater than their own hostility to the spouse.

Another way of ascertaining inter-spouse hostility, available only for the two week period prior to research interview, was provided by

Table 8-6
Summary Index of Verbal Hostility at Various Times (Sub 2)

	At Any Time (N = 102)		Before Separation Discussion (N = 102)		Since Separation Discussion (N = 102)		Last Two Weeks	
	To Spouse	From Spouse	To Spouse	From Spouse	To Spouse	From Spouse	To Spouse (N = 78)	From Spouse (N = 80)
Mean score	2.20	2.47	1.81	2.08	1.69	1.92	0.69	0.99
Median score	2.19	2.48	1.84	2.00	1.47	1.85	0.39	0.48

Table 8-7
Rater-Assessed Hostility in the Two Weeks prior to
Interview for Respondents in Contact (Sub 2)

Extent of Hostility	To Spouse ($N = 79$)	From Spouse ($N = 81$)
None	33	29
Little	17	20
Moderate	11	16
Considerable	13	10
Great deal	5	6

the *clinical raters' assessment* of whether the respondent either expressed hostility towards the spouse, or experienced hostility from the spouse. The question was asked of all respondents who were in contact. The results are found in Table 8-7.

According to the raters, 60 percent expressed or experienced little or no hostility in relation to the spouse in the last two weeks while about 40 percent experienced a moderate or larger amount of hostile interaction. These ratings are roughly comparable to the self-reports. Nearly two thirds of all respondents who were in contact with the spouse were rated as experiencing some hostility from the spouse in the last two weeks before interview; for about two fifths it was of moderate or greater intensity.

DISCUSSION

Does inter-spouse hostility peak before or after the separation discussion? Theoretically, a case could be made for both. On the one hand, mutual anger may lead to separation, and a lessening of tensions can then be expected. On the other hand, an impending or actual separation inflames anger. Our data do not give a clear-cut answer. While the post-separation discussion time interval may be shorter than the one preceding the separation discussion, we can take the incidence of hostile behavior in each time period at face value since these behaviors occur frequently enough to make it unlikely that they were absent due to a too-short time.

When we compare the incidence before and after the separation discussion we do not find a simple pattern. A great deal of anger, including some of murderous intensity, is reported as preceding the first serious discussion of marital separation. In other words, it occurred while the marriage was intact. That finding is consonant with the belief that hostility, even intense and prolonged, occurs in marriages over long periods of time, and is present in some that do not break up. Some manifestations of hostility, particularly verbal "putdown" and teasing, do not increase and may diminish after a separation discussion. Physical attacks also decrease. The divorce itself affords new opportunities for the expression of hostility. Almost 60 percent of the recently separated/divorced perceived the spouse as using financial and custody matters to express anger in the post separation discussion.

One finding suggests that the most serious kind of anger, death wishes, may increase after serious separation discussion, a finding compatible with the belief that murderous wishes and acts occur more around the time of separation and divorce than at other times. The evidence here, however, is not conclusive.

Overall, we are dealing with two phases of hostility: one preceding the divorce, and probably instrumental in bringing it about, which abates for one or both partners as the divorce becomes imminent or occurs; and another anger due to loss of the marriage and partner.

Inter-Spouse Hostility and Mental Health

Continued interaction between spouses after the separation process has begun, and particularly hostile interaction, may be significant in increased levels of disturbance among separated individuals. Further, the potentially most noxious factor may be the hostility a person is exposed to from the former spouse. How expressed hostility might affect the mental health of the individual expressing it is an important question about which no prediction was made.

HYPOTHESES

The following hypotheses were formulated prior to the beginning of the study: (1) the greater the degree of hostility expressed by the spouse to the respondent, as perceived by the respondent, the greater will be the rated mental health impairment. (2) The more likely the spouse is to have expressed death wishes to the respondent, as perceived by respondent, the greater will be the rated mental health impairment.* (3) The degree of hostility expressed by the respondent to

---

*The study as originally formulated dealt only with suicide potential. Prior to its beginning, the dependent variables were extended to include other aspects of mental health. Regarding the independent variables, the tests of the hypotheses reflect in general the intent of the proposal. They differ in a few specifics: The original proposal called

(Footnote continued on next page)

the spouse may be associated with either greater or less mental health impairment in the respondent.

GENERAL COMMENTS

The results of the correlation analysis of the hostility variables will be reported in the same order as were the findings on these variables, only for the separated/divorced (Sub 2). In each case respondents' mental health will be related first to respondent hostility as expressed *to* the spouse, and then to spouse hostility as experienced *by* the respondent. Because a prediction was made in regard to the latter but not the former, a one-tailed analysis of significance was performed regarding experienced spouse hostility and a two-tailed analysis was done regarding expressed respondent hostility.

All respondents were asked whether a given hostility behavior ever occurred. If the answer was yes, the question was asked whether it occurred before and/or after the separation discussion. If it occurred after the separation discussion, and if the respondent was in contact with the spouse in the two weeks prior to interview, the respondent was asked if the behavior occurred in the last two weeks. The greatest likelihood of finding an association between hostility and mental health existed if the behavior was recent. Therefore, those that could be asked about the last two weeks were selected first to analyze the relationship of mental health to hostility. In many instances, however, there was an insufficient number of respondents to allow such an analysis, i.e., $N < 30$ for all Sub 2 respondents. The second choice were those who reported the behavior since the separation discussion. If the number was still insufficient, the entire group was used for analysis and whether or not the behavior ever occurred constituted the hostility variable. When the number of respondents in the most recent group was sufficient to conduct a statistical analysis but was still small (less than 40 subjects), the next larger group was also analyzed. Whenever

---

for the individual analysis only of the death-related variables and for inclusion in the summary index of all hostility variables except for those involving physical hostility, which was to be separately analyzed. In the present analysis, all hostility variables are individually considered. Further, the summary index was reconstituted as described earlier in this chapter. The reason for both changes was that the items were sufficiently heterogeneous to warrant individual consideration. The summary index, as originally constituted, contained too many diverse items. Further, the original proposal called for three overall measures of hostility; two of these, the summary index and the rater's global hostility rating, were retained. A third, an overall self-rating of hostility, was dropped prior to the beginning of the study.

Table 8-8
Hostility Variables

Expressed Hostility				
Period of Event	M	F	M + F	Total
Last two weeks	0	1	3	4
Since separation discussion	1	3	5	9
Ever	2	2	3	7
Total	3	6	11	20
Respondent-Experienced Hostility				
Last two weeks	0	2	3	5
Since separation discussion	0	3	3	6
Ever	2	3	4	9
Total	2	8	10	20

the numbers were sufficient, correlations were obtained separately for men and women and for the group as a whole. Altogether, 20 hostility variables were related to 8 mental health measures, each in regard to respondent-expressed and respondent-experienced hostility. The breakdown is shown in Table 8-8.

In addition the group as a whole and men and women separately were analyzed in regard to two overall measures of hostility, both of which related to the last two weeks.

The answer to whether a particular behavior occurred was coded as "1" for "yes" and "2" for "no". A negative correlation, then, meant that increased hostility was associated with more disturbance, and a positive correlation indicated the reverse. Overall measures of hostility were scored "1" to "5" in increasing order of hostility; thus positive correlations indicate that greater hostility is associated with more disturbance. (The word "spouse" means present or former spouse throughout the discussion.)

EVERYDAY VERBAL HOSTILITY

This includes (1) putting the spouse down with words, (2) making the spouse feel wrong, and (3) teasing. The following relationships between expressed everyday verbal hostility and mental health measures were studied in the time periods and for the groups noted:

- Verbally putting down the spouse in the last two weeks: all of Sub 2 and women in Sub 2
- Making the spouse feel wrong in the last two weeks: all of Sub 2
- Making the spouse feel wrong since the separation discussion: all of Sub 2 and women in Sub 2
- Teasing the spouse since the separation discussion: all of Sub 2.

There were insufficient numbers for the remaining analyses for the reasons already stated. The results are shown in Table 8-9.

The data show a trend in women in the direction of better functioning associated with putting down the spouse verbally in the last two weeks. There is a significant relationship in this direction regarding social functioning. There were no significant associations in relation to making the spouse feel wrong in the two weeks before interview. In the period since the separation discussion, those that had said they made the spouse feel wrong showed significantly greater somatic discomfort, depression, and psychiatric disturbance (BPRS) than those who did not, both in the group as a whole and in women within that group. Teasing the spouse since the separation discussion is associated with increased somatic discomfort and depression.

These findings tell us that those who expressed verbal hostility showed increased somatic disturbance and depression on a number of mental health measures and increased psychiatric disturbance on one. The findings also suggest, however, that in some cases the opposite relationship may exist: expressed everyday hostility may be associated with better functioning. There is one statistically significant association of this kind: social functioning with verbal putdown of the spouse in women. The other associations, two of which involve measures of suicide potential, would have been significant had the relationship been predicted and a one-tailed test used. Caution is indicated in the interpretation, since only 3 of 21 correlations approach significance. The issue is worth further study, particularly since an association of decreased suicide potential with increased open expression of hostility as opposed to inwardly directed expression of hostility would theoretically be expected.

The following relationships between experienced everyday verbal hostility and mental health measures were studied in the time periods and for the groups noted:

- Being verbally put down by the spouse in the last two weeks; all of Sub 2 and women in Sub 2
- Being made to feel wrong in the last two weeks: all of Sub 2

Table 8-9
Relationship Between Expressed Everyday Verbal Hostility to Spouse and Mental Health Measures (Sub 2)[a]

| Mental Health Measure | Verbal Putdown In Last Two Weeks | | Making Spouse Feel Wrong | | | Teasing Spouse Since Separation Discussion (N=38) |
| | | | | Since Separation Discussion | | |
	F (N = 45)	All (N = 64)	Last Two Weeks (N = 32)	F (N = 34)	All (N = 47)	
SOMA	−.071	−.193	−.130	−.315c	−.253c	−.334c
ANX	.028	−.082	−.080	−.170	−.184	−.206
DEP	−.089	−.110	−.147	−.346c	−.319b	−.277c
SOC	.285c	.171	.162	−.124	−.112	−.037
BPRS	.223	.097	−.009	−.308c	−.309c	−.062
SPC 1	.230	.188	−.015	.301	.223	.098
SPC 2	.243	.140	−.019	.095	−.063	.091
ASP	.272	.195	−.030	.222	.157	.134

For explanation of mental health measures see Appendix 5-A.
[a]Measured by Kendall's tau, two-tailed analysis. Negative correlation indicates that hostility is associated with more disturbance.
[b]$p \leq .01$
[c]$p \leq .05$

Table 8-10

Relationship Between Experienced Everyday Verbal Hostility from Spouse and Mental Health Measures (Sub 2)[a]

Mental Health Measure	Experiencing Verbal Putdown Last Two Weeks		Being Made to Feel Wrong			Being Teased by Spouse Since Separation Discussion	
			Last Two Weeks	Since Separation Discussion			
	F (N = 44)	All (N = 63)	(N = 38)	F (N = 49)	All (N = 66)	F (N = 37)	All (N = 49)
SOMA	−.130	−.137	−.100	−.231[b]	−.047	−.268[b]	−.114
ANX	−.130	−.161	−.155	−.155	−.024	−.133	−.099
DEP	−.257[b]	−.233[b]	−.204	−.161	−.024	−.230	−.197
SOC	0.0	.007	.070	.077	.172[b]	−.088	−.050
BPRS	.035	.015	−.023	−.288[b]	−.052	−.273[b]	−.164
SPC 1	−.078	−.080	−.089	.032	.138	−.003	.052
SPC 2	−.186	−.220[b]	−.058	−.044	.020	.037	.099
ASP	−.214	−.266[b]	−.075	.093	.209[b]	−.087	−.016

For explanation of mental health measures see Appendix 5-A.

[a]Measured by Kendall's tau, one-tailed analysis. Negative correlation indicates that hostility is associated with more disturbance.

[b]$p \leq .05$

- Being made to feel wrong since the separation discussions: all of Sub 2 and women in Sub 2
- Being teased since the separation discussion: all of Sub 2 and women in Sub 2

The results are shown in Table 8-10.

Seeing oneself as a target of the spouse's everyday verbal hostility affects several of the respondents' mental health measures. Depression was significantly associated with experienced verbal "putdown" in the last two weeks for women and for the group as a whole. Somatic discomfort was significantly associated in women with being made to feel wrong and being teased since the separation discussion. Psychiatric functioning, as measured by the BPRS, was significantly associated in women with being made to feel wrong and being teased since the separation discussion. Perhaps most importantly, two of three suicidal measures were significantly associated with expressed verbal "putdown" in the last two weeks in women. Two findings are in the opposite direction. For the group as a whole, being made to feel wrong since the separation discussion is associated with better social functioning and less rater-rated suicide potential.

Though the three measures of verbal putdown were originally grouped together, it now appears as if there is a qualitative difference between experiencing verbal putdown, and being made to feel wrong and being teased. While all of these experiences tend to increase depression, experiencing verbal "putdowns" seems to increase suicidal potential. Being made to feel wrong does not, and indeed may have the opposite effect. Defining the spouse as actively hostile (i.e., making one feel wrong) involves fighting back and thus may lessen suicide potential. Overall, experiencing everyday verbal hostility is associated with depression and, in some instances, increased suicidal ideation, somatic discomfort, and increased psychiatric disturbance.

EXPRESSING DIVORCE-RELATED HOSTILITY

This includes turning the children against the spouse and using financial and custody matters against the spouse. Analysis of the relationship of mental health variables to turning the children against the spouse was not possible.* Analysis of using financial or custody matters against the spouse was carried out for the last two weeks and for

---

*Only the group that ever had the opportunity to do so ($N = 58$) would have been large enough for analysis, but the distribution was so lopsided (6 said they did and 52 said they did not) that Kendall correlation analysis would not have been meaningful.

Table 8-11

Relationship Between Expressed Divorce-Related Hostility to Spouse and Mental Health Measures (Sub 2)[a]

Mental Health Measure	Last Two Weeks ($N = 33$)	Using Financial and Custody Matters Against Spouse		
		Since Separation Discussion		
		M ($N = 32$)	F ($N = 70$)	Total ($N = 102$)
SOMA	−.189	−.262	−.222[c]	−.222[b]
ANX	−.162	−.209	−.189	−.192[c]
DEP	−.193	−.079	−.217[c]	−.184[c]
SOC	−.061	.152	−.121	−.054
BPRS	.036	−.182	−.245[c]	−.219[b]
SPC 1	.120	−.150	−.090	−.097
SPC 2	.130	−.132	−.077	−.087
ASP	.312	.011	.040	.033

For explanation of mental health measures see Appendix 5-A.

[a]Measured by Kendall's tau, two-tailed analysis. Negative correlation indicates that increased hostility is associated with more disturbance.

[b]$p \leq .01$

[c]$p \leq .05$

the period since the separation discussion. Results are shown in Table 8-11. That there is no significant association in the past two weeks may be due to the small number of subjects. Having used financial and custody matters against the spouse in the period since the separation discussion was significantly associated with greater somatic discomfort, anxiety, depression, and psychiatric disturbance for the group as a whole and for women. For women, however, the relationship with anxiety only approaches significance. For men, only the association with greater somatic discomfort approaches significance. The magnitude of the correlations suggests that with greater numbers some of the other indicators might also reflect a similar relationship in men.

Divorce-related hostility directed by spouse to respondent includes the respondent turning the children against the spouse and the spouse using financial and custody matters against the respondent. Correlation analysis was carried out in regard to the former for the group as a whole, and for females regarding whether or not respondents had ever had this experience. No later period was suitable for analysis on this variable. The most recent period suitable for correlation analysis of experiencing financial and custody matters used

Table 8-12

Relationship Between Experienced Divorce-Related Hostility from Spouse and Mental Health Measures (Sub 2)[a]

Mental Health Measure	Spouse Ever Turning Children Against Respondent		Spouse Using Financial/Custody Matters Against Respondent in Last Two Weeks	
	F $(N = 39)$	All $(N = 61)$	F $(N = 35)$	All $(N = 50)$
SOMA	−.282[b]	−.068	−.192	−.081
ANX	−.231[b]	−.002	−.065	−.090
DEP	−.084	−.035	−.272[b]	−.217[b]
SOC	−.028	.091	.068	.116
BPRS	−.215	−.005	.037	.111
SPC 1	−.007	.131	.067	.104
SPC 2	−.131	.047	.070	.075
ASP	.074	.165	.296[b]	.283[b]

For explanation of mental health measures see Appendix 5-A.

[a]Measured by Kendall's tau, one-tailed analysis of significance. Negative correlation indicates increased hostility is associated with more disturbance.

[b]$p \leqslant .05$

against the respondent was the last two weeks for the entire group and the women in it. The results are shown in Table 8-12.

Experiencing the spouse, at some time, as having turned the children against the respondent does not appear to have been a traumatic experience for the group as a whole but was associated in women with increased somatic discomfort and anxiety.

Experiencing the spouse as using financial and custody matters against the respondent was associated with depression. Here, however, also rater-rated suicide potential was less when the respondent reported spouse use of financial and custody matters in adversary fashion. Conceivably recognizing that the spouse was using financial and custody matters against the respondent might be associated with fighting back and therefore with less suicide potential.

DEATH-RELATED HOSTILITY

This includes telling the spouse to drop dead, wishing (whether expressed or not) that the spouse were dead, telling the spouse that he or she wished them dead, and encouraging suicide of the spouse. In regard to the last item, there were not enough respondents in this study to indicate that this occurred with enough frequency to warrant analysis of its relationship to mental health variables.

Only a limited number of analyses of expressions of death-related hostility toward the spouse were possible because for most time periods, either an insufficient number of persons could be asked the question or the distribution was skewed because very few acknowledged the behavior. Analyses were carried out relating mental health measures to telling the spouse to drop dead since the separation discussion, and if this ever occurred; wishing the spouse dead (whether expressed or not) in relation to whether this ever occurred and by males and females; and saying that one wished the spouse dead in relation to whether this ever occurred. The results are shown in Table 8-13. Significant associations are found with somatic discomfort, anxiety, depression, and increased psychiatric disturbance if one ever told the spouse one wanted him or her dead. The distribution, however, was so skewed (only 13 of 102 persons answered "yes") that the results need to be viewed with caution. The only other significant association is that of greater somatic discomfort with ever having told the spouse to drop dead. Overall, the results are inconclusive but suggest that there are probably some associations of expressing one's own death-related hostility with one's subjective discomfort, especially somatic disturbance and depression.

In regard to experiencing death-related hostility from the spouse, only the question of whether this *ever* occurred was analyzed, as there were not enough respondents who experienced death-related hostility since the separation discussion or in the last two weeks. Thus, the element of recency that probably would have given increased correlations is missing. Analysis by males and females was possible for two of the three variables, since the distribution was too skewed for the third. The results are found in Table 8-14.

Experiencing the spouse as expressing death-related hostility is clearly associated with impairment of mental health in a number of instances. The strongest associations were found for females, who showed significant associations of impairment with the experience of seeing the spouse as wishing them dead on seven of eight measures, including all three suicidal indicators. There were some, but fewer, significant relationships regarding being told to drop dead and the spouse's verbally wishing the respondent dead. Regarding the latter, caution is indicated because of the highly skewed distribution (15 yes; 86 no). In general, the findings tend to support the expectation that respondents, to some extent, see their own worth and right to live through the eyes of estranged and former spouses.

Table 8-13
Relationship Between Expressing Death-Related Hostility to Spouse and Mental Health Measures (Sub 2)[a]

Mental Health Measure	Since Separation Discussion (All, N = 32)	Telling Spouse to Drop Dead			Ever Wished Spouse Dead			Ever Said Wished Spouse Dead (All, N = 102)
		Ever						
		M (N = 32)	F (N = 70)	All (N = 102)	M (N = 32)	F (N = 69)	All (N = 101)	
SOMA	-.169	-.119	-.101	-.163[c]	.175	-.148	-.129	-.236[b]
ANX	-.018	-.131	.015	-.050	-.098	-.125	-.135	-.200[c]
DEP	-.081	-.253	-.034	-.102	-.067	-.132	-.125	-.213[b]
SOC	-.034	.012	-.017	-.029	-.175	-.011	-.053	-.110
BPRS	-.091	-.176	-.059	-.075	-.035	-.106	-.051	-.208[c]
SPC 1	.121	-.006	-.006	-.026	.030	.016	-.003	-.108
SPC 2	.065	-.050	-.006	-.031	-.064	-.013	-.038	-.016
ASP	.130	-.065	.054	.011	-.065	.169	.097	.038

For explanation of mental health measures see Appendix 5-A.

[a]Measured by Kendall's tau, two-tailed analysis of significance. Negative correlation indicates that increased hostility is associated with more disturbance.

[b]$p \leq .01$

[c]$p \leq .05$

Table 8-14

Relationship Between Ever Experiencing Death-Related Hostility from Spouse and Mental Health Mesures (Sub 2)[a]

Mental Health Measure	Spouse Telling Respondent to Drop Dead			Spouse Seriously Wishing Respondent Dead			Spouse Saying Wished Respondent Dead (N = 101)
	M (N = 32)	F (N = 70)	Total (N = 102)	M (N = 32)	F (N = 70)	Total (N = 102)	
SOMA	.090	−.228c	−.145c	−.063	−.188c	−.164c	−.029
ANX	.099	−.143	−.075	−.191	−.296b	−.262b	−.110
DEP	.034	−.175c	−.120	−.014	−.228c	−.169c	−.006
SOC	.116	−.030	.009	−.157	−.054	−.099	−.054
BPRS	−.043	−.087	.063	−.313c	−.190c	−.222b	−.090
SPC 1	.164	−.044	.015	.113	−.230c	−.131	−.097
SPC 2	.101	−.131	−.069	.220	−.240c	−.116	−.184c
ASP	.091	.010	.031	.223	−.264c	−.135	−.121

For explanation of mental health measures see Appendix 5-A.

[a]Measured by Kendall's tau, two-tailed analysis of significance. A negative correlation indicates that hostility is associated with more disturbance.

[b]$p \leq .01$

[c]$p \leq .05$

PHYSICAL HOSTILITY

This involves only two questions; "Did you physically attack your spouse?" and "Did your spouse physically attack you?" In both cases there were sufficient numbers of whom this question could be asked since the separation discussion to permit analysis for the recently separated/divorced as a whole and for women within that group. There was an insufficient number of men to permit a separate analysis. The relationship of respondents' mental health to their acknowledged physical attack on the spouse and to reported physical attack by the spouse on the respondent is found in Table 8-15.

Respondents who reported physical attacks on the spouse since the separation discussion did not show significant associations with mental health measures. The correlations, however, suggest that if the numbers were larger and an effect predicted, significant associations might appear regarding discomfort variables and perhaps one suicidal variable. There are significant associations of spouse attacks on re-

Table 8-15

Relationship Between Expression of Physical Hostility Since Separation Discussion and Mental Health Measures (Sub 2)[a]

Mental Health Measure	Attack by Respondent on Spouse		Attack by Spouse on Respondent	
	F (N = 33)	Total (N = 44)	F (N = 46)	Total (N = 57)
SOMA	−.224	−.216	−.234[b]	−.187[b]
ANX	−.159	−.088	−.254[b]	−.182
DEP	−.188	−.073	−.162	−.141
SOC	−.034	−.039	.062	.064
BPRS	.006	.034	−.141	−.016
SPC 1	−.120	−.219	−.062	−.096
SPC 2	−.057	−.084	−.083	−.102
ASP	.133	.021	−.057	−.076

For explanation of mental health measures see Appendix 5-A.

[a]Measured by Kendall's tau, two-tailed analysis of significance in regard to attack by respondent on spouse, one-tailed analysis of significance in regard to attack by spouse on respondent. A negative correlation indicates that increased hostility is associated with more disturbance.

[b]$p \leq .05$

Table 8-16

Relationship Between Overall Measures of Hostility of Respondent to Spouse in the Last Two Weeks and Mental Health Measures (Sub 2)[a]

Mental Health Measure	Summary Index of Verbal Hostility			Rater-Rated Hostility		
	M (N = 26)	F (N = 52)	Total (N = 78)	M (N = 25)	F (N = 54)	Total (N = 79)
SOMA	.036	.218[b]	.198[b]	.189	.207[b]	.220[b]
ANX	.103	.104	.137	.170	.065	.119
DEP	−.018	.211	.152	.111	.231[b]	.198[b]
SOC	−.031	−.247[b]	−.163	.036	−.100	−.043
BPRS	.027	−.142	−.086	.167	−.023	.036
SPC 1	−.190	−.208	−.191	−.086	−.142	−.112
SPC 2	.029	−.187	−.124	.119	−.163	−.073
ASP	−.112	−.195	−.170	.067	−.159	−.100

For explanation of mental health measures see Appendix 5-A.

[a] Measured by Kendall's tau, two-tailed analysis of significance. A negative correlation indicates that hostility is associated with more disturbance.

[b] $p \leq .05$

194

spondent, with somatic discomfort for the group as a whole and with somatic discomfort and anxiety for women.

OVERALL MEASURES OF HOSTILITY

These include the summary index of hostility (which includes the three everyday verbal hostility items and two verbal death-related items) and the overall assessment of the clinical raters of respondent and reported spouse hostility. Both pertain to the last two weeks before interview. The association of respondent hostility to spouse on mental health measures in relation to these two overall measures of hostility are shown in Table 8-16. Positive correlations indicate that greater hostility is associated with greater discomfort.

The relationships of the overall measures of respondent-expressed hostility to respondents' mental health are similar to those found regarding some of the individual items. Somatic discomfort and depression are associated with greater overall hostility by the respondent.

We next turn to the relation of spouses' reported overall hostility to the respondents' mental health (Table 8-17). Here again, positive correlations indicate that spouse hostility is associated with greater respondent disturbance. Depression is significantly associated with greater overall spouse hostility and somatic discomfort. Anxiety is significantly associated with the summary index.

OVERVIEW OF RESULTS

The wealth of data presented calls for an overview which allows us to look at the major trends. As seen in Table 8-18, significant associations of greater disturbance with greater self-reported hostility were found in 25 to 35 percent of the analyses relating to somatic discomfort, depression, and BPRS. There were two significant associations in the same direction with anxiety. Altogether, 20 out of 160 correlations, or 12.5 percent, showed a significant relationship between self-expressed hostility and greater disturbance; one correlation (SOC) was in the opposite direction. Near-significant associations ($p < .10$) are not included in the tabulation. Some suicidal variables were near significantly associated in the direction of less suicide potential with more self-expressed hostility.

Within the four hostility categories, findings were concentrated in the first two: 16.7 percent of the correlations regarding everyday verbal hostility were significant in the direction of association of hostility with dysfunction, as were 19.4 percent of divorce-related hostility, compared to only 7.8 percent of death-related hostility, and none in regard to physical expression of hostility.

Table 8-17
Relationship Between Overall Measures of Hostility of Spouse to Respondent in the Last Two Weeks and Mental Health Measures (Sub 2)[a]

Mental Health Measure	Summary Index of Hostility From Spouse			Rater-Rated Hostility From Spouse		
	M (N = 26)	F (N = 54)	Total (N = 80)	M (N = 26)	F (N = 55)	Total (N = 81)
SOMA	.019	.209[c]	.169[c]	−.032	.141	.102
ANX	.126	.145	.154[c]	.0	.064	.065
DEP	.063	.305[b]	.235[b]	.032	.275[b]	.195[c]
SOC	−.156	−.058	−.083	−.211	−.005	−.065
BPRS	−.054	.053	.002	−.021	.046	.028
SPC 1	−.201	.044	−.024	−.174	−.003	−.050
SPC 2	−.026	.068	.041	.112	.005	.036
ASP	−.137	.040	−.012	−.078	.056	.017

For explanation of mental health measures see Appendix 5-A.
[a]Measured by Kendall's tau, one-tailed analysis of significance. A negative correlation indicates that hostility is associated with more disturbance.
[b]$p \leq .01$
[c]$p \leq .05$

Table 8-18

Significance of Correlations of Respondent Hostility to Mental Health Measures (Sub 2)[a]

Mental Health Measure	Significant Association of Hostility with More Disturbance	Significant Association of Hostility with Less Disturbance	No Significant Association	Total
SOMA	7	0	13	20
ANX	2	0	18	20
DEP	6	0	14	20
SOC	0	1	19	20
BPRS	5	0	15	20
SPC 1	0	0	20	20
SPC 2	0	0	20	20
ASP	0	0	20	20
Total	20	1	139	160

For explanation of mental health measures see Appendix 5-A.
[a]Measured by Kendall's tau, two-tailed analysis of significance.

The significant correlations regarding hostility experienced as coming from the spouse, are summarized in Table 8-19. The overall pattern of experienced hostility is similar to that of expressed hostility, with some differences. Significant associations of greater experienced hostility with more disturbance are again found most frequently in relation to somatic discomfort, depression, and the BPRS, ranging from 25 to 45 percent. There were four (20 percent) significant associations with anxiety in the same direction. One correlation of social dysfunction and three involving suicidal variables, however, were significant in the direction of greater experienced hostility being associated with less disturbance. Altogether, 31 of 160 correlations (19.4 percent) showed a significant relationship between experienced hostility and greater disturbance, while 4 of 160 (2.5 percent) suggested the opposite.

The largest percentage of associations with greater disturbance is in regard to death-related hostility, where 28.6 percent of the items were so related. In comparison, 14.3 percent of everyday verbal hostility variables, 12.5 percent of divorce-related hostilities, and 18.8 percent of physical hostility variables were so associated.

Table 8-19

Significance of Correlations of Experienced Spouse Hostility to Mental Health Measures (Sub 2)[a]

Mental Health Measure	Significant Association of Hostility with More Disturbance	Significant Association of Hostility with Less Disturbance	No Significant Association	Total
SOMA	9	0	11	20
ANX	4	0	16	20
DEP	7	0	13	20
SOC	0	1	19	20
BPRS	5	0	15	20
SPC 1	1	0	19	20
SPC 2	3	0	17	20
ASP	2	3	15	20
Total	31	4	125	160

For explanation of mental health measures see Appendix 5-A.
[a]Measured by Kendall's tau, one-tailed analysis of significance.

There may be a complex relationship of perceived hostility to suicide potential. Two variables relating to spouse hostility (being made to feel wrong and spouse using financial and custody matters against the respondent) are associated with *less* suicide potential. On the other hand, *increased* suicide potential is associated with experienced verbal "putdown" and two death-related variables. This suggests that some actions, such as being made to feel wrong or believing that financial or custody matters are used against oneself may be perceived as actions against which one can fight back and thus not direct hostility inward. Others, such as verbal "putdown" and death-related hostility, cannot be responded to as readily with outward aggression and may increase suicide potential.

DISCUSSION

It is clear that reported expressions of hostility toward the spouse and hostility experienced as coming from the spouse are associated with some measures of impaired mental health, particularly depression. Statements about one's own or another's hostility are not objective measures. Techniques such as content analysis of speech samples, for example, might more accurately assess hostility. The present study measured the respondents' perceptions. Self-reports of hostility may be determined by a number of factors including the degree to which the respondent has insight into such hostile behavior and feels guilty about it. Conversely, reports of spouse hostility may reflect the true state of affairs, or may project the respondents' own hostility on the spouse. Perhaps the reason why depression is so frequently associated with expressed as well as experienced hostility is that hostility is more likely to be acknowledged when one feels guilty about it and turns some inward as well as outward.

The major difference in the patterns of impact on mental health between reported expressed and experienced hostility is regarding death-related hostility. Here, experienced hostility is more likely to result in disturbance than expression. This finding may mean that respondents find themselves more powerless to cope with their spouses' death-related hostility than with other forms of hostility against which they may feel more able to fight, such as spouses' hostile use of financial or custody matters. Conversely, expression of death wishes may be accompanied by feelings of power. It is also possible that those less guilty about death wishes will more readily acknowledge them.

This study includes both those who are still strongly attached to each other and those who are not. Future studies should compare former spouses who are attached to each other with those who are not, and examine whether hostility differs between these groups in regard to degree or kind. Future studies should also use more objective measures, such as observation or content analysis of speech, and relate the hostility determined in this manner to measures of mental health.

SUMMARY

This chapter has reviewed aspects of self-reported hostility as expressed to the spouse, and as experienced as coming from the spouse. Hostility has been divided into four specific subtypes: everyday verbal hostility, divorce-related hostility, death-related hostility, and physical hostility. Two summary measures of hostility were also used. Hostility is ubiquitous among separating and divorcing couples and occurs both before the first serious discussion of separation and after that event. While some aspects of hostility decrease after the separation discussion, others, particularly those that are divorce-related, increase.

Some of the more serious types of hostility, particularly the death-related kind, are more frequent after the separation discussion. There is a tapering off of hostility over time; however, some of the most serious types of hostility persist in a significant minority of individuals who remain in contact. For example, among individuals who have reported experiencing physical attack by the spouse since the separation discussion, and who were in contact in the two weeks prior to the first research interview, 30 percent had also experienced such attack in the last two weeks. Twelve percent of the respondents said the spouse tried to kill them at one time.

When the relationship of hostility expressed to the spouse and experienced as coming from the spouse was related to mental health measures, the results showed that some forms of reported hostility towards the spouse were associated with greater somatic discomfort, depression, and a higher score on the BPRS, but not with social dysfunction or suicide potential. Association with suicide potential may be in the opposite direction. The findings regarding perceived spouse hostility support the hypothesis that greater hostility is associated with increased impairment in the areas of somatic discomfort, depression, and to some extent other mental health measures. Perceived spouse hostility, particularly when it is death-related, may increase suicide potential.

REFERENCES

1. Fisher EO: Divorce: The New Freedom. New York, Harper and Row, 1974
2. Goode WJ: After Divorce. Glencoe, Ill, The Free Press, 1956
3. Hunt M, Hunt B: The Divorce Experience. New York, McGraw-Hill, 1977
4. Weiss RS: Marital Separation. New York, Basic Books, 1975
5. Hetherington EM, Cox M, Cox R: The aftermath of divorce. Read at the 54th annual meeting of the American Orthopsychiatric Association, New York, 1977
6. Simon W, Lumry G: Suicide of the spouse as a divorce substitute. Dis Nerv Syst 31:609–612, 1970
7. Brown G, Birley J, Wing J: Influence of family life on the course of schizophrenic disorders: A replication. Br J Psychiatry 121:241–258, 1972
8. Vaughn E, Leff J: The influence of family and social factors on the course of psychiatric illness. Br J Psychiatry 129:125–137, 1976

9. Bowlby J; Making and breaking of affectional bonds: I. Aetiology and psychopathology in the light of attachment theory. Br J Psychiatry 130:201–210, 1977

10. Parkes CM: Psycho-social transitions: A field for study. Soc Sci Med 5:101–115, 1971

11. Pollock GJ: Mourning and adaptation. Int J Psychoanal 42:341–361, 1961

9

Subjective Responses to Separation and Divorce: Feelings Toward the Spouse and Aspects of the Grief Process

This chapter deals with feelings towards the spouse, such as being in love with, missing, or resenting the spouse. It also addresses aspects of the grief process, which include sadness, anger, guilt, and memories and fantasies regarding the spouse. These variables differ qualitatively from those discussed in previous chapters: they are further removed from direct observation. The three types of variables that have been addressed, in order of being increasingly removed from direct observation, are:

1. Directly observable phenomena, such as number of contacts between the spouses.
2. Phenomena involving both events and their interpretation, such as relying on the spouse for being loved. This variable describes the respondent's perception of one aspect of his or her relationship to the spouse.
3. Respondent's feelings and fantasies, which may or may not be overtly expressed or manifested in behavior, such as thinking about the spouse.

The variables dealt with in this chapter belong to the third group. From a research standpoint, they are "softer" than those in other groups; from a clinical perspective they are important.

FEELINGS TOWARD THE SPOUSE

Other Studies

The categories used to characterize feelings toward the spouse are similar to those used by Goode: still in love with spouse; not in love but misses spouse very much; friendly but does not miss spouse very much; just as happy not to see spouse; actually dislikes spouse.[1] Goode asked the relevant questions both regarding the spouse's attitude to the respondent, as seen by the respondent, and regarding the respondent's feelings toward the spouse. Goode's groupings were slightly altered, and his respondents were required to make a forced choice between categories.

Goode reported his findings for both women who had not remarried ($N = 303$) and for all women ($N = 425$) in his samples. His findings suggest that remarried women tend to hold a more negative view of the ex-husband than women who have not remarried. He found that women with negative and positive attitudes had stronger affect towards their husbands[1] and that the attitude attributed to the husband and the attitude of the respondent were mirror images of each other. The association diminishes over time but remains significant.[1] Goode also found that negative feelings for the group as a whole were greater after two or more years after the separation than they were prior to that time. Negative feelings increased over time in individuals with high contact but not in those with low contact. Time did not affect the positives. With low contact, however, positive responses decreased but negatives did not increase.

Goode felt that trauma was greatest for women who had the most positive feelings towards the former husband. The high-trauma respondents included 51 percent of those with positive feelings, 44 percent of those with negative feelings, and only 36 percent of those who reported indifference.[1] Twenty percent of the high-trauma cases were willing to "wipe out" the divorce, as against 5 percent of the low-trauma respondents.

Weiss stated that the post-marital relationship tends to display a mixture of feelings, with positive and negative feelings either alternating or being present simultaneously.[2] Sometimes, he believed, former spouses "can almost choose whether to express anger or affection."[2] Weiss stated that continuing ambivalence is likely to defeat any attempt at complete resolution.[2]

Love, as Hunt and Hunt saw it, consists of "unbidden tormenting visions of tender moments . . . . " Some never expressed these feelings openly to the spouse, although they fantasized about doing so, but others expressed such feelings directly to the former spouse. Hunt and Hunt, by implication, considered such "leftover love" as maladaptive and referred to it as an "affliction" of the formerly married.[3] For the great majority, "leftover love and leftover desire wane quickly during the early months of separation," partly because of the anger and grieving and because the former partners establish new contacts.[3]

Hunt and Hunt distinguished between an "unfinal divorce" and a "final divorce", the latter occurring after about three to five years, when most ex-spouses reach the stage when they feel indifferent or mildly friendly towards each other.[3] Until that occurs, "loving feelings are a kind of captivity, but some divorced people fail to see that."[3] Some people are unable to tolerate demands and intensity of marriage and can enact a "charade of love-and-family life . . . at a safe distance."[3] These people may not progress to the "final divorce."

Present Study

The following questions were asked of each respondent: Are you in love with your (former) spouse? Do you/would you miss him/her? Do you feel friendly towards him/her? Are you just as happy not to be with him/her? Do you actually dislike him/her? Unlike Goode's study, this study asked separate questions, so that many possible combinations of replies were possible.

The answers to the question, "Are you in love with your (former) spouse?" and the relationship of the answers to marital dissolution status are shown in Table 9-1. Clearly, the number of respondents stating that they were in love with their present or former spouse diminished over time. Nearly two-thirds said so among those discussing separation. But only one fifth still felt this way one year after the last separa-

Table 9-1
Response to Question, "Are You in Love with Your (Former) Spouse?"

		Sub 2				
Response	Sub 1	Separated within Previous 13 mo	Filed within Previous 13 mo	Divorced within Previous 13 mo	Sub 3	Total
Yes	39	25	8	8	14	94
Don't know	3	6	1	2	1	13
No	20	13	19	20	54	126
Total	62	44	28	30	69	233

Table 9-2
Response to Question, "Do You/Would You Miss Your (Former) Spouse?"

		Sub 2				
Response	Sub 1	Separated within Previous 13 mo	Filed within Previous 13 mo	Divorced within Previous 13 mo	Sub 3	Total
Yes	55	35	15	14	24	143
Don't know	3	0	0	0	0	3
No	4	9	13	16	45	87
Total	62	44	28	30	69	233

tion event. The differences are highly significant ($X^2 = 47.25$, 8 df, $p < .0001$). Further, men as a group were more likely to state that they were in love with their (former) spouse than women were. Over half of the men (53.2 percent, $N = 77$) so stated, as compared to only 34 percent ($N = 156$) of the women ($X^2 = 8.01$, 2 df, $p < .02$). If only the recently separated/divorced are considered, however, there is no significant difference between the sexes.($X^2 = 2.24$, 2 df, $p > .05$). The turning point overall appears to be filing for divorce; until then more persons state that they were in love, but thereafter the majority did not. The sharpest decline occurred at the point of filing (from 56.8 percent to 28.6 percent). Thereafter, there is only a modest further decline to 20.3 percent among those who had the last separation event more than 13 months prior to the first interview. Stated love feelings in our population, if they survive the divorce filing, appear to be tenacious.

The next question posed was whether the respondent did or would miss the spouse. (Table 9-2). Again, the same pattern holds but is more marked; missing the spouse is far more frequent early on ($X^2 = 63.71$, 8 df, $p < .0001$). Almost 90 percent of these still living with their spouses would miss them, versus 67 percent of those who were still in love. There is no statistically significant difference between men and women. The reversal occurred at time of filing but was not dramatic; over a third still acknowledged missing the spouse 14 or more months after the last separation/divorce event.

The answers to the question dealing with whether or not the respondent feels friendly to the spouse in relation to marital dissolution status are shown in Table 9-3.

Here there is much less change over time. In fact, the differences between the marital separation subgroups do not achieve significance ($X^2 = 13.48$, 8 df, $p = .10$). To the extent that there is a trend, there is

Table 9-3

Response to Question, "Do You Feel Friendly Toward Your (Former) Spouse?"

Response	Sub 1	Separated within Previous 13 mo	Filed within Previous 13 mo	Divorced within Previous 13 mo	Sub 3	Total
			Sub 2			
Yes	48	40	20	24	45	177
Don't know	1	0	0	0	0	1
No	13	4	8	6	24	55
Total	62	44	28	30	69	233

a somewhat uneven tendency for friendly feelings to be higher among the recently separated/divorced. When the three components of this group are combined, the percentage of those friendly is 82.3, whereas it is 77.4 percent in those discussing separation/divorce, and 65.2 percent in those whose last separation/divorce event occurred 14 or more months earlier. It is hard to take this finding at face value; perhaps there is a greater denial of unfriendly feelings when the divorce process is at its most active. There is a difference between men and women that just misses statistical significance: more men (83.1 percent, $N = 77$) than women (72.4 percent, $N = 156$) say they are friendly ($X^2 = 5.93$, 2 df, $p = .051$). Perhaps cultural norms lead men to expect that it is appropriate for them to claim friendliness to their former wives. There is,

Table 9-4

Response to Question, "Are You Just as Happy Not to Be With Your (Former) Spouse?"

Response	Sub 1	Separated within Previous 13 mo	Filed within Previous 13 mo	Final within Previous 13 mo	Sub 3	Total
			Sub 2			
Yes	30	27	17	24	61	159
Don't know	8	0	1	0	0	9
No	24	17	10	6	8	65
Total	62	44	28	30	69	233

Table 9-5
Response to Question, "Do You Actually Dislike Your (Former) Spouse?"

Response	Sub 1	Separated within Previous 13 mo	Filed within Previous 13 mo	Divorced within Previous 13 mo	Sub 3	Total
			Sub 2			
Yes	24	13	11	8	19	75
Don't know	0	0	0	0	0	0
No	38	31	17	22	50	158
Total	62	44	28	30	69	233

however, no difference between men and women if only the recently separated/divorced group is considered.

The fourth question asked whether the respondent was just as happy not to be with the spouse (Table 9-4). There is a highly significant difference between categories ($X^2 = 39.76$, 8 df, $p < .0001$). Almost half of those not yet separated would just as soon not be with the spouse; the figure increased to 80 percent after the decree of divorce was final and almost 90 percent when more than one year had elapsed since the last separation event. There is no significant difference between men and women for the group as a whole or for the recently separated/divorced.

The last question was whether the respondent actually disliked the spouse (Table 9-5). The difference over time is not significant ($X^2 = 3.10$, 4 df, $p > .05$, NS). About a third of the respondents stated that they actually disliked the (former) spouse. There are no differences between men and women for either the sample as a whole or for the recently separated/divorced. There is a puzzling finding: more respondents answered affirmatively to the question if they disliked the spouse than answered negatively to whether they felt friendly in all categories except for the long-term separated/divorced. This may in part be due to a technical error* but it is also possible that these responses are a reflection of ambivalence.

Direct comparison of these findings with those of Goode is not

---

*The coding manual was developed to result in the higher score representing more positive feelings. Thus, the first three questions used coding of yes as 3 and no as 1; whereas the latter two called for coding yes as 1 and no as 3. It is possible that this may have resulted in some confusion on the part of the coders.

possible, since in Goode's work there was a forced choice between the options, whereas in my study respondents could and did respond affirmatively to two or more of the questions. We would expect, however, that the two questions about being in love and disliking the spouse could be comparable. In terms of being in love, all divorced individuals combined (the only relevant comparison group to Goode's work) respond affirmatively in 22 percent of the cases, compared to Goode's 13 percent. The difference is probably due to two factors: all of Goode's respondents were women, and more men than women in my study were still in love with the spouse. Further, it is likely, though not certain, that more time had elapsed for Goode's subject on the average since the divorce than was true in this sample. Twenty-seven percent of divorced individuals in this study, compared to 31 percent in Goode's study reported disliking the spouse. Unlike Goode, however, in this study there was no change over time, perhaps because less time had elapsed, on the average, between divorce and date of interview.

Table 9-6

Relationship Between Being in Love with (Former) Spouse and Mental Health Measures[a,b]

Mental Health Measure	Sub 2			Sub 3 (N = 69)
	M (N = 32)	F (N = 70)	All (N = 102)	
SOMA	.138	.239[c]	.181[c]	−.144
ANX	.168	.244[c]	.219[d]	−.194
DEP	.215	.276[d]	.251[d]	−.161
SOC	−.085	.053	.001	.035
BPRS	−.006	.141	.086	.004
SPC 1[e]	—	−.050	.042	−.004
SPC 2[e]	—	−.019	.059	.035
ASP[e]	—	−.100	.005	.095

For explanation of mental health measures see Appendix 5-A.
[a]Measured by Kendall's tau, two-tailed analysis of significance.
[b]No = 1, Don't know = 2, Yes = 3.
[c]$p \leq .05$
[d]$p \leq .01$
[e]There was an insufficient number of suicidal males to warrant computation of correlations.

RELATIONSHIP BETWEEN FEELINGS TOWARDS
THE SPOUSE AND MENTAL HEALTH VARIABLES

The feelings towards the spouse were related to mental health
measures (Tables 9-6 through 9-8). Positive correlations indicate that
being in love results in greater impairment on the mental health measures. For the recently separated/divorced and for women within that
group, all three measures of discomfort (SOMA, ANX, and DEP) are
greater for those who reported still being in love with the spouse. For
men, correlations are in the same direction and might reach significance if there were larger numbers. There is a suggestion that the opposite might be true for the longer term separated/divorced. Had such an
association been predicted, it would have been significant for anxiety
and would have approached significance for the other two. I have no
ready explanation for such a finding, should it be confirmed.

In the recently separated/divorced (Sub 2), five of eight measures
for women indicate that missing the spouse is significantly associated
with more disturbance (Table 9-7). In Sub 2 as a whole, three associa-

Table 9-7
Relationship Between Missing (Former)-Spouse and Mental Health
Measures[a,b]

Mental Health Measure	Sub 2		All ($N = 102$)	Sub 3 ($N = 69$)
	M ($N = 32$)	F ($N = 70$)		
SOMA	.006	.248[c]	.149	.006
ANX	−.055	.272[d]	.177[c]	.027
DEP	.051	.337[d]	.249[d]	.065
SOC	.044	.201[c]	.140	.101
BPRS	−.038	.368[d]	.227[d]	.092
SPC 1[e]	—	.030	.007	.219
SPC 2[e]	—	.186	.123	.207
ASP[e]	—	.104	.069	.273[c]

For explanation of mental health measures see Appendix 5-A.
[a]Measured by Kendall's tau, two-tailed analysis of significance.
[b]No = 1, Don't know = 2, Yes = 3.
[c]$p \leq .05$
[d]$p \leq .01$
[e]There was an insufficient number of suicidal males to warrant computation
of correlations.

tions are significant. For men, however, there are no significant associations. Perhaps, again, men will not acknowledge emotional involvement with an estranged or former spouse. In the longer-term separated and divorced, it is noteworthy that one measure of suicide potential is significantly associated with still missing the spouse and the other two approach significance, whereas there is no such trend in Sub 2. If this finding holds up, then the loss of the spouse may be more meaningful and possibly produce more despair in those longer-term separated/divorced persons who still maintain an attachment. In any event, clinicians need to be aware that the feelings toward a former spouse may be important, even if the last separation/divorce event occurred 14 or more months ago.

Feeling friendly is not associated with any disturbance. There are suggestions that not feeling friendly is so associated. One suicidal measure, SPC 1 (suicide potential at entry) is greater for Sub 2 as a whole (τ = −.281; $p \leq$ .01) if the respondent is unfriendly to the spouse. Except

Table 9-8

Relationship Between Being Just as Happy without Former Spouse and Mental Health Measures[a,b]

Mental Health Measure	Sub 2			Sub 3 ($N = 69$)
	M ($N = 32$)	F ($N = 70$)	All ($N = 102$)	
SOMA	.306[c]	.094	.095	−.067
ANX	.393[c]	.181	.223[d]	.018
DEP	.449[d]	.190	.255[d]	.066
SOC	.065	.129	.108	.080
BPRS	.238	.237[c]	.232[d]	.071
SPC 1[e]	—	−.028	.064	.178
SPC 2[e]	—	.079	.132	.068
ASP[e]	—	.022	.097	.265[c]

For explanation of mental health measures see Appendix 5-A.
[a]Measured by Kendall's tau, two-tailed analysis of significance.
[b]Yes = 1, Don't know = 2, No = 3.
[c]$p \leq$ .05
[d]$p \leq$ .01
[e]There was an insufficient number of suicidal males to warrant calculation of correlations.

for this one finding, feeling or not feeling friendly appears to be relatively neutral and not associated with disturbance.

The next item relates being just as happy not being with the spouse to mental health measures (Table 9-8). Because for this item, Yes was scored as 1, Don't know as 2, and No as 3, a positive correlation means that those who would *not* be as happy not to be with the former spouse are more disturbed. If we simplify by eliminating the double negative, a positive correlation means that the persons who would be happier *being* with the former spouse are more disturbed. Anxiety, depression, and the score on the BPRS are significantly associated with respondents' saying they would be happier if they were to be with the former spouse. These associations either are significant or approximate significance for both men and women. Perhaps men, while they cannot say they miss the former spouse, can acknowledge that they would rather be with her.

The last item relates to actually disliking the spouse. No significant associations were found.

DISCUSSION

In general these findings support Goode's contention that "trauma" (Goode's term) is greatest among those separating or divorcing who have positive feelings toward the former spouse.[1] Somatic discomfort, anxiety, and depression are generally associated with still being in love with or missing the spouse. This association is most marked for women. Similar findings exist regarding the association of preferring to be with the spouse with disturbance indicated by mental health measures, but for this item disturbance is more clearly present for men than for women. It is possible that men can acknowledge wanting to be with the spouse but not missing her.

There are also suggestions that disturbance may be associated with negative feelings towards the spouse, but the associations are less strong. Feeling unfriendly to the spouse is associated with suicide potential at entry for the recently separated/divorced.

In general, those with relatively neutral feelings towards the (former) spouse are least disturbed. These respondents are not in love with nor miss the former spouse and would just as soon not be with him or her but do not actively dislike him or her. In most cases, significant or near-significant associations are present only in regard to the recently separated/divorced. All three suicide measures approach significance, however, regarding still missing the spouse in the longer-term separated/divorced. A study involving larger numbers would be necessary to come to more definite conclusions.

ASPECTS OF THE GRIEF PROCESS

Other Studies

Sadness is universally accepted as part of a grief reaction. Anger has been described by Lindemann, Bowlby, Parkes, and Pollock.[4,5,6,7] Guilt is specifically referred to by Lindemann in relation to the reaction to bereavement.[4] Also, in regard to separation/divorce, Fisher noted a mourning process in divorce which includes, among other feelings, guilt, sadness, and hostility.[8] Bohannon stated that divorce may be more threatening than death to some people because they have perhaps wished it consciously.[9] Weiss wrote that those who left despite the spouse's plea may later be anguished by guilt activated by the spouse.[2]

Preoccupation with the lost person is generally related to "pining and yearning,"[2] analogous to pining, observed in bereavement by Lindemann and by Glick and Parkes.[4,10,11]

Recently, two attempts have been made to define the concept of attachment in measurable terms and to relate the result to distress and to other variables. Brown et al.[12] developed an index composed of three dichotomous variables including (1) "I feel free and relieved like a weight has been lifted off my shoulders" or "I feel empty inside like an important part of me is missing;" (2) "I've put the past behind me and I'm looking forward towards the future," or "The past is always on my mind,— I keep going over what happened in my marriage;" (3) "I feel like a person changing for the better all the time," or "I'm in a rut, my life isn't going anywhere." The index also included a 5-point scale indicating whether the respondent missed the spouse. A fifth item rated the affect towards the spouse as strong or mild, regardless of whether affect was positive or negative. Attachment scores based on these variables were divided into three parts: 47 percent of the respondents were in the lowest category, 31 percent in the middle category, and 22 percent in the highest category.

Distress was measured by 12 items pertaining to how often in the last two weeks respondents had felt blue, tense, worried, hopeless, etc., with responses ranging from "none of the time" to "all of the time." The correlation between attachment and distress was $r = .53$, $p < .001$, $N = 192$.[12] Attachment was found to be greater in males, although the authors qualify this finding by stating that the sample was drawn from a marriage counseling service, which might attract men who are more attached. Attachment was found to be less if more time had elapsed since divorce was considered, if there was more contact with the spouse, and if the respondent would prefer to remain married.

Kitson defined attachment in terms of four factors: wondering what the spouse is doing; spending a lot of time thinking about the spouse; disbelief that the couple is getting a divorce; and a feeling that the person will never get over the divorce.[13] Of the 177 respondents, 15.8 percent showed no attachment, 41.8 percent low attachment, 17.5 percent moderate attachment, and 24.9 percent high attachment. Distress was defined by items identifying depression–anxiety, daily routine leisure-time impairment, thoughts of suicide, and somatic concerns. Attachment and distress were positively correlated, i.e., the more attachment, the more distress ($r = .43$, $p < .001$). Attachment was found not to differ between men and women when zero-order correlations were used but to be greater in men when control for subjective distress was introduced. Attachment was greater for persons who reported a more difficult adjustment to living on one's own, who indicated a larger number of difficult adjustments to separation/divorce, who felt pressured to divorce, who did not feel a combination of relief and guilt, and who had lower self-esteem.

Present Study

The first objective in the present study was to confirm empirically the presence of manifestations of grief in the separated/divorced. The second objective was to try to determine whether these manifestations serve to maintain or give up the tie to the former spouse.

The four variables in the present study are sadness, anger, guilt, and preoccupation through memory and fantasy with the spouse.

ASPECTS OF THE GRIEF PROCESS

The four variables are based on ratings done by the clinician interviewers. In each case, inter-rater reliability will be reported.*

Sadness. All respondents were rated regarding whether sadness was present or absent. It was found to be present in 90.2 percent of the recently separated/divorced ($N = 102$) and in 90 percent of all subjects ($N = 232$). The inter-rater reliability in the matter of presence or ab-

---

*For method of determining inter-rater reliability, see p. 86.

sence of sadness was .93 ($p < .001$). The next question was whether sadness, if present, was related to the separation. The inter-rater reliability on this item was .84 ($p < .001$). Ratings were made regarding five possibilities: definitely; probably; not certain; probably not; and definitely not. The findings in relation to marital separation status are shown in Table 9-9.

Only those actually separated were included in this group. For the recently separated/divorced (Sub 2), more than half of those who indicated sadness were rated as having this sadness associated with the marital separation. The proportion decreases from over nine tenths of the recently separated to about three fifths of the recently divorced. The situation is reversed in the longer-term separated/divorced (Sub 3), only slightly more than one third of whom evidence separation-related sadness.

Lindemann discussed the sadness that accompanies the recall of someone lost by death and the recognition that one will never experience the relationship again.[4] Here, sadness is thought to be reversible and accompanied by fantasies and/or actions designed to reverse the loss through reconciliation. Clinical assessment of this phenomenon is difficult to prove. The two raters were not able to reliably assess this item. The inter-rater reliability was .06, NS. Given this, it is obvious that the results which were obtained must be treated with caution. Nonetheless it is of interest that regarding the recently separated/divorced, the raters believed that almost twice as many respondents' sadness was in the service of maintaining the relationship ($N = 43$) as was in the service of letting go of it ($N = 22$). Fifteen persons were

Table 9-9
Relationship of Sadness to Marital Separation

Question: Is Sadness Related to Separation?	Separated within Previous 13 mo	Filed within Previous 13 mo	Divorced within Previous 13 mo	Sub 3	Total
		Sub 2			
Definitely/ probably	37	17	16	19	89
Not certain	0	0	0	4	4
Probably/ definitely not	3	8	11	39	61
Total	40	25	27	62	154

rated as falling into an "other" category. Among the longer-term separated/divorced, only the 23 respondents whose sadness was definitely or probably related to the separation were rated, and they were virtually evenly divided, 11 rated as sad in the service of maintaining the relationship, 12 in the service of letting go of it. Overall, in spite of the problem that the lack of reliability poses, it appears that clinician raters felt that sadness in marital separation frequently differs from that of bereavement, with finality of the loss being less clearly associated with sadness in the former.

Anger.   The first question dealt with whether anger was present. Among the recently separated/divorced, 68.6 percent ($N = 102$) and 72.4 percent in the sample as a whole ($N = 232$) showed anger. The inter-rater reliability of this item was .86 ($p = .001$). The next question was whether anger was related to separation. Here inter-rater reliability was .83 ($p = .001$). The results are seen in Table 9-10.

Anger in relation to separation appears to be more persistent than sadness. Again, about nine tenths of the recently separated who were angry were so in relation to the separation. The ratio reverses only in the longer-term separated/divorced, but even here over two fifths were angry because of the separation.

The question was asked if anger was in the service of maintaining the relationship or letting go of it. Was the respondent angry about an irreversible loss or angry while trying to maintain the relationship in reality or fantasy? Unfortunately, the problem with reliability also re-

Table 9-10
Relationship of Anger to Marital Separation

Question: Is Anger Related to Separation?	Sub 2				
	Separated within Previous 13 mo	Filed within Previous 13 mo	Divorced within Previous 13 mo	Sub 3	Total
Definitely/ probably	29	12	14	21	76
Uncertain	0	0	0	2	2
Definitely/ probably not	3	6	6	26	41
Total	32	18	20	49	119

Table 9-11
Defense against Feelings of Anger

Question: Does Respondent Defend Against Feelings of Anger?	Sub 2				
	Separated within Previous 13 mo	Filed within Previous 13 mo	Divorced within Previous 13 mo	Sub 3	Total
Greatly/ considerably	9	2	7	9	27
Moderately	10	6	6	3	25
Quite limited or not at all	25	20	17	56	118
Total	44	28	30	68	170

curred ($-.21$, NS) and should be kept in mind. Fifty-six recently separated/divorced persons were rated on this issue.* Of these, 32 persons were rated as being angry in the service of maintaining the relationship, while 24 were seen as having this feeling in the service of letting go. Of Sub 3, 19 were rated regarding this issue: 13 were seen as being angry in the service of maintaining the relationship, 9 to let go of it. The raters appeared to believe that anger in relation to marital separation more commonly served the purpose of maintaining a bond rather than dissolving it.

Raters were also asked to indicate whether, in their view, respondents defended against feelings of anger regarding the separation (Table 9-11). On this question inter-rater reliability was .68 ($p < .001$). This question was asked to determine how frequently anger was apparent to the clinical rater but either not to or denied by the respondent. The concepts of repression or suppression derived from the psychoanalytic framework were used in the formulation of this question.

In this instance, anger was rated as defended against or not regardless of whether it was separation-related. Most respondents are not rated as defending against anger to an important degree. Three of ten respondents did so to a moderate or greater degree.

---

*This is one more than were rated as having anger definitely or probably related to separation. The difference is likely due to coding error.

Table 9-12
Relationship of Guilt to Marital Separation

Question: Is Guilt Related to Separation?	Sub 2			Sub 3	Total
	Separated within Previous 13 mo	Filed within Previous 13 mo	Divorced within Previous 13 mo		
Definitely/ probably	30	14	12	25	81
Uncertain	0	1	0	2	3
Definitely/ probably not	3	9	8	26	46
Total	33	24	20	53	130

Guilt. Raters were asked the same two questions that pertained to sadness and anger. In addition, the raters were asked whether or not guilt was appropriate.

The raters were asked to determine whether guilt was present. On this point inter-rater reliability was .84 ($p = .001$). Guilt was present in 75.5 percent of Sub 2 and in 72.4 percent of the whole sample ($N = 232$). The next question was whether guilt pertained to the separation. Here inter-rater reliability was .78 ($p < .001$). The results are shown in Table 9-12.

There is a decline in guilt over time, but even in the longer-term separated/divorced, the group seen as experiencing guilt is divided about evenly as to whether the guilt was seen as related to the marital separation.

An attempt was made to ascertain if guilt was in the service of maintaining or letting go of the relationship. In this case there was a negative correlation of $-.44$ between the raters. Clearly we did not establish adequate criteria as to conditions under which guilt served to maintain or let go of the relationship. Even so, it is worth noting that in Sub 2, the raters felt that in 43 out of 47 cases in which there was guilt, it was in the service of maintaining the relationship. A similar ratio was seen in Sub 3. The issue was relevant to only 20 of 70. Of these, 17 were seen as using guilt to maintain the relationship and 3 to let go of it.

The raters were also asked to assess the appropriateness of guilt (Table 9-13). It was considered appropriate if, in the opinion of the rater, the respondent's action in the separation hurt others. The raters

Table 9-13
Appropriateness of Guilt

Question: Is Guilt Appropriate?	Separation within Previous 13 mo	Filed within Previous 13 mo	Divorced within Previous 13 mo	Sub 3	Total
Definitely/ probably	29	15	24	44	112
Possibly	2	2	0	1	5
Probably/ definitely not	13	11	6	22	52
Total	44	28	30	67	169

were given considerable leeway in interpreting this variable. The reliability was .50 ($p = .006$).

The raters felt that guilt, which was rated whether or not it was considered connected to the marital separation, was appropriate in a majority of cases in all marital dissolution categories. Overall, two thirds of the observed guilt was felt by the raters to be probably or definitely appropriate. This may be due to the view that a certain amount of guilt over the failure of a marriage is realistic and perhaps inevitable.

Memory and fantasy regarding the spouse. Preoccupation with the image of the lost person is a central feature of the grief process. In this study, this phenomenon was represented by the question to the rater, "How much time does the respondent spend involving memory or fantasy about the spouse?" Answers on a 5-point scale ranged from none of the time to almost all of the time (Table 9-14). The inter-rater reliability on this item was .78 ($p < .001$).

The extent of preoccupation with memory or fantasy regarding the spouse declined with time. Those who spent at least some time in this pursuit amount to about 67 percent of those recently separated, to less than 25 percent of the recently divorced, and little more than 10 percent of the longer-term separated-divorced. Still, nearly half of the last group acknowledged such memories and fantasies at least a little of the time.

Table 9-14

Time Spent in Memory or Fantasy Regarding Spouse by Marital Dissolution Status

| Time Spent | Recently Separated/Divorced (Sub 2) | | | Longer-Term Separated/ Divorced (Sub 3) | Total |
	Separated Within Previous 13 Mo	Filed Within Previous 13 Mo	Divorced Within Previous 13 Mo		
None	8	9	13	36	66
Little	7	10	10	24	53
Some	11	6	5	6	27
Most	15	1	0	1	17
Almost all	3	2	2	1	7
Total	44	28	30	68	170

The question was also raised whether memory and fantasy served to maintain or to let go of the relationship. In this instance the inter-rater reliability was .46 ($p < .01$). This question was asked of the 72 in Sub 2 who spent at least a little time in such memory or fantasy. More than twice as many (46) were rated to use memory or fantasy to maintain the relationship as were rated to use it to let go ($N = 21$). Five were rated as using it for other purposes. In Sub 3, the question was asked of the 32 people who were rated as showing some memory or fantasy. Of these, four times as many (24) used this activity to maintain a relationship as did to let go of it (6). Clearly, in the opinion of the raters, memory or fantasy frequently do not function as Lindemann said they do in bereavement.[4] In the latter, the image of the lost person is invoked with the recognition that the remembered experience will not recur again. Here, the raters saw the phenomenon as more closely related to a wish-fulfillment fantasy, which implies a goal to satisfy the wish in real life. If this is true, the implicit pining and yearning is closer to that for the temporarily, but not necessarily permanently unavailable lover than it is for a spouse lost forever.

Gender analysis. Gender analysis regarding variables involving sadness, guilt, and memory and fantasy involving the spouse were carried out for Sub 2. The only variable in which there were significant gender differences was defense against anger, on which women were more likely to be rated high or low, while men tended to be rated in the intermediate ranges ($X^2 = 12.92$, 4 df, $p = .02$).

Overview.　In the respondent population the following phenomena were observed.

• The grief process, as commonly defined in the literature, is present in a population of separating and divorcing persons. Sadness, anger, guilt, and preoccupation with memory or fantasy of the spouse are present in the large majority of the recently separated and persist in a sizable minority in the longer-term separated/divorced.

• The study raises the possibility that while the phenomenology of grief appears to exist, its purpose in a number of respondents may be to maintain a relationship with the spouse, rather than give it up.

• Some variables that on psychodynamic grounds may be expected to be associated with mental health variables were described including the extent to which there is defense against anger, and the extent to which guilt is appropriate.

Table 9-15

Sadness Related to Separation and Mental Health Measures[a]

Mental Health Measure	Sub 2			Sub 3
	M ($N = 30$)	F ($N = 62$)	All ($N = 92$)	($N = 62$)
SOMA	.174	.118	.119	$-.070$
ANX	.114	.263[b]	.225[c]	$-.140$
DEP	.127	.184	.172[b]	.095
SOC	.051	.214[b]	.152	.067
BPRS	.032	.367[c]	.243[c]	$-.026$
SPC 1[d]	—	.094	.108	.121
SPC 2[d]	—	.290[b]	.286[c]	.268[b]
ASP[d]	—	.184	.215[b]	.234[b]

For explanation of mental health measures see Appendix 5-A.
[a]Measured by Kendall's tau, two-tailed analysis of significance.
[b]$p \leqslant .05$
[c]$p \leqslant .01$
[d]There was an insufficient number of suicidal males to warrant computation of correlations.

RELATION OF ASPECTS OF THE GRIEF PROCESS
TO MENTAL HEALTH MEASURES

The question was raised whether sadness, anger and guilt associated with the separation would be found to be associated with greater respondent disturbance than feelings not so associated. The results are shown in Tables 9-15, 9-16, and 9-17. For anger, sadness, and guilt, some of the mental health measures indicated that when the feeling under consideration was associated with marital separation, increased disturbance was found. The largest number of associations were found regarding sadness. Anxiety and depression, the BPRS, and two suicidal measures were all significantly higher when sadness was related to the separation in Sub 2, and in most cases this was also true for women. The longer-term separated/divorced (Sub 3) showed significant association of two suicide measures with connection of sadness with marital separation.

Anger showed a significant association of connection to marital separation regarding only the discomfort variables (somatic discomfort, anxiety, and depression) and only for Sub 2 as a whole. The association of guilt with marital separation, on the other hand, was related to increased anxiety and depression in the recently separated/divorced as a whole and for women in that group. There were not enough men in

Table 9-16

Anger Related to Separation and Mental Health Measures[a]

| Mental Health Measure | Sub 2 | | | Sub 3 |
	M ($N = 21$)	F ($N = 49$)	All ($N = 70$)	($N = 49$)
SOMA		.222	.311[b]	−.196
ANX		.121	.231[c]	−.232
DEP		.223	.230[c]	−.020
SOC	Insufficient for analysis.	.104	.142	.074
BPRS		.175	.179	−.028
SPC 1		.002	.104	.056
SPC 2		.004	.125	.114
ASP		.040	.138	.178

For explanation of mental health measures see Appendix 5-A.
[a]Measured by Kendall's tau, two-tailed analysis of significance.
[b]$p \leq .01$
[c]$p \leq .05$

Table 9-17

Guilt Related to Separation and Mental Health Measures[a]

Mental Health Measure	Sub 2			Sub 3 (N = 53)
	M (N = 26)	F (N = 51)	All (N = 77)	
SOMA	Insufficient for analysis.	.186	.121	−.023
ANX		.270[b]	.221[b]	−.005
DEP		.318[c]	.276[c]	.166
SOC		.108	.082	.135
BPRS		.335[c]	.161	.054
SPC 1		−.273	.014	.273[b]
SPC 2		.053	.126	.293[b]
ASP		.019	.105	.342[c]

For explanation of mental health measures see Appendix 5-A.
[a]Measured by Kendall's tau, two-tailed analysis of significance.
[b]$p \le .01$
[c]$p \le .05$

the group for an analysis. Guilt was significantly associated with suicide potential on all three measures in Sub 3, yielding one of the more consistent associations with suicide potential found in the study.

Sadness, anger, and guilt are more likely to be associated with discomfort variables, particularly anxiety and depression, if they are related to the marital separation in the recently separated/divorced than if they are not. They may be associated with psychiatric disturbance as measured by the Brief Psychiatric Rating Scale. There is an association with suicide potential in the recently separated/divorced in relation to separation-connected sadness and regarding both sadness and guilt in the longer-term separated divorced. Prolonged sadness and guilt regarding a marital separation seems to be particularly associated with suicidal risk.

Defense against anger. This variable was introduced on the basis of psychodynamic theory holding that anger held in (defended against) would increase disturbance, particularly depression and suicide potential. No specific prediction was made. The results are shown in Table 9-18.

There are a number of significant associations in the direction predicted by psychodynamic theory, but interestingly, they do not include depression, although such an association might have been predicted on theoretical grounds. In the recently separated/divorced they include

Table 9-18
Relationship Between Defense against Anger and Mental
Health Measures[a]

Mental Health Measure	Sub 2			Sub 3
	M (N = 32)	F (N = 70)	All (N = 102)	(N = 68)
SOMA	.070	−.009	−.029	−.095
ANX	−.054	.055	.013	−.002
DEP	.194	.042	.074	.103
SOC	.002	.254[b]	.171[c]	.108
BPRS	.061	.201[c]	.168[c]	.001
SPC 1[d]	—	.166	.172[c]	.086
SPC 2[d]	—	.310[b]	.261[b]	.137
ASP[d]	—	.325[b]	.298[b]	.117

For explanation of mental health measures see Appendix 5-A.
[a]Measured by Kendall's tau, two-tailed analysis of significance.
[b]$p \leq .01$
[c]$p \leq .05$
[d]There was an insufficient number of suicidal males to warrant computation of correlations.

social functioning (SOC), the BPRS, and all three suicidal measures. Most of these associations also hold for women; one suicidal measure is significantly associated in the case of men and the other approaches significance. These associations are not found regarding the longer-term separated/divorced. This finding, however, must be viewed with caution in light of the highly skewed distribution of responses in the latter group. In addition, the psychodynamically oriented clinician-raters may have had a bias in rating individuals who defended against anger as more disturbed than those who did not. The fact that the associations appear only on the mental health measures of the clinicians and not the self-ratings underlines the problem. The raters, however, were at least internally consistent in seeing defense against anger as related to impairment. In sum, rater-rated defense against anger is associated with multiple measures of disturbance, including suicidal indicators, but not with self-rated mental health measures.

Appropriateness of guilt. This issue was raised because of the possibility that inappropriate guilt might be associated with more disturbance. No etiologic hypothesis was implied here: irrational guilt could be a cause or effect of disturbance or both. No prediction was made. The results are shown in Table 9-19.

Table 9-19

Appropriateness of Guilt and Mental Health Measures[a]

Mental Health Measure	Sub 2			Sub 3
	M (N = 32)	F (N = 70)	All (N = 102)	(N = 67)
SOMA	−.249	−.127	−.160[b]	.010
ANX	−.216	−.192[b]	−.212[c]	−.138
DEP	−.464[c]	−.154	−.251[c]	−.116
SOC	−.243	−.232[c]	−.227[c]	−.196[b]
BPRS	−.214	−.347[c]	−.299[c]	−.186
SPC 1[d]	—	−.086	−.126	−.110
SPC 2[d]	—	−.123	−.223[b]	−.166
ASP[d]	—	−.175	−.216[b]	−.215

For abbreviations of mental health measures see Appendix 5-A.
[a]Measured by Kendall's tau, two-tailed analysis of significance.
[b]$p \leq .05$
[c]$p \leq .01$
[d]There was an insufficient number of suicidal males to warrant computation of correlations.

There is indeed an association across a wide range of mental health measures for the recently separated/divorced, and in a number of instances for women and men in this sub-group. Since inappropriate guilt is coded as 1 and appropriate guilt as 5, negative correlations indicate that inappropriate guilt correlates with more disturbance. There is a significant association with somatic discomfort, anxiety, depression, social functioning, the BPRS, and two of three suicidal measures in the recently separated/divorced. In the longer-term separated/divorced, only social functioning, is significantly associated, though the association with the BPRS and one suicidal measure approaches significance.

Thus, the more inappropriate the guilt, the greater discomfort, social dysfunction, BPRS scores, and suicidal ideation in the recently separated/divorced. There are trends towards association with social function, BPRS, and one suicidal variable in the longer-term separated/divorced as well. Guilt, and especially guilt which clinicians see as inappropriate, is likely to be associated with greater difficulty in a separating/divorcing group.

Memory and fantasy regarding the spouse. Memory and fantasy about a "lost" person is widely accepted as pathognomonic of bereave-

Table 9-20
Memories and Fantasies Regarding Spouse and Mental
Health Measures[a]

Mental Health Measure	Sub 2			Sub 3
	M (N = 32)	F (N = 70)	All (N = 102)	(N = 68)
SOMA	.274[c]	.305[b]	.231[b]	.031
ANX	.254	.435[b]	.355[b]	−.013
DEP	.254	.450[b]	.363[b]	.100
SOC	.094	.245[b]	.185[c]	.055
BPRS	.136	.355[b]	.274[b]	.048
SPC 1[d]	—	.149	.120	.150
SPC 2[d]	—	.284[b]	.230[b]	.218
ASP[d]	—	.147	.132	.210

For explanation of mental health measures see Appendix 5-A.
[a]Measured by Kendall's tau, two-tailed analysis of significance.
[b]$p \leq .01$
[c]$p \leq .05$
[d]There was an insufficient number of suicidal males to warrant computation of correlations.

inent and plays an important role in marital separation/divorce. Whether this phenomenon is related to mental health is shown in Table 9-20.

There is a consistent association of the presence and degree of memory and fantasy regarding the spouse with disturbance as indicated by the mental health measures. All but two suicidal variables are significantly associated with memory and fantasy in the recently separated/divorced, and in the women in that group.

DISCUSSION

This chapter has compared two kinds of psychological variables. The first deals with feelings and fantasies, mainly related to marital separation, and the second with variables indicative of the level of mental health. Doing so has added another level to the overview of the relationship of the divorce process to mental health—participants' responses to events, and the relationship of that dimension to mental health. Not only the events themselves but the manner in which they are filtered through intra-psychic processes ultimately determine their impact.

There was another consideration of interest. While anger is clearly associated, to some extent, with disturbance of mental health, this association tends to be less strong than that connected with the more obvious attachment-related variables, i.e., being in love with the (former) spouse, sadness about the separation, and memories and fantasies regarding the spouse.

Do the data then indicate that anger is less important than attachment as an explanation of the disturbances in divorce? I do not think so. In this study the respondents have been asked only about conscious anger. Psychodynamic theory suggests that in the presence of an actual or threatened loss, anger is likely to be repressed. Indeed, our raters stated that about two out of five of the respondents showed evidence of moderate or greater defense against anger. Some indirect support for the importance of unacceptable anger for mental health comes from the demonstrated association of guilt, especially inappropriate guilt, to mental health measures including, in some instances, suicide potential. It is possible that it is not so much overt anger that is associated with difficulty but that which is not consciously acknowledged. Future studies designed to deal with some of the methodological problems will be needed to resolve the question. As it is, we can say that overt anger plays a role, though not as great as the one played by overt attachment in the mental health of those undergoing marital dissolution.

SUMMARY

In this chapter the feelings of our respondents to the former spouse have been examined in some detail and related to mental health. The focus has been on *feelings associated with the separation,* rather than on events.

A majority of those seriously discussing separation and those recently separated but who have not filed for divorce said that they are still in love with the spouse. Over three-quarters in these two groups say they do or would miss the spouse. Being in love with and missing the spouse decline over time, though one-fifth of the respondents say that they are in love with the (former) spouse 14 or more months after the last separation event and about one-third state they still miss the spouse at that time.

Friendly feelings, which may coexist with other feelings, are claimed by about three-fourths of the respondents overall. Not wishing to be with the (former) spouse increases over time, reaching almost 90 percent in the long-term separated/divorced. About one-third actually dislike the spouse and there is no consistent change over time.

Feelings were related separately to respondents' mental health measures among both the recently and longer-term separated. In general, disturbance so measured in the recently separated/divorced was greatest among those who are in love with and do or would miss the former spouse and would prefer to be with the spouse. There were few associations in the longer-term separated/divorced, although suicidal measures tended to be related to missing the spouse in that group. There are also suggestions that disturbance may be associated with negative feelings toward the spouse, such as feeling unfriendliness or dislike, but the associations are less strong. In general, those with relative neutral feelings toward the (former) spouse are least disturbed.

Various aspects held to be indicative of the grief process in marital separation/divorce were studied. These included sadness, anger and guilt in relation to the separation, and the amount of time respondents spend in memory and fantasy involving the (former) spouse. The grief process as commonly defined in the literature was found to be present: separation-related sadness, anger, and guilt were found in the large majority of the recently separated and persist in a sizable minority of the longer-term separated/divorced. Further, the study raised the possibility that while the phenomenology of grief appears to exist, its purpose may often be to maintain a relationship with the (former) spouse rather than to give it up. It was also found that about three in ten respondents were seen by clinical raters as defending against anger to a moderate or extreme degree and that the raters believed that guilt feelings were probably or definitely appropriate in two of three instances.

Those respondents whose sadness, anger, and guilt are associated with marital separation were distinguished from those for whom these feelings had other origins. The two groups were compared regarding mental health measures. Those whose feelings were linked to the marital separation were more likely to report greater discomfort than the others and in some instances showed greater psychiatric disturbance on the BPRS, and increased suicide potential. The differences were most frequently found in the recently separated/divorced group but some, including suicidal variables, were also found in the longer-term separated/divorced.

Further, those who defend against anger and who were rated as being inappropriately guilty tended to show increased disturbances. Finally, there is a consistent association of the presence and degree of memory and fantasy regarding the spouse with disturbance on most mental health measures. The associations are most pronounced in the recently separated/divorced, and in women in that group.

REFERENCES

1. Goode WJ: After Divorce. Glencoe, Ill, The Free Press, 1956
2. Weiss RS: Marital Separation. New York, Basic Books, 1975
3. Hunt M, Hunt B: The Divorce Experience. New York, McGraw-Hill, 1977
4. Lindemann E: Symptomatology and management of acute grief. Am J Psychiatry 101:141–148, 1944
5. Bowlby J: Making and breaking of affectional bonds: I. Aetiology and psychopathology in the light of attachment theory. Br J Psychiatry 130:201–210, 1977
6. Parkes CM: Psycho-social transitions: A field for study. Soc Sci Med 5:101–115, 1971
7. Pollock GJ: Mourning and adaptation. Int J Psychoanal 42:341–361, 1961
8. Fisher EO: Divorce: The New Freedom. New York, Harper and Row, 1974
9. Bohannon P: The six stations of divorce, in Bohannon P (Ed): Divorce and After. New York, Doubleday, 1970, pp 33–62
10. Glick IO, Weiss RS, Parkes CM: The First Year of Bereavement. New York: Wiley-Interscience, 1974
11. Parkes CM: Bereavement. Studies of Grief in Adult Life. New York, International Universities Press, 1972
12. Brown P, Felton BJ, Whitman V, et al: Attachment and distress following marital separation. J Divorce 3(4):303–316, 1980
13. Kitson GC: Attachment to the spouse in divorce: A scale and its application. J Marriage Family 44:379–393, 1982

10

Supports, Rivalries, and New Loves

Relationships with others are essential to everyone, but they are especially important for those who are undergoing the breakup of a marriage and turn to family and friends for support. The former spouse may continue to be involved with the same persons to whom his or her marital partner turns, creating the opportunity for triangles, rivalries, and alliances. Similarly, most separating/divorcing individuals eventually reach out to new romantic or sexual partners. In this sphere also, the former spouse often remains an involved participant, at least in the early phases of the separation process.

This chapter deals with relationships to family and friends, and subsequently with new love partners. In each instance there will be special attention to the role of the (former) marital partners in the patterns of interaction.

INTERACTION WITH FAMILY AND FRIENDS

Previous Studies

Others' attitudes toward the divorce is an important aspect of the interaction with family and friends. Goode noted that in divorce cases, 61 percent of the wife's family approved, 17 percent were indifferent, and 20 percent disapproved. The wife's friends mostly approved, while the husband's family and friends tended to be more indifferent.[1] Trauma was found to be most severe in those whose family disapproved, next in those whose family approved, and least in those whose family was indifferent.[1] Goode also discussed social adjustment after divorce. Over half of his respondents claimed to have kept their old friends throughout the separation and divorce period. The divorcees felt that their new friends were "about the same 'quality' as their old circle, or better."[1]

Raschke[2] studied 277 members and guests of Parents without Partners group. Her findings strongly supported the hypothesis that the greater the social interaction of divorcing persons with relatives, friends, and organizations, the lower will be the stress associated with separation and/or divorce. (The zero-order correlation was .38 when other variables were controlled; $p = .001$.) At the same time, a hypothesis that stress would be less for persons active in the formerly married subculture was not supported. Raschke also found that men participate socially in new roles more than women; older men participate more than younger men; and men with more children participate more than men with fewer children.

Hunt and Hunt saw a "proliferation of helping hands" reaching out to the formerly married, including Parents without Partners, mental health centers, and religious groups.[3] Within the first six months of postmarital life, roughly three quarters of male respondents and one half of female respondents had begun going to parties, public events, and organization meetings.[3]

Chiriboga et al. considered variations in the use of social supports in their study based on interviewing 330 men and women aged 21 to 79.[4] Respondents most frequently turned to friends, spouse (sic), and counselors for help. Women and younger respondents sought support more frequently than men and older persons. For all respondents, the perceived degree of divorce-related stress was a major factor behind the quantity and quality of social supports that were sought. Kitson also found that divorcing persons who had a friend with whom to talk over confidential matters were more distressed than those who did not.[5]

Gongia studied 400 women with children who had filed for divorce in the Cleveland metropolitan area.[6] She found that in-law relationships were considerably more likely to worsen than relationships with blood kin. With the husband removed, the access to in-laws was also removed. Most friendships were perceived as not changing after separation, although friendships with males were more likely to worsen than friendships with other females. Gongia concluded that the major finding is the lack of change apparent for most relationships after marital separation.

Kitson et al. found, on the basis of data drawn from several studies, that divorcees have a greater sense of restricted relationships with others than do widows. The authors believed this finding is due to the greater clarity of the status of a widow. Based on this analysis, if a widow or divorcee were of the same age, one might expect that the divorcee, because of her sense of restricted relationship with others, would receive less support from them, making her adjustment more difficult.[7]

Some authors deal with specialized support systems. Bernard reported that a Unitarian minister designed a religious "rite of passage" for divorcing individuals.[8] Similarly, a rabbi has also developed a divorce ceremony.[9] A different type of support is women's centers, which, according to their advocates, offer a logical basis for developing a wide variety of continuing supports.[10]

Present Study

The present study did not address the issue of family and friends as social supports as such. Instead it focused on only one aspect of relationships with family and friends: those that specifically and pointedly exclude the former spouse, because such relationships may be associated with disturbance.

Respondents were asked if they had ever formed an emotional alliance with relatives, children, or others which shut the spouse out. If so, further details were obtained. Respondents were also asked if the spouse ever formed an emotional alliance which shut out the respondent and if so, more details were obtained.

FINDINGS

Findings will be reported first in regard to respondent alliances and then in regard to spouse alliances.

Respondent alliances.   A minority of all respondents stated that they entered into any alliances which shut out the spouse. Of the entire sample ($N = 231$), 85 persons (36.8 percent) said they had entered into alliance, while 146 (63.2 percent) said they had not. There was no significant difference between marital dissolution categories. Women ($N = 154$) were significantly more likely to enter into an alliance than men ($N = 77$). Forty-two percent of the women compared to 27 percent of the men, had done so (corrected $X^2 = 3.91$, 1 df, $p = .034$).

Typically, respondent alliances were with respondents' family and friends. This was true in 76 cases (88.4 percent). Seventeen respondents reported alliances with the mother and/or father, 4 with brothers and sisters, and 9 with a son or daughter. Another 11 said their alliances involved combinations of these family members. Thus 41, over half of the respondents, allied themselves exclusively with blood relatives. Another 14 were involved with blood relatives in alliances that also included others. Only 22, just over one-quarter, reported non-family alliances. There were no differences related to marital dissolution status categories or sex. A small number (17) said they had entered into an alliance with the spouse's family or friend. The spouse's mother or father was the most common ally. Respondents were asked whether the alliances occurred before or after the separation discussion. For 36 persons (41.9 percent) they occurred before and after; for 42 persons (48.8 percent) after only; and for 8 persons (9.3 percent) before only. There were no differences between marital dissolution status categories or sex.

Alliances tended to be somewhat ephemeral. When asked whether the alliances were active in the two weeks prior to the interview, only 33 persons (41.3 percent) said they were; 47 said they were not (58.8 percent). There was a highly significant difference in effective alliances in the last two weeks between marital dissolution categories ($X^2 =$ 27.34, 4 df, $p = .0001$), with fewer alliances in the latter categories. This is due to the fact that as time passes, the spouse is seen less and less as the focus on one's relationships and alliances. There are no sex differences on this item.

Spouse alliances. More respondents said that the spouse had ever entered into an alliance from which they were excluded than acknowledge their own alliances. One hundred fourteen (48.9 percent) said such was the case. There was a trend, which just missed significance, for those in the later marital dissolution categories to report spouse alliances less frequently ($X^2 = 9.46$, 4 df, $p = .051$). Men perceived women as entering into alliances more often than women perceived this of men, but the difference was not statistically significant. Reported alliances were with the spouses' family or friends in 89 cases (78.9 percent). Of these, 19 involved the spouse's mother and/or father, 5 involved the brother and/or sister, 6 involved the son and/or daughter, 18 involved various combinations of blood relatives, 18 involved both blood relatives and others, and the remainder involved others only. Spouse alliances were reported to be with the respondent's family and friends in 43 of 114 cases (37.7 percent). Of these, 13 involved the son and/or daughter. The respondent's parents were designated in 7 cases, brother and/or sister in 4, multiple alliances including family members in 10, and alliances involving others in 9 cases.

There were some trends toward sex differences: men tended to be more likely than women to see their (former) spouses allied with the spouse's family and/or friends (corrected ($X^2 = 3.03$, 1 df, $p = .082$). Women more often than men believed their (former) spouse was involved with the respondents' family and/or friends (corrected $X^2 = 3.03$, 1 df, $p = .082$). In both instances, wives' family and friends were seen as the more likely alliance partner of the spouse. Fifty-three of these reported alliances (slightly under half) began before the separation discussion. Of these, 12 continued after that discussion, 61 occurred after the discussion only. As in the case of respondent alliances, only a minority (39) of reported spouse alliances were ongoing in the two weeks prior to interview. Four respondents did not know if there was a spouse alliance, and 65 respondents said the spouse alliances were not currently active. Six respondents did not reply.

Summary and discussion. Alliances that shut out the spouse are probably quite common. The true incidence is probably closer to the 49 percent who said that the spouse had entered into such an alliance than it is to the 37 percent who admitted engaging in alliances themselves. On this basis it is probable that alliances that shut out the spouse occur in about half of the separation/divorcing group.

Women may be more likely than men to acknowledge entering into alliances. It is possible that women, in fact, enter into more alliances than men. It is socially more acceptable for women than for men to return to their original family. Support for this thesis is suggested by the finding that men saw women entering into alliances more frequently than women saw men doing so, though the difference did not reach significance.

Alliances are very likely to involve blood relatives only or mainly. For respondents, alliances with the family of origin are most frequently mentioned, while spouses' alliances with children are mentioned first. Respondents may ally with children more often than they admit, because of the general taboo on making alliances with children against the spouse. Probably alliances with both the family or origin and with children are common.

Alliances tend to precede discussion of separation in about half of the cases. If this information is correct, then alliances are as likely to be a potential cause of as a result of marital difficulties. Alliances are not likely to be long-lasting; only a minority continued to the time of the research interview.

RELATIONSHIP TO MENTAL HEALTH MEASURES

No predictions were made regarding the relation of respondent and spouse alliances to respondent mental health. Either positive or negative impact is possible. Alliances may be associated with feeling supported by others, but it is also possible that shutting out the spouse could be disturbing to the respondent. Spouse alliances could not be expected to have any supportive function, since they are directed against the respondent but may well have adverse effects.

Respondent alliances. Mental health measures were related to whether or not the respondent ever entered into an alliance which shut out the spouse. Those who did report such alliances were significantly more anxious than those who did not. This finding was true for the total group, combining all marital status categories ($\tau = -.155, p < .01$, $N = 231$) and for Sub 2 ($\tau = -.184, p < .05, N = 100$). For the group as a whole, depression showed a trend toward association ($\tau = -.106, p = .054, N = 233$) and the same was true for somatic disturbance in Sub 2 ($\tau = -.157, p = .062$).

Whether those who allied with their own family and/or friends were better off than those who allied with spouse's family and/or friends could not be adequately tested due to lopsided distribution in both instances. In the former, 88 percent of those who had alliances at all had them with their own family and/or friends. Conversely, only 20 percent reported alliances with spouses' family and/or friends.

The groups that reported alliances both before and after the separation were compared with those whose alliances occurred after the separation only for Sub 2. The results are shown in Table 10-1. Those who were part of alliances both before and after the separation discussion were compared with those whose alliances occurred only after that discussion. The latter group showed higher scores (more disturbance) on all items, and the differences were significant for the BPRS and all three suicidal measures.

The findings suggest that stable alliances pre-dating the beginning of dissolution of the marriage may serve a more supportive function than those forged in the throes of the crises of the ending marriage. It is possible that the alliance causes disturbance, because some aspect of the alliance is distressing and/or because the respondent is in conflict about shutting out the spouse. It is also possible that the greater the level of emotional disturbance resulting from the marital crisis, the more likely persons are to seek out alliances with their families. Both factors probably play a role.

Spouse alliances. There were no associations of respondents' mental health measures with whether or not the spouse had ever formed an alliance which shut the respondent out. Nor was the respondents' mental health affected if the spouse allied with the spouses' family and/or friends.

Table 10-1

Relationship Between Alliances Beginning Before and After
Separation Discussion and Mental Health Measures (Sub 2)

Mental Health Measure	Time Alliance Began	No. of Cases	$\overline{X}$	SD	t	df
SOMA	Before and after	15	1.575	0.514	−.128	33
	After only	20	1.794	0.492		
ANX	Before and after	15	1.967	1.030	−0.98[b]	22
	After only	20	2.263	0.626		
DEP	Before and after	15	2.689	0.970	−0.93	33
	After only	20	2.958	0.741		
SOC	Before and after	15	1.780	0.633	−1.81	33
	After only	20	2.182	0.662		
BPRS	Before and after	15	1.546	0.275	−2.38[a]	33
	After only	20	1.825	0.387		
SPC 1	Before and after	15	0.0	0.0	−2.68[a]	33
	After only	20	1.285	1.853		
SPC 2	Before and after	15	0.180	0.697	−2.07[a,b]	28
	After only	20	1.000	1.578		
ASP	Before and after	15	1.000	0.0	−2.27[a]	33
	After only	20	1.400	0.681		

For explanation of mental health measures see Appendix 5-A.

[a] $p \leq .05$

[b] F-test for homogeneity of variances indicates significant differences in
variances of the two groups. Therefore, separate variance estimate is reported
and t-test subsequently adjusted.

There were, however, associations with whether or not the spouse
was believed to have entered into alliances with the respondent's family and/or friends (Table 10-2). In Sub 2, respondents who believed that
the spouse had entered into alliance with the respondent's family and/
or friends had significantly more somatic disturbance and showed
more anxiety than those who did not.

Summary and discussion. There are only a few significant relationships between alliances and respondents' mental health measures.
Alliances that shut out the spouse are associated with increased anxiety and, in some circumstances, with a trend toward increased depression or somatic discomfort. The support function that such alliances
may have for the respondent appear to be outweighed by the psycho-

Table 10-2
Spouse Alliance with Respondent's
Family and/or Friends in Relation to
Respondents' Mental Health Measures[a,b]

Mental Health Measure	All Marital Status Subgroups (N = 114)	Sub 2 (N = 54)
SOMA	−.089	−.244[c]
ANX	−.143	−.298[c]
DEP	−.070	−.172
SOC	−.044	−.033
BPRS	−.096	−.197
SPC 1	−.193[c]	−.212
SPC 2	−.154	−.247
ASP	−.135	−.206

For explanation of mental health measures see Appendix 5-A.

[a]Measured by Kendall's tau, two-tailed analysis of significance.

[b]Yes = 1, No = 2. A negative correlation means that spouse alliance is associated with greater disturbance.

[c]$p \leq .05$

logical conflicts due to hostility toward the spouse. It is also possible that the alliances, occurring at a time of marital strain, involve strained relationships of their own. There is another finding which makes such reasoning plausible: The recently separated/divorced who form alliances only after the separation discussion are more disturbed on the BPRS and on all three suicidal measures than those whose alliances were in effect both before and after the separation discussion. The latter group appeared to obtain more beneficial effect from alliances not forged during turbulent period of the marital dissolution. An alternative explanation of these findings is that persons more disturbed by the marital breakup may seek out more alliances.

Spouse alliances as such did not relate to respondents' mental health. However, when Sub 2 spouses entered into alliance with the respondents' family and/or friends which shut out the respondents, those respondents were more anxious and depressed and tended to score higher on the BPRS and on two suicidal measures.

NEW LOVE PARTNERS

The majority of the separated and divorced ultimately find new love partners. In this section we will be concerned with two aspects of this topic: the respondents' and spouses' romantic and sexual involvements and the respondents' new relationship.

Other Studies

Goode saw frequency of dating as a function of three independent factors: age, opportunity for meeting people, and attitudes towards remarriage.[1] He stated that "the steps from the bitterness of a marital conflict to a new marriage do not occur at random,"[1] and those who try to move toward a new marriage take clear-cut steps toward that end by exposing themselves most often to the chance to do so. Of particular interest from the standpoint of the present work is Goode's finding that affect toward the ex-husband is important in determining whether a respondent was dating steadily, considering marriage, or claiming that remarriage had a fair chance of occurring. Those who expressed antagonistic or loving attitudes toward their former husband had the lowest frequency of steady dating, the lowest frequency of potential spouses among their close male friends, and the lowest frequency of claiming that there was a fair chance that a marriage might actually take place. Those who expressed friendly or indifferent attitudes had a higher score on all three variables.[1]

Weiss discussed "dating and related matters," using the term "dating because no better one is available, even though it at times seems incongruous when applied to people who have been married and have children."[11] Most separated people, he believed, enter into dating at some point. According to Weiss, the possibility of new attachments is the most important reason people date, and the role of sexual need in the initiation of dating is secondary in most instances.[11] For those who have a special relationship with an existing spouse and in persons not divorced, sexual relations may at times be interpreted as adultery.[11] Dating may be seen as revenge on, or constitute distancing from the spouse. Generally, spouses tolerate each other's dating, though a few become intensely jealous.[11]

Weiss described three stages of new attachment: "going together," living together, and marriage. He considered the likelihood of making the same mistake again, i.e., marrying a person similar to the former spouse, as a worry that divorced people often express. While individuals seem able to become attached only to people with a limited range

of characteristics, new attachment figures will be different in significant respects from the former figure.[11]

Hunt and Hunt similarly noted that the crisis of the marital breakup may disrupt habitual modes of thinking and feeling. This disruption
can become manifest in new dating relationships.[3] They reported that
nearly 6 of every 10 women in their survey said that most or all of the
men they had dated made a sexual approach on the first or second
date, while only four of ten men acknowledged making such an approach.[3] Nearly three quarters of the men and nearly two thirds of the
women had at least some casual sex after their marriage terminated[3]; 6
men and 5 women out of 10 had only friendly or moderately affection-
ate feelings for most of their sex partners. Once sexual activity begins,
the majority of the formerly marrieds remain active: only one man in
six and one woman in three said they had a year or more of celibacy
since the end of marriage.[3] Most formerly marrieds find post-marital
sexual experiences more satisfying than marital ones.[3] Hunt and Hunt
stated that their belief—"If the sexual behavior of the formerly married is hedonistic in intent, it is rehabilitative in effect",[3]—is shared by
the majority of the formerly married. As relationships progress, the
formerly married are slow to speak of "love." They prefer to speak of
having a "serious involvement" or "a relationship".[3] Only gradually is
greater intimacy acknowledged, followed—for some—by living together and getting married.

Present Study

The issue of new involvements was addressed by asking the respondents about their own and their spouse's romantic and sexual relationships and new dating and/or love partners.

FINDINGS

The findings will be given first, followed by a description of the
relationship of the findings to respondents' mental health variables.

Respondents' romantic and sexual involvement. Respondents
were asked whether they were ever or currently romantically or sexually involved with someone other than their spouse. The answer was
positive for 181 respondents (78.0 percent, $N = 232$), ranging from 31
of 61 of those still married but discussing separation to 68 of 69 of those
whose last separation event occurred more than 13 months prior to the
interview. For all groups who had filed for divorce or had a final decree, over 90 percent answered affirmatively. There was no difference
between men and women.

Respondents were asked whether the spouse knew the new partner personally. Only a minority, 70 persons, did (38.7 percent). This
was true regardless of marital dissolution category, there being no significant differences between them. There was also no difference between the sexes for the group as a whole, but if only the recently sepa-
rated/divorced were considered, 45.5 percent of the women ($N = 55$)
but only 18.5 percent of the men ($N = 27$) said their spouse knew the
other person (corrected $X^2 = 4.56$, 1 df, $p = .03$).

Those who stated their spouse knew the other person were asked
by what route the acquaintenceship was made. This was asked to determine whether a special and triangular relationship existed involving
the respondent, spouse, and new person. Two questions were asked
that would indicate such special relationships: Was the new partner a
relative of either spouse? Was the new partner a best or close friend of
the respondent, known as such to the spouse? Only 12 of 70 (17.2 percent) fell into either category. Three were relatives; nine were close
friends. The remaining 58 persons knew the spouse by other routes.

Respondents were asked when the involvement(s) occurred. Of
the 181 who had ever had an involvement, 99 said it had occurred before the separation, 153 after the separation, and 111 two weeks before
the interview. (The answers were not mutually exclusive.) In terms of
degree of involvement, of 142 who said they were involved at time of
interview, 26.9 percent were minimally involved, 16.9 percent somewhat involved, 53.6 percent very much involved. Those with greater
degree of involvement were more frequently found in the later marital
dissolution states ($X^2 = 19.55$, 8 df, $p = .012$). There was no difference
by sex.

The majority of respondents (71.5 percent, $N = 179$) said the
spouse had found out about the involvement. There was no difference
between marital dissolution categories or between sexes. Of the spouses who found out, 53 did so before the separation, 98 after the separation, and 13 in the two weeks prior to interview. (These figures are not
mutually exclusive.)

Respondents were asked how involved the spouse was in the respondent's other romantic or sexual relationship(s). Of the 117 who
answered the question, 46 said the spouse was not at all involved, 16
minimally so, 14 somewhat, and 41 very much involved. There was
more spouse involvement in the early dissolution categories ($X^2 =
28.29$, 12 df, $p = .005$). There were no differences between the sexes.

Spouses' romantic and sexual involvement. Respondents were
asked if the spouse was at the time or had ever been romantically or
sexually involved with another person. Of 233 respondents, 152 said

yes, 13 did not know, and 68 said no. Thus, a total of 65.2 percent said their spouses had been or is involved with another at some point, which is slightly lower than the four fifths who attributed such involvement to themselves. As expected, the number of involved spouses was significantly greater in the later dissolution categories (X^2 = 57.91, 8 df, p = .0001). There were no differences by sex.

As to whether or not the respondents knew the person with whom the spouse was involved, 41.4 percent, (N = 152) did. There was no difference between marital dissolution categories. Men were clearly more likely to know the person with whom their (former) wife was involved (58.7 percent, N = 46) than wives were to know the person with whom the (former) husband was involved (34.0 percent, N = 106) (corrected X^2 = 7.10, 1 df, p = .008). The same finding holds if only the recently separated/divorced are considered (corrected X^2 = 4.33, 1 df, p = .04, N = 73). Of the 63 persons with whom the spouse was involved and who were known to the respondent, 4 were relatives of either respondent or spouse and 11 were best or close friends of the respondent; the remainder fell into other categories.

Respondents were asked when the spouse involvement began. Of the 152 instances in which spouse involvement was reported, it occurred before the separation in 88 instances, after the separation in 119 cases, and in the last two weeks in 76 cases. (The figures are not mutually exclusive.)

One hundred thirty-eight respondents were asked about the degree of the spouse's involvement. Minimal involvement was reported in 42 cases, moderate involvement in 15 cases, and much involvement in 63 cases. Degree of involvement was not known in 18 instances. Involvement was significantly greater in the later marital dissolution categories (X^2 = 39.27, 12 df, p = .0001). There were no differences by sex.

Respondents were asked whether the spouse's involvement in the last two weeks was more, the same, or less than in previous periods, as it was thought that increased spouse involvement might be troubling to the respondent. Of 140 spouses about whom the question was answered, 29 (20.7 percent) were more involved, 12 (8.6 percent) less involved. The remainder either reported no change or did not know.

Respondents were asked about when they found out about the spouse involvement. Eighty-one found out before the separation; 94 since the separation; and 22 in the last two weeks. (The numbers are not mutually exclusive.)

Finally, respondents (N = 152) were asked about their involvement in the spouse's new romantic and sexual relations. Slightly less than half (71), claimed not to be involved at all; 23 said they were mini-

Table 10-3
Dating Since Separation by Marital Status

Marital Status	Have Dated Since Separation		Have not Dated Since Separation		Total
	Ever	At Time of Interview	Never	Not at Time of Interview	
Still living with spouse[a]	27	(10)	35	(52)	62
Separated within previous 14 months; have not filed for divorce	18	(14)	26	(30)	44
Filed for divorce within previous 14 months; no final decree	26	(20)	2	(8)	28
Final divorce within previous 14 months	29	(23)	1	(7)	30
Last separation/divorce event 14 or more months previous	67	(44)	2	(25)	69
Total	167	(111)	66	(122)	233

[a]Refers to dating since separation discussion.

mally involved, 22 somewhat involved, and 36 very much involved. Thus, slightly less than two fifths said they were meaningfully (somewhat or very much) involved. Those in the later marital dissolution categories were less involved ($X^2 = 40.44$, 12 df, $p = .0001$). Women exceeded men both among those very much involved and those not at all involved at a level approaching significance ($X^2 = 6.95$, 3 df, $p = .07$). For Sub 2, women were more likely than men to report little or no involvement ($X^2 = 12.13$, 3 df, $p = .007$).

*General dating patterns.** Respondents were asked if they had dated someone other than the spouse at all since the separation or, for those still living with the spouse, since the separation discussion.

---

*Most of the new relationships involved partners of the opposite sex. In the entire sample, however, 2 of 59 men and 9 of 123 women reported that they had been romantically or sexually involved with one or more persons of the same sex at some time since the separation. Same held true among the recently separated/divorced for 1 of 27 men and 4 of 57 women.

Those who ever dated were also asked whether they were dating at the time of interview. The results are shown in Table 10-3. In all but the first two categories, 90 percent had dated at one time. The data suggests that there is a very high proportion of re-establishment of dating relationships following the breakup of the marriage. The majority in the later separation categories also dated at time of interview. There were no differences by sex.

Dating tended to begin quickly after the separation (or separation discussion for those still living with the spouse). Of the respondents who were dating at the time of interview ($N = 109$), 67.9 percent started dating within one month or less after separation, and 13.8 percent began dating within two or three months. These findings suggest that those who continue dating start early. Those who were dating at time of interview also dated often. Thirty-three persons (31.7 percent), dated daily, and 51 persons (49.0 percent) dated more than once a week. Only 20 persons (19.2 percent), dated weekly or less often.

Those respondents who were dating at the time of interview were asked whether they began dating before the separation or, in cases of those still living with their spouses, before the separation discussion. The results are shown in Table 10-4. Slightly over half (55.9 percent) of those dating at time of interview began doing so before the separation discussion. Those dating were asked if they had ever dated more than

Table 10-4

Dating Before Separation by Marital Status, for All Persons Dating at Time of Interview

Marital Status	Dated Before Separation	Did not Date Before Separation	Total
Still living with spouse[a]	7	3	10
Separated within previous 14 months; have not filed for divorce	9	5	14
Filed within previous 14 months; no final decree	12	8	20
Final decree within previous 14 months	9	14	23
Last separation/divorce event 14 or more months previous	25	19	44
Total	62	49	111

[a]Refers to dating since separation discussion.

Table 10-5
Dating One or More Persons, for All Persons Dating at Time of Interview

Marital Status	Dated More than One Person		Did not Date More than One Person		Total
	Ever	At Time of Interview	Ever	At Time of Interview	
Still living with spouse	6	(2)	4	(8)	10
Separated within previous 14 months; have not filed for divorce	6	(1)	8	(13)	14
Filed within previous 14 months; no final decree	17	(12)	3	(8)	20
Final decree within previous 14 months	20	(8)	3	(15)	23
Last separation/divorce event 14 or more months previous	39	(13)	5	(31)	44
Total	88	(36)	23	(75)	111

one person and if so, if they were dating more than one person at the time of interview. (Table 10-5). The overwhelming majority of those in the separation process did not immediately restrict themselves to one partner, but tended to be dating only one person at time of interview. Those separated and divorced who said they were dating at the time of interview were asked if they lived with the new partner. This was true of 14 of 56 (25.0 percent) of Sub 2 and of 12 of 44 (27.3 percent) of Sub 3.

Emotional involvement. Those who were dating at the time of interview were asked if they were emotionally involved with someone other than their (former) spouse, and if so, were they in love (Table 10-6). There was a tendency for emotional involvement to occur more frequently in the later dissolution categories ($X^2 = 9.20$, 4 *df*, $p = .056$). There were no differences by sex regarding emotional involvement and no differences between marital status category or by sex regarding being in love. Clearly, the respondents who had started dating did not, for the most part, see their involvement as casual: over four-fifths saw

Table 10-6

Emotional Involvement and Being in Love, for All Persons Dating at Time of Interview, by Marital Status

Marital Status	Emotionally Involved	In Love
Now living with the spouse (N = 10)	5	4
Separated within previous 13 months; not filed for divorce (N = 14)	11	7
Filed within previous 13 months; no final decree (N = 20)	15	9
Final decree within previous 13 months (N = 23)	21	13
Last separation/divorce event 14 or more months ago (N = 44)	38	27
Total (N = 111)	90	60

themselves as emotionally involved and over half said they were in love with a new partner.

Respondents were asked if they allowed themselves to behave in a warm and loving way to their new partners. The overwhelming majority—92 of 107 (86.0 percent) of those who were dating—said they did. There was no difference in marital dissolution categories or between the sexes. If the separation experience did interfere with closeness with new partners, respondents were not ready to acknowledge it. By a similar margin, the majority of respondents—75 of 107 (75.7 percent)—said they could trust their new partner, and 8 (7.5 percent) said they did not know. Again, there were no differences between dissolution categories or the sexes.

Quarreling. A majority (67 of 106, or 63.2 percent) acknowledged that they sometimes quarreled with the new partner. Those later in the separation process said that quarrels occurred more often (X^2 = 11.41, 4 *df*, p = .022). Seventeen persons (16.0 percent) acknowledged physical fights with their new partners; there were no marital dissolution status or differences by sex, though there was a trend towards more physical fights in men. The figure is of the same magnitude as the 12- to 16-percent incidence of physical violence in intact families[12,13] but much less than the 44- to 55-percent incidence in separating and divorced couples. Intensity of quarrels was rated as mild by 25 of 67 respondents (37.3 percent); moderate by 16 (23.9 percent); and intense by 26 (38.8 percent). There were no differences between marital dissolution categories or by sex.

Sexuality. All respondents, whether they dated or not, were asked if they had any interest in sex. The five categories and the percentage of respondents in each ($N = 233$) were as follows: no obvious interest, 11.4 percent; only fantasies, 3.1 percent; can take it or leave it, 16.6 percent; sometimes strong interest, 24.9 percent; frustrated without it, 44.1 percent. There were no differences by marital status. There was a trend approaching significance indicating less interest in sex by women ($X^2 = 8.62$, 4 *df*, $p = .072$, $N = 229$).

Respondents were asked how often they felt sexual satisfaction in their current relationships. Of those 168 persons who had sexual relations, 24 (14.3 percent) said never; 14 (8.3 percent) said rarely; 23 (13.7 percent) said occasionally or sometimes; 46 (27.4 percent) said most of the time; and 61 (36.3 percent) said always. Thus, about two thirds of those sexually active said they were satisfied. There was no difference by marital dissolution status or by sex.

Comparison to (former) spouse. Some questions were asked to determine how the respondents consciously saw the similarities and differences between the new partner and the former spouse. Respondents ranked the new partner on a five-point scale on the question of how different the spouse is from the new partner. Of the 106 who answered the question, 56 (52.8 percent) said the new partner was practically the opposite and 29 (27.4 percent) said the new partner was very different. Twelve (11.3 percent) said the new partner was somewhat different and 9 (8.5 percent) said there was either a slight difference or none.

To assess the same dimension, respondents were asked if they sometimes engaged in behavior with the new partner which they realized was appropriate instead to the former spouse. Of 105 persons, 66 (62.9 percent) denied this ever occurred; 14 (13.3 percent) said it happened occasionally; 16 (15.2 percent) indicated it occurred sometimes; and 9 (8.6 percent) said it happened very often or practically all of the time.

Continued involvement with someone known before separation. It is of interest how frequently involvement with someone dated before the separation discussion continues. Of 54 separated or divorced persons who dated before the separation, 20 (37.0 percent) dated someone at time of interview whom they knew before the separation. That figure may understate persons known before the separation and dated at time of interview, since it was possible to date someone at time of interview whom the respondent knew but did not date before the separation. Perhaps more relevant is the number of persons emotionally involved: 25 of 85 separated or divorced persons who said they were emotionally involved were involved with someone they knew before the separation (29.4 percent). Of these, 18 persons said they were in love with someone they knew before the separation and 8 said they were currently living with such a person. If we compare those involved with someone they knew before separation with the *total* separated and divorced group ($N = 171$), about one in seven (14.6 percent) were emotionally involved at the time of interview with someone they knew before the separation. Thus, the incidence of lasting romantic involvements with persons whom separating/divorcing individuals knew before the separation is relatively low in our sample.

Summary and discussion.   The extent to which our respondents become involved with others was striking. Almost four fifths were at one time involved romantically or sexually with another, and this was true of about half of those still married. Respondents were asked whether the spouse knew about the involvement; about 70 percent did. In about 40 percent the spouse knew the new partner personally. Of the spouses who knew about the involvement, somewhat over 40 percent were said to be very much involved emotionally in the respondent's new relationship.

How respondents saw their former spouses' romantic and sexual involvement was also considered. About two thirds said their former spouse was romantically and/or sexually involved with another man or woman. About two fifths of these respondents knew the spouse's new partner personally. Regarding their own emotional involvement in the spouses' new relationship, slightly less than two fifths said they were either somewhat or very much involved emotionally. Respondents were also asked whether spouse involvement had changed in the last two weeks: about 20 percent of the spouses had become more involved.

Slightly under one-half of the respondents were dating someone other than the spouse at the time of interview. Over half of those dating at the time of interview had begun dating before the separation (or separation discussion if they were still marrried). This finding suggests that involvements with new partners are common in the terminal stages of a marriage, although it cannot be necessarily concluded that they are causal in nature. About 70 percent had dated at some time since the separation discussion, whether or not they were dating at the time of interview. Of those dating at the time of interview, over two thirds started dating within one month of the separation; about half dated once a week, and a third daily. About eight in ten had dated more than one person, though only about one in three was dating more than one person at the time of interview.

Respondents readily become emotionally involved with the persons whom they date: over four in five said they were so involved, and over half said they are in love. Over four in five claimed that they allowed themselves to behave in a warm and loving way with their new partners. At the same time, about two thirds acknowledge that they quarreled, and in one quarter of these physical fights occurred. Sexual interests were prominent: over two thirds said they sometimes had strong interest in sex or were frustrated without sex, and close to two thirds said they achieved sexual satisfaction.

Respondents stated that they saw their new partners as quite different from their spouse. Over half said the new partner was practically the opposite from the (former) spouse and more than one quarter say the two were very different. Similarly, about two thirds of the respondents denied that they act towards the new spouse in ways that would more befit the (former) spouse.

While over half of the respondents started dating before the separation (or discussion), fewer continued relationships begun at that time. About one in three of those currently separated or divorced who were emotionally involved were involved with someone they knew before the separation. Those emotionally involved with someone known before the separation, compared with all separated and divorced respondents, represent only about one in seven.

Our respondents did not withdraw, nor did they grieve alone. With few exceptions, they developed new relationships quickly, though not without at times creating triangles involving the (former) spouse. Nonetheless, respondents claimed to be emotionally involved and sometimes in love with a new partner, to be able to relate warmly and to be sexually active and satisfied, while acknowledging quarrels and, in a substantial minority, physical violence. New partners commonly entered the lives of persons whose marriages were ending, but much less frequently did they become long-term love objects. Our findings confirm the impression in the existing literature that those whose marriages are dissolving eagerly reach out for new relationships, and that these relationships meet many needs but tend to be time-limited.

RELATIONSHIPS TO MENTAL HEALTH MEASURES

Romantic and sexual involvement. The relationship of romantic and sexual involvements to mental health measures was considered only for those who were separated or divorced. Of the respondents who were asked whether they had ever been romantically or sexually

Table 10-7

Relationship Between Ever Being Romatically or
Sexually Involved with Someone Other than
Spouse and Mental Health Measures (Sub 2)[a,b]

Mental Health Measure	M (N = 32)	F (N = 70)	All (N = 102)
SOMA	−.060	.148	.073
ANX	.016	.182	.137
DEP	.202	.274[c]	.249[c]
SOC	.089	.303[c]	.229[c]
BPRS	.067	.239[d]	.173[d]
SPC 1[e]	—	.131	.097
SPC 2[e]	—	.220	.188
ASP[e]	—	.147	.129

For explanation of mental health measures see Appendix 5-A.

[a]Measured by Kendall's tau, two-tailed analysis of significance.

[b]Yes = 1, No = 2. Positive correlations indicate that not being involved is associated with more disturbance.

[c]$p \leq .01$

[d]$p \leq .05$

[e]There was an insufficient number of suicidal males to warrant computation of correlations.

involved with another, 80.3 percent said yes. Keeping the lopsided distribution in mind, there were a number of significant associations, as shown in Table 10.7. For Sub 2 as a whole, and for women in that group, those who had ever been romantically or sexually involved with someone other than the spouse, or were so at the time of interview, were less depressed, less socially dysfunctional, and less disturbed on the BPRS than those who had not been or were not at the time so involved. There were no significant associations for men which may or may not be due to the small size of the sample together with the skewed distribution.

Degree of respondent involvement was not consistently related to respondents' mental health measures for either the recently separated/divorced as a whole or for women in the group. There were not sufficient cases to allow such an analysis regarding men. In the longer-term separated/divorced, however, the more involved respondents were, the lower was their score on the BPRS ($\tau = -.341$, $p < .01$). The findings suggest that in the longer-term separated/divorced, the degree of emotional involvement correlates inversely with psychiatric dysfunction.

Spouses' romantic and sexual involvement. It was anticipated that spouses' romantic and sexual involvement might be disturbing to respondents. This was tested through correlation with respondents' mental health measures in the recently and long-term separated/ divorced.

Only a few associations were found. Whether or not the spouse had ever been romantically or sexually involved was associated with social dysfunction only in Sub 2. Those whose spouses were not so involved were more dysfunctional than the others ($\tau = .173$, $p < .05$, $N = 102$). There were neither significant associations nor trends regarding either discomfort, psychiatric, or suicidal variables, however. Overall, it did not seem to matter much whether the spouse was romantically or sexually involved with anyone else. Too few spouses were not involved with someone in Sub 3 to make analysis meaningful. Nor was respondents' mental health related to whether they knew the person with whom the spouse was involved, nor with the reported degree of the spouses' involvement.

There was, however, a relationship between the extent to which respondents reported they were involved in their spouse's romance and the respondents' mental health measures. The relationships are shown in Table 10-8. The more involved the respondent in the spouse's

Table 10-8
Relationship Between Respondents' Feelings about Spouse's Romantic or Sexual Involvement and Mental Health Measures[a]

Mental Health Measure	Sub 2 F (N = 52)	Sub 2 All (N = 73)	Sub 3 (N = 60)
SOMA	.226[b]	.100	.112
ANX	.248[b]	.150	.065
DEP	.260[b]	.214[b]	.141
SOC	.160	.106	.189
BPRS	.261[b]	.205[b]	.184
SPC 1	.084	.095	.154
SPC 2	.161	.140	.288[b]
ASP	.120	.147	.243[b]

For explanation of mental health measures see Appendix 5-A.
[a]Measured by Kendall's tau, two-tailed analysis of significance.
[b]$p \leq .05$

romantic and sexual affairs, the more depressed the respondent and the higher the score on the BPRS in Sub 2 as a whole. Significant associations in the same direction are found in Sub 2 women regarding somatic discomfort, anxiety, depression, and the BPRS. There were insufficient men in the Sub 2 group for analysis. In the longer-term separated/divorced, there are significant associations in the same direction regarding two suicidal variables. The findings suggest that it is a person's involvement in the spouse's affairs rather than the affairs themselves that affects level of functioning.

New dating and love partners. A number of variables dealing with respondents' new dating and love partners were studied in relation to respondents' mental health measures in the separated/divorced. Did respondents who had ever dated fare better than those who had not? The question could be asked only to those who were separated but had not filed, since in all other categories those who had dated outnumbered those who had not by such lopsided margins that statistical analysis was not possible. Among the separated persons who had not filed ($N = 44$), those who had ever dated were significantly less depressed ($\tau = .251, p < .05$), less socially dysfunctional ($\tau = .281, p < .05$), and less disturbed on the BPRS ($\tau = .300, p < .05$).

Similarly, those who were dating at the point of interview were significantly less disturbed on a number of mental health measures, as shown in Table 10-9. Those currently dating among Sub 2 were less depressed, less socially dysfunctional, and had lower scores on the BPRS than their non-dating counterparts. In Sub 3, social dysfunction and depression showed parallel relationships.

There was no relationship between frequency of dating and mental health status for Sub 2 as a whole ($N = 54$) or for Sub 2 women ($N = 38$). There were not enough men in Sub 2 to analyze the relationship. However, in Sub 3 ($N = 42$), those dating more frequently were less psychiatrically disturbed as measured by the BPRS ($\tau = -.248, p < .05$) and less socially dysfunctional ($\tau = -.283, p < .05$).

Whether or not respondents' mental health would be affected by dating before the separation could theoretically be answered in two opposing ways. On the one hand, dating before venturing a separation could be seen as avoiding the loss of heterosexual contacts; on the other hand, there could be guilt or other conflict regarding marital infidelity. The data do not provide a clear-cut answer. In Sub 2 ($N = 57$), however, correlations are in the direction of greater disturbance if the respondent dated before the separation, though only the score on the BPRS is significant ($\tau = -.225, p < .05$). Associations are in the same direction in Sub 2 women ($N = 44$) but do not reach significance. There are no meaningful associations in Sub 3.

Table 10-9
Relationship Between Dating at Time of
Interview and Mental Health Measures[a,b]

Mental Health Measure	Sub 2			Sub 3
	M ($N = 32$)	F ($N = 70$)	All ($N = 102$)	($N = 69$)
SOMA	.169	.097	.075	.032
ANX	.219	.123	.143	−.027
DEP	.353	.173	.213[d]	.042
SOC	.190	.203[d]	.195[d]	.330[c]
BPRS	.141	.167	.161[d]	.266[c]
SPC 1[e]	—	−.035	.100	−.001
SPC 2[e]	—	.022	.048	−.027
ASP[e]	—	.042	.062	.078

For explanation of mental health measures see Appendix
5-A.

[a]Measured by Kendall's tau, two-tailed analysis of significance.

[b]Yes = 1, No = 2. Positive correlations means that those not dating are more disturbed.

[c]$p \leqslant .01$

[d]$p \leqslant .05$

[e]There was an insufficient number of suicidal males to warrant computation of correlations.

The relationship between emotional involvement and mental health measures was not testable because too large a proportion of respondents said they were involved. No correlations were found in Sub 2 ($N = 54$) between being in love and mental health measures. For Sub 3, being in love was associated with less disturbance on the BPRS ($\tau = .331$, $p < .01$, $N = 43$).

There was no association between quarreling and mental health measures for Sub 2 ($N = 55$). In Sub 3 those who said they quarreled with their new partner were less disturbed on the BPRS ($\tau = .266$, $p < .05$, $N = 42$).

There was no connection between presence and absence of physical fights and mental health measures in either Sub 2 ($N = 30$) or Sub 3 ($N = 33$). Intensity of quarrels was associated with increased disturbance in Sub 2 ($N = 31$) on two suicidal measures (SPC 1: $\tau = .320$, $p < .05$; ASP: $\tau = .353$, $p < .05$). There are no significant associations in the longer-term group ($N = 33$). Interest in sex was selectively associated with disturbance, as shown in Table 10-10. There were no significant associations for Sub 2 as a whole ($N = 102$). There was a sugges-

Table 10-10

Relationship Between Interest in Sex and Mental Health Measures[a]

Mental Health Measure	Sub 2			Sub 3 (N = 69)
	M (N = 32)	F (N = 70)	All (N = 102)	
SOMA	.234	.028	.039	−.052
ANX	.210	−.001	.042	−.061
DEP	.288[c]	.016	.077	−.110
SOC	.194	−.180[c]	−.064	−.349[b]
BPRS	.243	−.124	−.017	−.319[b]
SPC 1[d]	—	.063	.111	−.199
SPC 2[d]	—	−.006	.035	−.141
ASP[d]	—	.033	.102	−.190

For explanation of mental health measures see Appendix 5-A.

[a]Measured by Kendall's tau, two-tailed analysis of significance.

[b]$p \leq .01$

[c]$p \leq .05$

[d]There was an insufficient number of suicidal males to warrant computation of correlations.

tion, however, that this finding was due to opposite associations for men and women. For men, depression was significantly associated with more interest in sex. For women, the associations tended to be in the opposite direction, i.e., greater interest in sex was associated with less disturbance, reaching significance in the case of social dysfunction. In Sub 3, on the other hand, the results were more clear-cut, with sexual interest being associated with less disturbance for the group as a whole, significantly so, in the case of social dysfunction and the BPRS. There were not enough men in this group to examine separately.

Table 10-11 shows associations with mental health measures to the frequency with which respondents attained sexual satisfaction. In Sub 2 as a whole, respondents who reported greater sexual satisfaction were significantly less depressed than those who reported less sexual satisfaction. There were not sufficient cases to analyze men. For women, there were significant associations regarding depression, social dysfunction, the BPRS, and two suicidal measures. In Sub 3 as a whole, the associations were in the same direction and were significant for social dysfunction and the BPRS.

Table 10-11
Relationship Between Frequency of Sexual
Satisfaction and Mental Health Measures[a]

| Mental Health Measure | Sub 2 | | Sub 3 |
	F (N = 48)	All (N = 70)	(N = 53)
SOMA	−.090	.001	−.113
ANX	−.212	−.120	−.171
DEP	−.231[c]	−.184[c]	−.122
SOC	−.275[c]	−.087	−.250[c]
BPRS	−.289[b]	−.099	−.346[b]
SPC 1	−.181	−.132	−.001
SPC 2	−.262[c]	−.196	.092
ASP	−.293[c]	−.223[c]	.013

For explanation of mental health measures see Appendix 5-A.

[a]Measured by Kendall's tau, two-tailed analysis of significance.

[b]$p \leq .01$

[c]$p \leq .05$

Similarities and differences between the present partner and the former spouse were not examined in relation to mental health measures, nor was whether the respondent was involved at the time of interview with someone known before the separation.

Summary and discussion. Our findings tend to confirm the belief that involvement with new partners mitigates the trauma of marital separation and divorce. Persons who had ever been romantically or sexually involved with a partner other than the former spouse showed better functioning on several mental health measures than those who had not, as did respondents who were dating at time of interview compared to those who were not. Interest in sex, however, is not associated with mental health in either direction in the recently separated and divorced as a whole, although the findings suggest that men may be more disturbed if they have greater sexual interest, while women may be less disturbed. In the longer-term group as a whole, however, greater sexual interest was associated with better functioning. The findings regarding emotional involvement were not clear-cut although there was a suggestion that being in love may have a positive effect on the long-term separated/divorced. *These findings are compatible with the view that while new romantic and sexual relationships generally are positive factors in the separated/divorced, this is not necessarily true for all aspects of such involvement or for both sexes.* The suggestion that greater sexual interest appears to be related to more disturbance in men, for instance, is intriguing and unexpected. If these findings are replicated, they suggest that for men whose marriages are dissolving, sexual relations may be perceived as more shallow and mechanical and therefore disturbing, whereas for women, they may be seen as reassuring and comforting.

The findings also confirm the expectation that the spouse's involvements have a bearing on the respondent's mental health. It is not, however, the spouse's new romantic and sexual relationships as such, but the respondent's involvement in these attachments, that is associated with greater disturbance, particularly for recently separated/divorced women.

SUMMARY

This chapter deals with the relationships that individuals undergoing marital dissolution maintain or establish with persons other than the former spouse; focuses on the characteristics of these relationships, with special interest both in their potentially beneficial effects and in the triangles and alliances that may ensue; and explores the patterns involving new dating and love partners.

Interactions with family and friends involving alliances that shut out the spouse are acknowledged to occur in about one third of the respondents. The true incidence is probably closer to the about 50 percent reported for spouses. Women are more likely than men to acknowledge entering into alliances. Alliances most commonly involve members of the family of origin and children of one or both spouses. Alliances tend to precede the separation in about half of the cases and may therefore be considered a possible cause as well as a possible consequence of marital difficulties.

Respondent alliances that shut out the spouse are associated with increased anxiety and a trend towards increased depression and somatic discomfort in some circumstances. The recently separated/divorced who form alliances only after the separation discussion are more disturbed on the Brief Psychiatric Rating Scale and on all three suicidal measures than those whose alliances occur both before and after the separation discussion. Spouse alliances affect respondents' mental health only when they are with respondents' family or friends, in which case respondents are more anxious and depressed and tend to score higher on the BPRS and on two suicidal measures.

About four fifths of the respondents were at one time involved romantically or sexually with another man or woman, as were about half of those still married. About two thirds of the respondents said their (former) spouse was romantically or sexually involved with another man or woman. Respondents varied in how much they cared about the (former) spouse's other partners. Slightly less than two fifths said they were either somewhat or very much involved emotionally in their spouses' relationships.

Slightly less than half of the respondents were dating at the time of interview, about 70 percent had dated at some time since the separation, or since the separation discussion if they were still living with the spouse. Over half of those dating at the time of interview had begun dating before the separation or separation discussion. After the separation, dating begins quickly. Over two thirds of the respondents started dating within one month after separation. Of those dating, over four fifths said that they were emotionally involved, and over half said they are in love. Over two thirds said they achieved sexual satisfaction with their partners. Of those emotionally involved at the time of interview, only about one in seven were involved with someone known before the separation. The findings suggest that those whose marriages are dissolving reach out for new relationships, which may meet many needs though they may also be time-limited.

There were some association of new involvement with respondents' mental health. Persons who had ever been romantically or sexually involved with a partner other than the (former) spouse showed better functioning on several mental health measures than those who had not, and the same association holds for those dating at the time of interview. Not all associations are clear-cut, however. Among the recently separated/divorced, men may be more disturbed if they have greater sexual interest while women may be less disturbed. In the longer-term group, greater sexual activity is associated with better functioning for men and women combined. In general, romantic and sexual involvements appear to be positive factors for the separated/divorced, though this is not necessarily true for all aspects or for both sexes. The spouses' new relationships do not appear to be related to the respondents' mental health as such; however, the respondents' degree of emotional involvement in the spouses' new attachment is associated with greater disturbance, especially among recently separated/divorced women.

In conclusion, new relationships are important in those whose marriages are dissolving. Alliances with relatives and friends may not have a positive effect if a major aspect is shutting out the spouse. New dating and love relationships are generally, but not always, associated with positive effects on mental health. Involvement with the spouses' new relationships adversely affects respondents. The findings suggest that to view all relationships with persons other than the spouse as necessarily supportive is to oversimplify. Some new relationships, especially with romantic and sexual partners, are generally helpful, but all relationships, with family, friends, and new partners, must be understood within the context of the general turbulence that characterizes a marital breakup.

REFERENCES

1. Goode WJ: After Divorce. Glencoe, Ill, The Free Press, 1956
2. Raschke HJ: Social and psychological factors in voluntary marital dissolution adjustment. Dissertation Abstracts International, 1975, p 5594A
3. Hunt M, Hunt B: The Divorce Experience. New York, McGraw-Hill, 1977
4. Chiriboga DA, Coho A, Stein J, et al: Stress and social supports: A study in helpseeking behavior. J Divorce 3:121–136, 1979
5. Kitson GC: Attachment to the spouse in divorce: A scale and its applications. J Marriage Family 44:379–393, 1982
6. Gongia PA: Social relationships after marital separation and divorce, in Raschke H, Raschke V (Eds): Computer Printout of Update of Divorce Research Summaries, Chesapeake, VA, 1979
7. Kitson GC, Lopata JZ, Holmes WM, et al: Divorcees and widows: Similarities and differences. Am J Orthopsychiatry 59(2):291, 1980
8. Bernard J: No news, but new ideas, in Bohannon P (Ed): Divorce and After, New York, Doubleday, 1970
9. Grollman EA: Interview, in Marriage and Divorce Today 3:1, 1978
10. Brown CA: Feldberg R, Rox EM, et al: Divorce: Chance of a new lifetime. J Soc Issues 32:119–133, 1976
11. Weiss RS: Marital Separation. New York, Basic Books, 1975
12. Saunders DG: Marital violence: Dimension of the problems and models of intervention. J Marriage Family Counseling 3:43–49, 1977
13. Straus MA: quoted in MD Magazine, January 1980, p 55

11

Regression Analysis

Previous chapters of this volume reported significant associations of a number of independent variables with dependent mental health measures. Which independent variables continue to relate significantly to the dependent mental health measures when the other independent variables are held constant? Unless otherwise stated, findings will pertain to the recently separated/divorced, i.e., those who within the last 13 months have been separated, have filed for divorce, or have obtained a final decree. The number òf variables previously reported is sizable: 55 independent and 8 dependent variables were included in the tables in the preceding chapters. Thus a total of 440 correlations are possible for Sub 2 as a whole. Of these, 125 or 28.4 percent were significant at the $p \leq .05$ level.

METHOD OF SELECTION OF VARIABLES*

In brief, the variables reported were grouped according to their general characteristics into demographic, non-separation/divorce–related, separation/divorce-related, and other categories. The separation/divorce variables were in turn broken down into subgroups on the basis of the aspects of the separation/divorce process which they describe. The subgroups were hostility, attachment and loss, ambiguity, separation-related anger and guilt, new love relationships, initiation of sepa-

---

*The details of the selection of variables to be included in the regression equations reported in this chapter will be found in Appendix II at the end of the book.

ration, and triangles. Each group consisted of from two to six varia-bles. A regression analysis was done for all variables in each group. The results of the regression analyses were examined, and one or more variables were selected for subsequent analyses. While there is a logi-cal process to this culling of variables, judgment was necessarily in-volved, and it is therefore conceivable that alternate approaches would have resulted in a different final set of variables.

Two regression analyses will be reported for the recently sepa-rated/divorced (Sub 2). The first, a general regression analysis, was based on prior regression analyses involving all eight dependent mental health measures. The second was based only on prior findings pertain-ing to the three suicidal measures.

GENERAL REGRESSION ANALYSIS: RECENTLY SEPARATED/DIVORCED (SUB 2)

Variables Selected

The dependent variables include the eight mental health measures (somatic discomfort, anxiety, depression, score on the Social Func-tioning Rating Scale (SOC), score on the Brief Psychiatric Rating Scale (BPRS), suicide potential retrospectively assessed at time of entry (SPC 1), suicide potential at time of interview (SPC 2), and rater's as-sessment of suicide potential (ASP).

The independent variables selected fall into four groups: demo-graphic variables, variables not related to marital separation and/or di-vorce, variables related to marital separation and/or divorce, and other variables.

DEMOGRAPHIC VARIABLES

These are age, sex (0 = female; 1 = male), and socioeconomic status (two-factor index of social position, 1 to 5).

VARIABLES NOT RELATED TO MARITAL
SEPARATION AND/OR DIVORCE

These variables have not been previously reported. They were in-cluded here to investigate the net effects of variables not related to separation and divorce in a regression equation with variables related to marital separation and/or divorce. The underlying assumption is that while divorce-related factors are important, they are not the sole determinants of mental health.

The items included in the regression equations were adapted from the Social Assets Scale[1] based on Langner and Michael's work.[2] They are all childhood stress factors and have been shown in other studies to be predictive of the presence of physical and psychological symptoms. Since they preceded marital separation, they are by definition independent of it, if accurately reported. The items are:

• Respondent's answer to the question, My health between the ages of 16 to 20 was _____. (childhood health). Answers were 10 = poor; 30 = fair; 40 = good.

• Respondent's answer to the question, When you were growing up, were either of your parents in poor health? (parent's health). Answers were 10 = yes, all of the time; 20 = yes, frequently; 30 = yes, but rarely; 35 = no, never.

VARIABLES RELATED TO MARITAL SEPARATION/DIVORCE

• Respondent's answer to the question: Do you think that your (former) spouse ever seriously wished you dead? (death wish by spouse). Answers were yes = 1, don't know = 2, no = 3.

• The question to the mental health professional rater: How much time does the respondent spend involving memory or fantasy about the (former) spouse? (memory/fantasy). Answers ranged from 1 = none, to 5 = almost all of the time. This variable was applied to Sub 2 as a whole and to women in that group.

• The respondent's answer to the question: Are you just as happy not being with the spouse? (not with spouse). Answers were yes = 1, don't know = 2, no = 3. This variable was substituted for the prior item, memory/fantasy, for Sub 2 men.

• Respondent's answer to the question: How frequently do you say one thing and do another relative to contacts with the (former) spouse? (consistency). Answers ranged from 1 = almost never, to 5 = almost always.

OTHER VARIABLES

Two other variables were included in the general regression equation. In order to limit the number of independent variables, they were added one at a time rather than together. They are:

• Respondent's answer to the question: Did you have financial difficulties since the separation? (financial). Answers were 1 = yes, 2 =

Table 11-1

Correlation Between Variables Included in Overall Regression Analysis (Sub 2)

	Non-Separation-Related Factors					Separation-Related Factors			Other Factors
	Socio-economic Status	Sex	Age	Child-hood Health	Parents' Health	Death Wish by Spouse	Memory/ Fantasy about Spouse	Consist-ency of Spouse Contacts	Financial
Socioeconomic status	1.000								
Sex	−0.090	1.000							
Age	0.154	0.032	1.000						
Childhood health	−0.222[b,d]	0.124	0.083	1.000					
Parents' health	−0.109	0.080	−0.141	0.177	1.000				
Death wish by spouse	−0.012	0.064	0.075	0.175	0.211[b,d]	1.000			
Memory/fantasy about spouse	0.130	0.133	−0.009	−0.182	−0.163	−0.096	1.000		
Consistency about spouse contacts	0.387[a,f]	−0.114	−0.031	−0.198	−0.164	−0.232[b,e]	0.211[c,e]	1.000	
Financial matters	−0.105	0.048	0.076	0.032	−0.005	0.111	−0.212[b,d]	−0.078	1.000

[a] $p \le .001$ (two-tailed)
[b] $p \le .05$ (two-tailed)
[c] $p = .056$ (two-tailed)
[d] $N = 102$
[e] $N = 84$
[f] $N = 82$

no.* This variable was included because greater financial difficulties might adversely affect mental health.

• The question to the mental health professional rater: Is there lack of friends, social contacts? Answers ranged from 1 = not at all, to 7 = very severe.† This item was included because of the widely held view that a network of friends and social contacts is associated with better functioning and therefore may be associated with lower scores on measures of disturbance.

Correlation Matrix

The correlation matrix of the variables is shown in Table 11-1. Socioeconomic status is related to childhood (adolescent) health ($r = -.222$, $p \leq .05$), with lower status linked to poorer health. This finding is congruent with the generally accepted link of social class to health. Less obvious is the correlation of low socioeconomic status with less consistency, ($r = .387$, $p \leq .001$).

Poor parental health is associated with presence of death wish by spouse ($r = .211$, $p \leq .05$). Less consistency is associated with presence of death wish by spouse ($r = -.232$, $p \leq .05$). Financial problems since the separation are associated with memory/fantasy ($r = -.211$, $p \leq .05$). Less consistency is associated with more memory/fantasy ($r = .211$, $p = .056$).

Non-separation/divorce-related factors, which, as will be shown, affected mental health measures in our study, also appear to be linked to separation/divorce-related factors. This suggests the existence of a pattern of interaction between non-separation/divorce factors, separation/divorce factors, and measures of mental health.

Regression Analysis

FINDINGS

The results of the general regression analysis are shown in Table 11-2. The number of men reporting any suicide potential was too small to make meaningful calculations of the association of independent vari-

---

*In Sub 2 as a whole ($N = 106$), responses were 1 = yes (65.1 percent), 2 = no (34.9 percent). Greater anxiety was related to presence of greater financial difficulties by Kendall's tau, two-tailed analysis of significance ($\tau = -.177$, $p = .034$).

†In Sub 2 as a whole ($N = 102$) responses were: 1 (not present) = 79.4 percent; 2 (very mild) = 2.9 percent; 3 (mild) = 4.9 percent; 4 (moderate) = 10.8 percent; 5 (severe)
(Footnote continued on next page)

ables with the suicidal measures SPC 1, SPC 2, and ASP, and they have not been computed.

Of the basic demographic variables, only *socioeconomic status* was significantly associated with any dependent mental health variables; these were anxiety and the Social Functioning Rating Scale in Sub 2 as a whole, and in men, but not in women in that group. Of the variables not related to separation and divorce, the following showed significant relationships: *Parents' health* was associated with somatic discomfort in Sub 2 as a whole and in women in that subgroup and with anxiety in Sub 2 as a whole; *childhood health* was associated with somatic discomfort, the Social Functioning Rating Scale, and the BPRS in Sub 2 men. Childhood Health was also associated with two suicidal measures (SPC 1 and SPC 2) in Sub 2 as a whole. Of the separation/divorce related variables, the following showed significant relationships: *consistency* with somatic discomfort in Sub 2 men and Sub 2 as a whole, *death wish by spouse* with anxiety in Sub 2 women and Sub 2 as a whole; *memory/fantasy about spouse* with somatic discomfort in Sub 2 as a whole and with anxiety and depression in Sub 2 women and Sub 2 as a whole, and *not with spouse* with anxiety and depression in Sub 2 men. There were no significant associations with the *financial* variable, nor with *lack of friends/social contacts* when it was substituted for it, except for the Social Functioning Rating Scale.

COMMENTS ON FINDINGS

This section will deal with a comparison between the number and kind of significant associations found when variables entered in the regression equation were individually related to mental health measures using Kendall's tau and the number and kind of significant associations found in the regression analysis. It will also include some other comments.

Demographic Variables. There were no significant correlations involving age and only one involving sex: women were more likely than men to report somatic discomfort. It is not surprising that *there were no significant relations involving age and sex in the regression equation. The findings regarding age may be due to the narrow range into which these respondents fall,* and as older persons become divorced in large numbers this finding may change. There may in fact be no differences between the sexes regarding overall disturbance, except

---

= 2.0 percent; 6 (very severe) = 0.0 percent. Greater lack of friends was associated with more disturbance on the Social Functioning Rating Scale from which the item was taken (τ = .374, p = .002 [two-tailed]), and on the BPRS (τ = .191, p = .018 [two-tailed]).

Table 11-2
Overall Regression Equation (Sub 2)

Dependent Variable	Independent Variable	Beta, F			R^2			F			N. Int		
		M	F	M/F	M	F	M/F	M	F	M/F	M	F	M/F
SOMA	Financial	−.054,0.19	−.063,0.25	−.045,0.26	.740	.397	.478	7.10[a]	3.62[a]	7.34[a]	28.2.70	52.2.09	81.2.30
	Socioeconomic status	.173,1.84	.081,0.33	.122,1.60									
	Sex	NA	NA	−.173,3.85									
	Age	−.029,0.06	−.123,0.92	−.043,0.23									
	Childhood health	−.587,13.74[a]	−.021,0.03	−.176,3.70									
	Parents' health	−.167,1.16	−.296,5.42[b]	−.338,13.86[a]									
	Death wish about spouse	.101,0.65	−.083,0.42	−.034,0.14									
	Memory/fantasy[c]	.066,0.31	.264,3.94	.195,4.47[b]									
	Consistency	.300,6.04[2]	.223,2.41	.220,5.11[b]									
ANX	Financial	.065,0.18	−.132,1.23	−.045,0.25	.596	.455	.458	3.68[a]	4.59[a]	6.76[a]	28.1.09	52.2.44	81.1.94
	Socioeconomic status	.390,6.05[b]	.169,1.58	.239,5.94[b]									
	Sex	NA	NA	−.138,2.37									
	Age	−.086,0.32	−.079,0.42	−.056,0.38									
	Childhood health	−.162,0.67	.045,0.14	.012,0.02									
	Parents' health	−.056,0.84	−.193,2.54	−.189,4.16[b]									
	Death wish about spouse	.050,0.10	−.261,4.61[b]	−.209,5.12[b]									
	Memory/fantasy[c]	.312,4.44[b]	.393,9.70[l]	.384,16.65[a]									
	Consistency	.278,3.34	.010,0.01	.089,0.79									

(continued)

263

Table 11-2 (continued)

Dependent Variable	Independent Variable	Beta, F			R^2			F			N, Int		
		M	F	M/F	M	F	M/F	M	F	M/F	M	F	M/F
DEP	Financial	.160,0.89	−.030,0.05	.043,0.18	.518	.352	.317	2.69[b]	2.98[a]	3.71[a]	28,1.10	52,2.60	81,2.33
	Socioeconomic status	.391,5.10[b]	.009,0.00	.131,1.42									
	Sex	NA	NA	−.122,1.46									
	Age	−.062,0.14	−.085,0.40	−.073,0.52									
	Childhood health	−.132,0.38	.028,0.05	−.008,0.01									
	Parents' health	.048,0.05	−.087,0.44	−.103,0.98									
	Death wish about spouse	.030,0.03	−.118,0.79	−.105,1.01									
	Memory/fantasy[c]	.449,7.70[a]	.491,12.72[a]	.441,17.40[a]									
	Consistency	.064,0.15	.082,0.30	.073,0.42									
SOC	Financial	−.118,0.48	.073,0.28	−.031,0.08	.509	.265	.262	2.59[b]	1.99	2.84[a]	28,2.34	52,0.80	81,1.28
	Socioeconomic status	.394,5.09[b]	.226,2.09	.302,6.90[b]									
	Sex	NA	NA	.079,0.57									
	Age	−.006,0.00	.063,0.20	.068,0.42									
	Childhood health	−.548,6.35[b]	.070,0.25	−.050,0.21									
	Parents' health	.309,2.12	−.104,0.55	−.074,0.47									
	Death wish about spouse	.041,0.06	.047,0.11	−.000,0.00									
	Memory/fantasy[c]	−.052,0.10	.224,2.34	.108,0.97[a]									
	Consistency	.155,0.86	.251,2.50	.208,3.21									
BPRS	Financial	.057,0.13	.025,0.03	.015,0.02	.591	.263	.295	3.61[a]	1.97	3.34[a]	28,2.46	52,1.43	81,1.72
	Socioeconomic status	.274,2.94	.071,0.21	.215,3.68									
	Sex	NA	NA	.147,2.07									

Age	−.099,0.41	.074,0.27	.014,0.02
Childhood health	−.608,9.37[a]	.052,0.14	−.090,0.71
Parents' health	.209,1.15	−.170,1.46	−.176,2.80
Death wish about spouse	−.217,1.90	−.087,0.38	−.174,2.70
Memory/fantasy[c]	.125,0.70	.253,2.97	.186,3.00
Consistency	.086,0.32	.277,2.05	.116,1.04

SPC 1[d]

Financial	Not computed	.023,0.03	.037,0.10	—	.206	.145	1.43	1.36	—	52,1.98	81,1.23
Socioeconomic status		.183,1.27	.155,1.57								
Sex		NA	−.056,0.25								
Age		.104,0.50	.101,0.80								
Childhood health		−.275,3.55	−.258,4.84[b]								
Parents' health		.095,0.42	.092,0.63								
Death wish about spouse		−.266,3.27	−.122,1.10								
Memory/fantasy[c]		0.96,0.40	.118,0.99								
Consistency		−.171,1.07	−.101,0.65								

SPC 2[d]

Financial	Not computed	−.005,0.00	.072,0.43	—	.233	.195	1.67	1.94	—	52,0.29	81,−0.16
Socioeconomic status		.136,0.73	.182,2.30								
Sex		NA	−.037,0.11								
Age		.173,1.42	.138,1.56								
Childhood health		−.215,2.25	−.236,4.32[b]								
Parents' health		.103,0.52	.065,0.33								
Death wish about spouse		−.212,2.17	−.076,0.46								
Memory/fantasy[c]		.232,2.41	.225,3.86								
Consistency		−.060,0.14	−.041,0.11								

(continued)

265

Table 11-2 *(continued)*

Dependent Variable	Independent Variable	Beta, F			R^2			F			N, Int		
		M	F	M/F	M	F	M/F	M	F	M/F	M	F	M/F
ASP[d]	Financial	Not computed	.052,0.12	.058,0.25	—	.117	.110	—	0.73	0.99	—	52,1.54	81,1.31
	Socioeconomic status		.158,0.86	.129,1.04									
	Sex		NA	−.013,0.01									
	Age		.073,0.22	.122,1.11									
	Childhood health		−.162,1.11	−.213,3.17									
	Parents' health		.018,0.01	−.012,0.01									
	Death wish about spouse		−.214,1.90	−.061,0.26									
	Memory/fantasy[c]		.092,0.32	.073,0.37									
	Consistency		−.125,0.52	−.018,0.02									

[a] $p \leq .01$

[b] $p \leq .05$

[c] "Not with spouse" was used in place of "memory/fantasy" for males.

[d] There were not enough suicidal males to warrant computation of the correlation coefficient.

perhaps in the case of somatic discomfort. This does not mean that there is no difference between men and women as to what aspects of the separation/divorce process are associated with disturbance in each. This point will be further discussed.

Regarding *socioeconomic status,* significant correlations were found for all dependent mental health measures except for SPC 1 and ASP. In the regression analysis, only the relations to somatic discomfort and the Social Functioning Rating Scale remained significant. The association with the BPRS approached significance. The correlations reported above of lower socioeconomic status with poorer health and less consistency may be a factor in the reduced number of significant relations. Socioeconomic status affects mental health in the recently separated/divorced, and there may be interactions with other variables which mediate the relationship.

Non-separation/divorce related variables. Two variables, *childhood health* and *parents' health,* were included in this group. In the instance of parents' health there were two significant correlations— somatic discomfort and anxiety—and the same two are also significant in the regression equation. For childhood (adolescent) health, there were significant correlations with somatic discomfort and all three suicidal measures. In the regression analysis, two of the suicidal measures remained significantly related and the other two associations approached significance. These data suggest that the two variables exert their influence on mental health measures largely independently of each other and of other variables included in the regression equation.

Separation/divorce related variables. Three subgroups were included in the general regression analysis: attachment and loss, represented by memory/fantasy; interspouse hostility, represented by death wish by spouse; and ambiguity, represented by consistency. In all instances, there are fewer significant associations in the regression equation than were found in the Kendall correlations. In the latter, all three independent variables were significantly related to somatic discomfort, anxiety, depression, and at least one other mental health measure. In the regression analysis, only *memory/fantasy* remained significant for three dependent variables. The others are significant only in relation to one each.

Prior regression equations (Appendix II) indicate that the difference between significance in Kendall correlations and the regression equation is largely due to interaction between the variables of the separation/divorce process, rather than to the interaction of these with other variables in the regression equation. Aspects of the separation/divorce process are related to mental health, but interactions between variables describing the process limit our ability to identify the contribution of each component to mental health measures.

Other variables. Financial difficulties showed no significant associations when included in the regression equation. Individual Kendall correlations were significant with anxiety. Rated lack of friends and social contacts showed significant associations in the regression equation only with the Social Functioning Rating Scale, while Kendall correlations were significant also with the BPRS. In this study financial difficulties and lack of friends have some significant individual correlations with mental health measures, but net effects are minimal.

REGRESSION ANALYSIS WITH DEPENDENT VARIABLES INDICATIVE OF SUICIDE POTENTIAL FOR SUB 2

As noted in relation to the overall regression equation (see Table 11-2), there were only two significant associations involving the three suicidal dependent measures. These involved childhood health and suicide potential at entry (SPC 1) and suicide potential at interview (SPC 2). However, the overall F value for the regression equation was not significant in relation to any of the three measures of suicide potential.

For this reason, a separate regression analysis was done, including only demographic characteristics and those independent variables shown in previous regression analyses to be significantly associated with two or more suicidal measures for Sub 2. The marginal distribution in all three suicidal measures is skewed due to the fact that the majority of respondents did not have any suicide potential. For SPC 1 (suicide potential retrospectively assessed to time of admission), 73 of 102 respondents had zero suicide potential (71.6 percent). For SPC 2 (suicide potential at time of interview), the corresponding figure was 81 respondents (79.4 percent) and for ASP (assessment of suicide potential by mental health raters), it was 82 (80.4 percent).

Variables Selected

Demographic variables were age, sex, socioeconomic status, and presence or absence of children. They were included because they either showed significant associations with suicide potential in this study, and/or have been reported in the literature to be so associated.

Non-separation/divorce–related variables included respondent's health between ages 16 and 20 *(childhood health)*. In the general regression analysis, poor childhood health was associated with more suicide potential in two out of three suicidal measures.

Separation/divorce related variables did not include any of the variables in this category which were included in the general regression equation, since none met the criteria for inclusion. Two variables were included: reality testing and defense against anger. Reality testing is defined as the difference between the degree of likelihood of reconciliation as estimated by the respondent on a scale of 1 to 5, and by the rater, similarly estimated. The higher the score, the poorer the reality testing. Defense against anger is defined by the mental health professional's response to the question: to what extent does respondent appear to be defending against feelings of anger associated with separation from the spouse? Responses ranged from 1 = not at all to 5 = extremely great. Poorer reality testing and greater defense against anger had been shown to be associated with increased suicide potential on two or three suicidal measures in Kendall correlation and preliminary regression analyses (see Chapters 7, 9, and Appendix II).

Correlation Matrix

Items included are sex, age, socioeconomic status, presence or absence of children,* childhood health, reality testing, and defense against anger. Correlations are for Sub 2 as a whole. Correlations reported in connection with the general regression analysis will not be repeated. Significant correlations were as follows:

• Presence of children is related to older age ($r = -.290$, $p \leq .01$, $N = 106$).

• Presence of children is possibly related to less defense against anger ($r = .167$, $p = .094$, $N = 102$).

• Poorer reality testing is related to greater defense against anger ($r = .192$, $p = .054$, $N = 102$).

Significant correlations with variables in the general regression equation (Table 11-2) are:

• Poorer reality testing is related to more memory/fantasy ($r = .329$, $p \leq .001$, $N = 102$).

• Poorer reality testing is related to less consistency ($r = .497$, $p \leq .001$, $N = 84$).

• Greater defense against anger is related to more memory/fantasy ($r = .295$, $p \leq .01$, $N = 102$).

---

*Presence of children: yes = 1, no = 2.

Table 11-3

Variables Related to Suicidal Dependent Measures (Sub 2)

Dependent Variable	Independent Variable	Beta, F			R^2			F			N, Int		
		M	F	M/F	M	F	M/F	M	F	M/F	M	F	M/F
SPC 1[c]	Sex	Not computed		−.052,0.30	—	.253	.214	—	3.39[a]	3.53[b]	—	66,−0.20	98,−0.24
	Age		.244,3.75	.150,2.25									
	Socioeconomic status		.022,0.03	.116,1.39									
	Presence/absence of child		.307,6.37[a]	.207,4.26									
	Reality testing		.062,0.27	.086,0.75									
	Defense against anger		.144,1.36	.197,3.99[b]									
	Childhood health		−.306,6.76[b]	−.246,6.26[b]									
SPC 2[c]	Sex	Not computed		−.036,0.16	—	.389	.326	—	6.37[a]	6.30[a]	—	66,−1.28	98,−1.25
	Age		.308,7.29[a]	.178,3.70									
	Socioeconomic status		.022,0.04	.181,3.93									
	Presence/absence of child		.337,9.35[a]	.231,6.22[b]									
	Reality testing		.171,2.50	.216,5.57[b]									

270

Defense against anger	.268,5.74[b]	.245,7.19[b]				
Childhood health	−.280,6.94[b]	−.226,6.17[b]				
ASP[c]						
Sex	Not computed	−.041,0.20	.260	—	3.52[a]	66,−0.51
Age	.221,3.08	.175,3.29	.269		4.71[a]	98, 0.47
Socioeconomic status	.001,0.00	.126,1.74				
Presence/absence of child	.298,6.04[a]	.230,5.65[b]				
Reality testing	.142,1.44	.204,4.61[b]				
Defense against anger	.242,3.90	.236,6.15[b]				
Childhood health	−.190,2.64	−.190,4.02[b]				

[a] $p \leqq .01$
[b] $p \leqq .05$
[c] There were not enough suicidal males to warrant computation of the correlation coefficient.

Regression Analysis

The results of the regression analysis are shown in Table 11-3, which includes Sub 2 and women in that subgroup. Findings are not reported for men, since only five to seven men were reported to exhibit any suicidal potential.

It is clear that the independent variables which influence the suicidal variables are somewhat different from those that affect other dependent mental health measures. Of the demographic variables, age is significantly associated with suicide potential on one measure in women. More associations would probably be found if the age range were wider. Socioeconomic status was previously found to be significantly associated with SPC 2 when Kendall correlation analysis was used and just fails to reach the .05 level of significance with SPC 2 in the regression analysis. Sex was not significantly associated. *Absence of children* is related to suicide potential for Sub 2 as a whole and for women on all three measures, probably related to the greater likelihood that women without children live alone, and living alone is generally considered to be a risk factor for suicide.[3]

The *non-separation/divorce–related variable,* health between the ages of 16 and 20 *childhood health,* was significantly associated with all three suicidal measures. This finding confirms that suicide potential in the recently separated/divorced is also related to factors existing prior to the marital dissolution.

Both *separation/divorce related variables—defense against anger* and *poor reality testing* regarding likelihood of reconciliation—were significantly associated with two or three measures of suicide potential. The former is generally recognized to be associated with suicide potential, while the latter has not previously been reported. Both can be useful in alerting clinicians to possible suicidal risk.

Thus, *recently separated/divorced persons are more likely to be suicidal if they are older, report poor health between ages 16 and 20, have no children (for women), tend to misjudge reality in terms of possible reconciliation* (typically in the direction of underestimating its likelihood), *and defend against anger regarding the separation.*

SEX DIFFERENCES IN THE RECENTLY SEPARATED/DIVORCED

A number of differences between the findings regarding Sub 2 men and women were apparent in the regression analyses. In the general regression analysis (Table 11-2), women had a significant association between poorer parents' health and greater somatic discomfort, while men but not women had a significant relationship between their own poorer health between ages 16 and 20 (childhood health), greater somatic discomfort, and poorer adjustment on the Social Functioning Rating Scale. Men showed a relationship between lower socioeconomic status and more anxiety.

Extent of memory and fantasy regarding the spouse was included in the general regression equation for Sub 2 women only, since it was previously shown that more memory and fantasy was significantly related to more disturbance as indicated on several mental health measures in women but not in men. Conversely, not being happy not being with the spouse was associated with more disturbance in men only, and was therefore included in the general regression analysis for men instead of memory/fantasy. Perceiving the spouse as wishing respondent dead related to greater anxiety in women but not in men.

One of the limitations of this study is that the number of Sub 2 men was relatively small ($N = 32$ for most analyses) compared to women ($N = 80$ for most analyses). As a result it is difficult to determine to what extent differences between the sexes are generalizable to other populations. The data obtained suggest that men who are most disturbed in the separation/divorce process may be those who entered marriage with a poorer health history and who are concretely dependent on the spouse. They do not demonstrate a relationship of mental health measures to the relatively more subtle emotional phenomena of spending time in memory or fantasy about the spouse and/or perceiving a death wish in the spouse. Conceivably, men are less likely to conceptualize their experience in emotional terms. This is not to say that they do not experience these phenomena; only that they may not integrate that experience into their awareness or relate it to discomfort or disturbance.

Women, on the other hand, appear to be more disturbed if they report poorer health in their parents, if they experience and acknowledge spending more time in memory and/or fantasy about the spouse, and experience a death wish from the spouse.

REGRESSION ANALYSIS IN OTHER SUBGROUPS

No attempt was made to systematically cull the independent variables that had maximum impact on the dependent variables for persons seriously discussing separation/divorce but not separated (Sub 1) and the longer-term separated/divorced (Sub 3) for whom the last separation-related event occurred more than 14 months prior to date of interview. The variables identified as significant for Sub 2, were, however, applied to Sub 1 and Sub 3, to see to what extent, if any, they were significant.

Persons Seriously Discussing Separation or Divorce but not Separated (Sub 1)

A regression analysis was done for Sub 1, using the same variables included in the general regression equation of Sub 2 (Table 11-2), with the omission of the consistency variable, which was irrelevant since the spouses lived together and were in daily contact. Further, the variable relating to lack of friends or social contacts replaced financial difficulties, because the latter applies to the time after separation. Lack of friends or social contacts was significantly associated in Sub 1 with increased disturbance as indicated by the Social Functioning Rating Scale ($\tau = .376$, $p < .01$) and also with the higher scores on the Brief Psychiatric Rating Scale ($\tau = .267$, $p = .01$). Other Kendall correlations were not significant.

The results of the regression equation are shown in Table 11-4. Regarding demographic factors, *sex* differences were found to be more important in those married and seriously discussing separation/divorce than in the recently separated/divorced. Women indicated higher degrees of subjective disturbance before the separation discussion than men, but men indicated increasing disturbance after the separation, and therefore the difference between the sexes is diminished after that event.

Of the non-separation/divorce–related variables, *poorer childhood health* was related to greater somatic discomfort. It is not clear why only one association (childhood health) is significant for this group, and why it is particularly associated with somatic discomfort, while there are more associations with childhood health and some associations with parents' health in the recently separated/divorced.

Of the separation/divorce-related variables only *perceived death wish by spouse* was associated with disturbance in the married but seriously discussing separation/divorce group, though this finding must be treated with caution due to the skewed distribution.* Such an association might be expected, since death wishes from someone with whom

---

*Responses to the question: Did your (former) spouse ever seriously wish you dead? in Sub 1 were: yes = 9, don't know = 2, no = 51. Thus 82.3 percent denied perceiving death wishes in the spouse.

Table 11-4
Overall Regression Equation, All Categories, Males and Females Combined (Sub 1)[a]

Dependent Variable	Independent Variable	Beta	F	R^2	F	N	Int
SOMA	Sex	−.379	7.84[b]	.295	2.51[c]	56	2.57
	Age	−.130	1.01				
	Socioeconomic status	−.087	0.46				
	Childhood health	−.275	4.25[c]				
	Parents' health	.047	0.14				
	Death wish by spouse	.199	2.56				
	Memory/fantasy about spouse	−.050	0.15				
	Lack of friends	−.045	0.12				
ANX	Sex	−.385	7.43[b]	.233	1.82	56	2.13
	Age	−.127	0.88				
	Socioeconomic status	.010	0.01				
	Childhood health	−.014	0.01				
	Parents' health	.058	0.19				
	Death wish by spouse	−.178	1.89				
	Memory/fantasy about spouse	.136	0.98				
	Lack of friends	.118	0.75				
DEP	Sex	−.396	8.18[b]	.264	2.15[c]	56	−0.69
	Age	.169	1.62				
	Socioeconomic status	−.112	0.74				

(continued)

275

Table 11-4 *(continued)*

Dependent Variable	Independent Variable	Beta	F	R^2	F	N	Int
	Childhood health	−.082	0.36				
	Parents' health	−.031	0.06				
	Death wish by spouse	−.145	1.29				
	Memory/fantasy about spouse	.139	1.07				
	Lack of friends	.014	0.01				
SOC	Sex	.048	0.15	.400	4.00[b]	56	2.22
	Age	.053	0.20				
	Socioeconomic status	−.010	0.01				
	Childhood health	−.007	0.00				
	Parents' health	.045	0.14				
	Death wish by spouse	−.323	9.72[b]				
	Memory/fantasy about spouse	−.074	0.37				
	Lack of friends	.474	15.50[b]				
BPRS	Sex	−.194	2.19	.336	3.04[b]	56	1.70
	Age	.160	1.61				
	Socioeconomic status	.062	0.25				
	Childhood health	.084	0.42				
	Parents' health	.016	0.02				
	Death wish by spouse	−.415	11.82[b]				
	Memory/fantasy about spouse	−.076	0.35				
	Lack of friends	.355	7.87[b]				
SPC 1	Sex	−.087	0.39	.254	2.05	56	2.57
	Age	−.069	0.27				

	Variable						
	Socioeconomic status	.011	0.01				
	Childhood health	-.156	1.29				
	Parents' health	.095	0.53				
	Death wish by spouse	-.401	9.79[b]				
	Memory/fantasy about spouse	.206	2.32				
	Lack of friends	-.056	0.19				
SPC 2	Sex	-.230	2.33	.124	0.85	56	-0.70
	Age	-.005	0.00				
	Socioeconomic status	-.034	0.06				
	Childhood health	.133	0.79				
	Parents' health	.118	0.69				
	Death wish by spouse	-.078	0.31				
	Memory/fantasy about spouse	.224	2.32				
	Lack of friends	.047	0.10				
ASP	Sex	-.179	1.40	.123	0.84	56	0.57
	Age	.030	0.04				
	Socioeconomic status	.065	0.21				
	Childhood health	.152	1.05				
	Parents' health	.089	0.39				
	Death wish by spouse	-.187	1.81				
	Memory/fantasy about spouse	.101	0.47				
	Lack of friends	.213	2.15				

[a]Separate regression analyses for women and men are not reported, since the small number of cases in each group makes interpretation of the findings difficult.

[b]$p \leqslant .01$

[c]$p \leqslant .05$

one lives could be of particular significance. It is plausible that variables indicative of lost attachment—*memory/fantasy* and *not being happy not being with the spouse*—would not be significant in people still living together.

Of the other variables, *lack of friends** was associated in this subgroup with more disturbance not only on the Social Functioning Rating Scale, but also on the Brief Psychiatric Rating Scale. In comparison to the recently separated/divorced, in whom the only significant association was with the Social Functioning Rating Scale, this finding suggests that lack of friends may be more significant in those still married.

The relationship of spouse interaction to mental health in couples still married but seriously discussing separation and/or divorce may have more in common with the situation involving marital pairs in general than with that of separated and/or divorced persons.

Longer-Term Separated and/or Divorced (Sub 3)

The regression analysis for Sub 3 used independent variables which had been shown to be significant for Sub 2. The purpose was to determine to what extent these same variables were still significant for Sub 3. The total number of respondents was 56, too small to allow separate analysis by males and females.

Variables included were *sex, age, socioeconomic status, childhood (adolescent) health, parents' health, death wish by spouse, memory and/or fantasy regarding spouse,* and *lack of friends.* The analysis was done first without and then with the *consistency* variable. This variable, which relates to former spouse contacts is meaningful only to respondents who were in contact with each other in the two weeks prior to interview. The number of those in contact is 30. Because of the small number of findings, only the positive findings will be noted. These findings must be interpreted with caution, since the *F* value for the regression equation was significant only for the Social Functioning Rating Scale, when the consistency variable was excluded, and that is to be expected because of the inclusion of the "lack of friends" item which is part of that scale.

Of the demographic variables, the association of *lower socioeconomic status* with more suicide potential on SPC 1 was significant. Neither of the non-separation/divorce–related variables was signifi-

---

*Regarding lack of friends, 72.6 percent were rated as having no significant lack of friends, while the remainder were reported to have various degrees of such lack.

cant; only the relationship of less *consistency* regarding spouse contact was significantly associated with higher scores on the BPRS. The *F* value for the regression equation was not significant. Further, the skewed distribution of the responses to the consistency question in Sub 3 must be kept in mind.* Because of the limitations, it is possible that this association is due to chance, but it is also possible that for longer-term separated or divorced who were still in contact, inconsistency may in fact prove to be associated with greater disturbance. Further studies are required to resolve this point. Of the other variables, *lack of friends* was significantly associated with higher scores on the anxiety and depression measures, on the Social Functioning Rating Scale, and on the Brief Psychiatric Rating Scale. The findings suggest that lack of friends plays a more important role in the long-term separated/divorced than it does in the recently separated/divorced. It is of interest to note that these factors differ substantially from those applying to the recently separated/divorced. Sub 3 does not differ in overall disturbance from Sub 2. Thus, longer-term separated or divorced people who seek help in a crisis clinic are as disturbed as those who have recently experienced separation/divorce, but the specific factors related to the separation appear to differ.

Some factors relating to the former spouse, i.e., memory/fantasy about the spouse and perceived death wish by spouse may become less important as time goes on. The suggestion that inconsistency regarding spouse contacts may be associated with greater disturbance raises the possibility that what goes on between former spouses may affect the mental health of each in the long run. Some of the individual correlations reported earlier also suggest this possibility.

SUMMARY

In this chapter, variables that had previously been shown to have an effect on mental health measures were re-analyzed to determine whether they continued to have an impact when other variables were held constant. Two regression analyses were carried out for the recently separated and/or divorced (Sub 2). The first of these was based on findings regarding the relationship of independent variables to all eight mental health measures. The second was based on findings regarding the three suicidal potential measures only.

_____

*The distribution was as follows: 1 = *Almost never* says one thing and does another regarding spouse contacts, 19; 2 = *Rarely*, 4; 3 = *Sometimes*, 4; 4 = *Frequently*, 2; 5 = *Almost always*, 1.

In the first analysis variables that were significantly associated with higher scores on one or more of the eight mental health measures were: lower socioeconomic status, poorer parental health, poorer adolescent health, greater time spent in memory and/or fantasy about former spouse, respondent's perception that the former spouse wished him or her dead, and respondent's greater inconsistency in arranging contacts with the former spouse.

In the second analysis, variables that were significantly related to greater suicide potential on two or three of the three measures of suicide potential were absence of children, poorer adolescent health, poor reality testing, and greater defense against anger.

In the recently separated/divorced group, there were differences between men and women. Since the number of men was much smaller than that of women, the findings must be interpreted with caution. Findings regarding suicidal measures could not be analyzed for men because of the small number of men who were suicidal. As to the analysis based on all mental health measures, variables that were significantly associated with higher scores on one or more mental health measures in men were lower socioeconomic status, poorer adolescent health, and respondent's statement of not being as happy without the spouse. In women, the variables associated with higher scores on one or more mental health measures were poorer parental health, greater amounts of memory and/or fantasy regarding the spouse, and respondent's perception that former spouse ever wished him or her dead. The findings suggest that in men disturbance is more likely to be associated with concrete dependence on spouse, whereas more subtle emotional factors, such as memory and fantasy about the former spouse, may be more important in women.

A regression analysis was also carried out for the group still married but seriously considering separation and/or divorce. No attempt was made to select the variables which have the greatest impact on the mental health of this group as such. Instead, the analysis used variables selected for Sub 2 to determine which, if any, also impacted Sub 1. Variables associated with higher scores on one or more mental health measures in Sub 1 were female sex, poorer adolescent health, and respondent's perception that former spouse ever wished him or her dead. The latter finding must be treated with caution due to a skewed distribution. Those still married but discussing separation/divorce may be more similar to the married group as a whole than to the separated or divorced population, in that factors unrelated to marital discord may play a larger role than factors associated with the potential end of the marriage.

A similar analysis was carried for Sub 3. Few significant associations were found, but the findings suggest that lack of friends may be more important for this group than for the recently separated/divorced. While the overall level of mental health did not differ between Sub 2 and Sub 3, the specific factors related to disturbance in Sub 2 were not found to be related to disturbance in Sub 3, except, perhaps, for consistency regarding spouse contacts. This finding suggests that while the relationship with the former spouse may still be significant, determinants of mental health in the longer-term separated/divorced group differ from those relevant to the recently separated/divorced.

REFERENCES

1. Luborsky L, Todd TC, Katcher A: A self-administered social assets scale for predicting physical and psychological illness and health. J Psychosom Res 17:109, 120, 1973
2. Langner TS, Michael ST: Life stress and mental health. London, Collier-MacMillan Ltd., 1963
3. Zung WWK: Index of potential suicide (IPS). A rating scale for suicide prevention, in Beck AT, Resnik HLP, Lettieri DJ (Eds): The Prediction of Suicide. Bowie, MD, Charles Press Publishers, 1974, pp 221–249

12
Concluding Comments

This chapter will highlight the findings of several topics which have been previously discussed.

RELATIONSHIP TO FORMER SPOUSE

Similarities between loss of spouse by death and loss by separation/divorce include the presence of grief and the possibility of an adaptive or maladaptive outcome. Differences are due, first, to the continued existence of the living former spouse. In addition, the relationship between former spouses at the time of divorce is typically less-satisfactory and angrier, overtly or covertly, than that between spouses at the time of death of one of them.

This section will deal with the relationship between the former spouses in three areas. The first is the actual interaction as described by the respondents. The second concerns wishes, feelings and fantasies about the former spouse, regardless of the presence or quality of any real interaction. The third addresses the ambiguity which often characterizes the inter-former spouse relationship.

Interaction Between Former Spouses

There is a connection between what goes on between members of intact families and the mental health of each member. The same is true of the interaction between former spouses so long as their lives continue to impact on one another. The relationship between two people rarely ends suddenly and completely after separation or divorce. In our study, the recently separated, by a ratio of 11:1, had some form of contact with the former spouse in the two weeks prior to interview, and about a third of those divorced or separated for longer had some contact with the former spouse during the same period. A significant minority of the recently separated/divorced continued to rely on their former spouse emotionally and for practical matters, and about one in seven acknowledged some form of sexual contact with him or her in the prior two weeks. While interaction was often because of children, childless couples also frequently maintained contact, and those who had children often related to each other regarding other matters as well.

One of the hypotheses of this study was that in the recently separated and/or divorced, the more frequent the contacts between former spouses, the greater the disturbance as indicated by the chosen mental health measures. We felt that contact between former spouses is likely to be associated with frustration of emotional needs and/or guilt, which was predicted to result in measurable changes in the mental health measures. The findings, however, did not result in a clear-cut confirmation or refutation of the hypothesis. It is possible that there is a U-shaped relationship between former spouse contact and mental health, with greater disturbance associated with no contacts and many contacts, and less disturbance with a middle range of contacts.

Another hypothesis of our study was that in the recently separated and/or divorced, the greater the emotional reliance on the former spouse in the two weeks prior to interview, the greater the disturbance on the mental health measures. Emotional reliance, as observed by a professional rater, was associated with more disturbance on several measures. Self-reported emotional reliance, however, was not so associated. This finding suggests that reliance evident to a trained observer, but not necessarily conscious or admitted by the respondent, is likely to be disturbing.

A parallel hypothesis was proposed regarding everyday reliance. There were some significant associations in the expected direction for the recently separated/divorced as a whole. Breakdown by gender showed that this association was present in men but not in women. Women were more likely to show an association of emotional reliance with disturbance, a point to which we will return.

An important and potentially destructive aspect of the continued interaction of former spouse is that of hostility. Hostility is common and takes a variety of forms, some of which are specifically related to separation and divorce, such as using financial and custody matters against the spouse, and others of which relate to death wishes, both expressed and implied. Physical expressions of hostility are common and sometimes life-threatening. Hostility both directed toward the former spouse and reported as coming from former spouse were associated with more disturbance on a number of mental health measures, and with less disturbance on a few (see Chapter 8). The issue of hostility was not addressed in relation to the longer-term separated/divorced group.

The findings indicate that contacts between former spouses are common, and that under some circumstances they are disturbing for the recently separated/divorced.

Wishes, Feelings and Fantasies about Former Spouse

Whether or not there is an actual relationship between former spouses, wishes, feelings, and fantasies about the former spouse plays an important role in the psychological life of the separated and/or divorced.

In the recently separated and/or divorced, less than a quarter definitely wanted a reconciliation; slightly more were uncertain, and just under one half said that they probably or definitely did not want a reconciliation. Persons contacted earlier in the separation process were more likely to want a reconciliation than those further along. Strong feelings on the subject were common: only about a third had no or mild affect; the balance had moderate, strong, or extremely strong affect, regardless of whether they did or did not wish a reconciliation. Wanting reconciliation was significantly related to disturbance on several measures in the recently separated/divorced. In the longer-term separated/divorced group, this association was not found; on the contrary, those still wishing to reconcile actually showed less disturbance on two measures. This finding must be considered with caution, because only a few persons in the longer-term group still wished to reconcile, and no explanation for this finding was readily apparent.

Slightly less than one half of all respondents said they were still in love with the former spouse or were uncertain, but those still in love were concentrated in the earlier stages of the separation process. In the longer-term group, only one in five was still in love. Somewhat more—about six in ten overall—missed the former spouse. Again, fewer missed the spouse in the later stages of the separation/divorce process. Almost seven out of ten respondents overall were just as happy not being with the former spouse.

Being in love with or missing the former spouse, and not being just as happy without the spouse, are all associated with more disturbance on a number of non-suicidal measures in the recently separated/divorced. In the longer-term group, there are only a few significant associations, but these involve variables indicative of suicide potential. Because of the smaller number of persons having such feelings and because of the small number of suicidal individuals in the longer-term group, these findings need replication. If they are replicated, then continued missing and wanting to be with the spouse in the longer-term group could be an indicator of increased risk of suicide.

The presence of sadness, anger, and guilt about the separation, and preoccupation with memory or fantasy about the former spouse, parallel grief following bereavement. All of these were shown to be common in the recently separated and/or divorced, being present in four to seven out of each ten of our respondents. In the longer-term group, they were less frequent, occurring in between one and under three in ten. All these aspects of the grief process were significantly related to two or more mental health measures in the recently separated/divorced. There were not as many associations in the longer-term group, but those that were present included some with suicidal measures. Anger turned against the self and unrealistic guilt are also associated with disturbance in the recently separated/divorced, but the finding in the longer-term group is not conclusive.

Increased disturbance associated with feelings about the former spouse does not necessarily imply that the absence of such feelings is desirable. When there has been a real loss, the complete absence of grief and its associated disturbance may foreshadow greater difficulties in the long run. As with grief following bereavement, it is likely that there is an optimal amount of painful feeling related to the former spouse, and that both less and more than that amount may create difficulty at a later date.

Ambiguity in the Relationship Between Former Spouses

One aspect of the proposed model of separation and divorce dealt with persons going back and forth between desires for separation and reconciliation. The model suggests that this situation will occur when absence of the former spouse is associated with a high level of disturbance and psychological pain, and action may be taken to resume the relationship with the former spouse. Unfortunately, this step may result in a recurrence or intensification of the conflict that brought about the separation in the first place. Separation occurs again, and the cycle starts over.

The research, since it does not follow persons over time, cannot address this issue directly. Three variables in the study, however, dealt with how consistent, clear and realistic respondents were on issues related to the separation. Together these three variables represent ambiguity. The greater the ambiguity, the more likely it is that the respondents will alternate between being together with and apart from the former spouse. The three variables are (1) vacillation, defined as the number of times respondent and spouse vacillated about separation since the first decision to separate; (2) consistency, defined as the extent to which respondent says one thing but does another about contacts with the former spouse; and (3) reality testing, defined as the extent to which the respondent differs from the rater in estimating the likelihood of reconciliation. It is assumed that the rater is more realistic than the respondent.

Vacillation was the most commonly observed variable. Among the recently separated/divorced, 70 percent changed their mind at least once; as did 40 percent of the longer-term separated/divorced group. Lack of consistency was acknowledged by 40 percent of the recently separated/divorced who were in contact with the former spouse. There was a difference between raters and respondents as to the likelihood of reconciliation in slightly less than half of the respondents.

More vacillation, less consistency, and poorer reality testing were all associated with greater disturbance in the recently separated/divorced. In the longer-term group there were no associations regarding vacillation. The association was not tested regarding the other two variables.

Raters were asked to assess whether preoccupation with the spouse (i.e., memory/fantasy) was in the service of giving up the relationship or maintaining it. The recently separated/divorced were considered to use memory/fantasy to hold on to the relationship more than twice as often as those who used it to let go. Thus, ambiguity about the extent and nature of the separation is frequent in the separation/divorce process and is associated with greater disturbance.

Relationship Between Former Spouses: Summary

The overall findings confirm that the relationship between former spouses is important. There are a number of significant associations of various aspects of this relationship with mental health measures. The findings suggest that disturbance will be less when there is a moderate amount of contact between the spouses and when emotional reliance is acknowledged when it exists. Other factors associated with less disturbance are the absence of most forms of overt hostility between the former spouses, and the absence of wishes for reconciliation. Persons not missing the former spouse and not likely to spend considerable time in memory and fantasy about the former spouse will tend to be less disturbed. The same is true of those who are clear about the status of separation and are consistent about contact with the former spouse.

RELATIONSHIPS WITH OTHERS

While the relationship to the former spouse is significantly associated with mental health, it is plausible that other interpersonal relationships also play a role. This subject was addressed by exploring the presence or absence of friends or social supports, involvement with relatives and friends in alliances that shut out the spouse, and the relationships with new love partners.

The issue of social supports was not a major focus of the present study, and was addressed by way of the Social Functioning Rating Scale (SFRS). This required a determination by the professional rater as to whether there was lack of friends or social contacts. Only 20 percent among the recently separated/divorced were rated as having any such lack. Lack of friends or social contacts in the recently separated/divorced was significantly related to the SFRS from which it was drawn and the BPRS. In the longer-term group, lack of friends or social contacts was also associated with anxiety and depression. This finding suggests that lack of friends may be more important to the longer-term than to the recently separated/divorced. Alliances with family members and friends that shut out the former spouse were common and tended to be associated with more rather than less disturbance, particularly if they were formed after the separation. This finding suggests that some relationships with others can have negative rather than positive implications for the respondent's mental health.

New love partners were common. About 80 percent of the respondents had dated at one time since the separation. Over half of those still living together but discussing separation were romantically and/or sexually involved with another person, and this was also true of 90 percent of those who had filed for or received final decree of divorce. In general, this involvement appeared to be beneficial, with persons who had ever been romantically/sexually involved outside of their marriage having lower scores on several measures of disturbance. This finding needs to be viewed with caution, however, because so few of those in our study were *not* involved outside of the marriage. However, in recently separated/divorced men, increased interest in sex was associated with more, not less depression.

FACTORS NOT RELATED TO SEPARATION/DIVORCE

The separation/divorce process could not account for all of the variances in mental health measures. No claim is made for spreading so wide a net as to try to include all determinants of mental health. Thus a limited number of factors unrelated to divorce were also considered. Variables selected were parents' health and respondent's health between the ages of 16 and 20, factors which cannot be the result of marital dissolution, since they preceded it. The main purpose for including these variables was to enter them in a regression equation to show how factors related to and not related to separation and divorce would impact mental health measures when the others were held constant. It was found that in each group some measures were affected in the presence of the other group, confirming that neither pre-existing nor divorce-related factors alone account for the mental health level of the separated/divorced.

Demographic Factors

These include sex, age, socioeconomic status, and presence and absence of children. There was greater disturbance in women on several measures, but the differences were largely confined to the group still married but discussing separation. Disturbance in men increased relative to that in women after the separation, so that the sexes differed on only one measure in the recently separated/divorced and on none in the longer-term group. Increasing age was associated with more disturbance on one suicidal measure. Lower socioeconomic status was associated with seven of eight measures of disturbance (all but depression) in the group as a whole, and analysis by marital subgroups showed that its impact was greatest in the recently separated/divorced. Absence of children was associated with more suicide potential.

OVERVIEW OF FACTORS ASSOCIATED WITH MENTAL HEALTH

A regression equation was used to consider the net effect of variables related to the former spouse, to persons other than the former spouse, to factors preceding separation/divorce, and to demographic variables. Three variables pertaining to the relationship to the former spouse were significant in relation to one or more mental health measures: the amount of time spent in memory/fantasy regarding the spouse; the fact that the spouse was thought at one time to wish the respondent dead; and the respondent's saying one thing but doing another regarding spouse contacts. These findings confirm that several aspects of the inter-former spouse relationship are important when other variables are held constant. Two variables pre-dating divorce— parents' health and respondents' health between ages 16 and 20, and socio-economic status—were also significant on one or more measures. Lack of friends and new love partners were either not entered into the regression equation or were not significant.

A separate regression analysis considered only the relationship of the independent variables to the three measures of suicide potential. Two factors related to the former spouse were associated with more suicide potential: defense against anger, and less-adequate reality testing regarding the likelihood of separation. Also associated were parents' health, poor health between ages 16 and 20, and lower socioeconomic status.

The findings can be interpreted as contradicting the theory that disturbance in the separated/divorced is entirely the result of pre-existing pathology. On the other hand, they do not support the view that disturbance is entirely explained by the stress of divorce, since pre-existing factors and socioeconomic status play a role. Relations to others may be less important than is commonly thought, regarding mental health in the recently separated/divorced.

Special Considerations Involving Suicide and Homicide

Because they constitute a threat to life, suicide and homicide risks are particularly important in relation to separation and divorce. Depending on the subgroup and measure, two to three of ten respondents were considered to have any degree of suicide potential. While this is much higher than the potential in the general population, it was somewhat lower than originally expected in light of the belief that the loss of a major relationship will heighten suicidal risk. (The popular concept of "dying of a broken heart" comes to mind in this context.)

The statistical measures of association of suicidal potential with other variables must be viewed with caution because of the relatively small proportion of respondents with this potential. A number of independent variables were so associated in the recently separated/divorced. In addition to poor reality testing regarding the likelihood of reconciliation and greater defense against anger, a number of variables were significant in relation to one or more of the three suicidal variables when individually correlated. These include (1) spouse initiation of separation, (2) lack of clarity as indicated by more frequent vacillation, (3) discrepancy between wish for and likelihood of reconciliation, (4) spouse hostility (particularly verbal), (5) death wish by spouse (also related to one measure in the longer-term group), and (6) failure to be romantically/sexually involved with someone other than the former spouse. The findings suggest that suicide risk is probably not a common accompaniment of separation/divorce, but is of real concern in special circumstances.

Another issue on which the present study could shed only limited light is that of homicide risk in the context of separation or divorce. Crime reports suggest that homicide is commonly a family matter, and a review of newspaper clippings indicates that situations involving separation are commonly mentioned in stories about homicide. Three of our 102 respondents reported that they did try to kill the (former) spouse at one time, and 12 indicated that the spouse had tried to kill the respondent. Ten of these 12 reported that the attempts occurred after the separation discussion. In addition, four respondents said they encouraged the (former) spouse to commit suicide, three said they did so after the separation discussion, and six respondents reported that their former spouse encouraged them to commit suicide. These data suggest that homicide is a greater risk than is generally believed in the separation/divorce situation. In future studies, *homicide potential should be assessed and related to other variables in the separation/divorce situation.*

Sex Differences

The responses for men and women have been separately reported whenever there were a sufficient number of cases to make this possible. In the recently separated/divorced group, there were 32 men and

70 women for whom responses on most variables were available. Caution must be used in interpreting findings for men for two reasons. First, the number of men studied was smaller than the number of women, and second, the sample was drawn from a population of applicants to a crisis clinic. Since women tend to use helping resources more readily than men do, it is possible that they are more representative of women in general than the men in this sample are of men in general.

Men and women differed by the type of reliance associated with disturbance. In women, emotional dependence was related to disturbance; in men everyday reliance was so related. The explanation may be that men in our study defined the meaning of the relationship practically, while women defined it emotionally.

Women were more disturbed than men when they reported that the former spouse initiated the last separation. This finding may not indicate any actual difference in responses to initiation. It may be due to men denying that women initiated separations. This explanation is supported by the fact that men in the population as a whole were significantly less likely than women to say that the women initiated the last separation. The same trend exists, but is no longer statistically significant, for the recently separated/divorced.

A relationship between the number of times respondents changed their mind about separation and disturbance was found in women but not in men. It is unclear whether there is a real difference in how disturbing vacillations are, or whether men are more likely to deny that they vacillate since this may be perceived as weakness. Findings regarding the relationship of reconciliation wishes to mental health measures generally ran parallel for men and for women. Men tended to show less clear patterns of association between hostility behaviors and mental health measures than women did. It is not definite whether and to what extent this relates to the smaller number of men, to less readiness in men to admit to the existence of hostility behaviors, or to actual differences in responses to hostility behavior between men and women.

There were differences between the sexes regarding the association of feelings about the former spouse and mental health. In women, the items which were associated with disturbance were being in love with the former spouse and missing the former spouse. In men, disturbance was associated with a negative answer to the question, "Are you just as happy not being with your spouse?" For men, the concrete reality of not being with the spouse may be more important than feelings they may not be aware of or may not wish to acknowledge.

Both men and women were more suicidal if they defended against anger and if they evidenced inappropriate guilt. Both men and women showed correlations between the amount of memory and fantasy about the former spouse and disturbance, but there are more correlations in women, and only in women does this variable remain significant in the regression equation. We may again be dealing with the tendency in men to be less aware of feelings and fantasies, and therefore to be less likely to show an association with disturbance.

Women but not men were more disturbed if they were not romantically or sexually involved with someone other than the former spouse, suggesting that at least on the conscious level, such relationships are more important to women. Both were less disturbed, however, if they were dating at the time of interview. There is a trend towards more depression in men and not women if they were interested in sex, but only women scored better on a scale of social functioning if they were sexually interested. If these findings are confirmed, sexuality may be neutral or disturbing to separated/divorced men, but supportive to women.

It should be kept in mind that *except for the somatic discomfort measures, there were no differences between recently separated/ divorced men and women in level of disturbance*. There are, however, differences in the factors associated with disturbance.

CLINICAL CONSIDERATIONS

Research deals in probabilities and cannot substitute for a careful individualized approach to the single patient. At the same time it can help in assessment and treatment. In assessment, knowledge of probabilities can alert the clinician to areas which need investigation. In treatment, telling the patient what is "par for the course" can help the patient feel less alone or abnormal.

There has been a tendency among clinicians, to disregard marital separation and divorce unless it occurred recently or constituted the presenting problem. Separation and divorce, however, may affect the patient's psychological state for months or years afterward, even though it may not be spontaneously mentioned. It is important to know the frequency and nature of the contacts with the former spouse. The clinician should gain a clear understanding of the status of the legal action, if any, since such events as filing for divorce and obtaining a final decree may have considerable psychological significance. While it is most important in early separations to be aware of the contacts, in situations of remarriage and step-families, contact with the former spouse often has many ramifications months and years later.

It is easy to overestimate pathology in persons undergoing a major life change such as separation and divorce. Only when the sequelae of such a change have been mastered can one clearly ascertain the underlying long-term level of functioning. In the recently separated/divorced and those who have been separated or divorced longer but for whom the issues are still active, it is important to allow sufficient time to deal with the current problem. Exploring earlier antecedents, such as those relating to the family of origin, too soon may result in therapist and patient avoiding the most important issue in the patient's current life—separation and divorce.

The patient is dealing with the issues surrounding the breakup of the marriage. *What went wrong with the marriage may be a tempting subject for both patient and therapist, but its investigation shortly after separation is more likely to increase the patient's self blame than be helpful.* There is time for this later when learning from the experience can be useful in thinking about future relationships.

It is not uncommon for both clinician and patient to be uncomfortable when dealing with divorce. The clinician may be unfamiliar with the subject, or may find that personal feelings about the subject intrude. The patient may avoid the subject lest he or she reveal continued attachments that may no longer be ego-syntonic or be required to deal with hostile interchanges or emotionally charged subjects related to the separation. Allowing this material to emerge may result in considerable relief for the patient.

Therapists are often taken by surprise by the extent of the ambiguity that characterizes divorce. Divorce is on a continuum that has at one end former spouses who have total absence of contact, and on the other former spouses who regularly sleep in the same bed. Therapist awareness and non-judgmental attitudes towards the range of possibilities will make it easier for patients to discuss the situation.

Clinical management of clients involved in a divorce are discussed in more detail elsewhere.[1]

RESEARCH CONSIDERATIONS

It is important to recognize that the interactions with significant others, and the psychological phenomena associated with these interactions, can be defined in terms of specific variables, and that a correlation between these variables and measures of levels of mental health can be demonstrated using statistical techniques. The present trend in psychiatric research is to focus on the delineation of specific diagnostic categories, and on organic (including genetic) etiologies. Interpersonal relations, not only biological factors, are measurably related to dysfunction, or, using medical model terminology, to disease. For this reason, studies of interpersonal relationships, including those dealing with separation and loss, complement those involving classification and the search for biological explanations. Research in both areas of inquiry should be pursued on an equal basis.

In the research under discussion in this book, there are two kinds of variables: independent, pertaining to interactions with others and to associated psychological phenomena; and dependent, measuring the level of mental health. Theoretically, there should be no overlap between them. In practice, however, some overlap is inevitable because of the nature of existing tests of psychiatric disturbance. There are no problems with scales measuring somatic discomfort, anxiety, and depression, since none of these relate to interpersonal behavior. Both the Social Functioning Rating Scale and the Brief Psychiatric Rating Scale, however, contain a few items that do, such as items pertaining hostility. Fortunately, there are only a few such items, and there is a difference between a general assessment of hostility intended to measure an attitude towards people in general, and the presence of hostile behavior towards one person. The presence of a fairly large number of items in each test, and the presence of some measures that have no overlap, indicate that we were not, by and large, measuring the same thing by our independent and dependent variables. Nevertheless, it is important to minimize the potential for overlap.

An additional problem could arise if independent variables are defined as psychological states that, by their very nature, involve distress. For this reason, the answer to the question, Is sadness present? was not included in the analysis, because it is very similar to the definition of depression. On the other hand, the question whether existing sadness is or is not due to the marital separation was included, since it defined something different from depression.

It is apparent but should be mentioned that *the existence of a relationship does not tell us anything about etiology.* It is necessary to look at each association and consider whether one caused the other or whether the relationship is reciprocal. It could not, for example, be said with certainty whether recently separated and/or divorced persons spend more time in memory/fantasy about the former spouse because they are depressed, or whether the reverse is true.

The State of the Art and Future Research

A discussion of the relationship of separation and divorce to mental health has also been published recently by Kitson and Raschke.[2] Any conclusions as to which findings can be considered generally accepted and which need further work is a matter of judgment. The following statements, however, represent a consensus of workers in the field:

• Evidence of psychological disturbance is present in a significant proportion of individuals undergoing marital separation and divorce. This disturbance cannot be entirely explained in terms of pre-existing pathology, although such pathology may play a role in some instances.

• Facts and feelings regarding the relationship with the former spouse are correlated with the degree of disturbance. Attitudes towards reconciliation, preoccupation with the thought of the former spouse, hostility between former spouses, and ambiguity about the situation surrounding the separation, are among the factors associated with disturbance.

• Relationships with new partners are significantly related to mental health, but it is unclear whether these remain significant in the recently separated/divorced if variables pertaining to the relationship to the former spouse are held constant. The same question exists regarding the presence of friends and social supports. New partners, friends and social supports are probably more significant in the longer-term separated/divorced.

• There is little, if any, difference in the overall adjustment of men and women to divorce. Also, no clear-cut relationship to age has been established. Persons of lower class and/or with less income tend to be more disturbed. The evidence regarding the impact of the presence or absence of children on disturbance is not conclusive, except that absence of children probably increases suicide potential in women.

The following represent the major unresolved issues to which future research needs to be addressed:

• There needs to be a better understanding of the difference between short-term and long-term phenomena associated with separation/divorce. Some studies have suggested that maximum disturbance is associated with the period preceding and shortly following the separation. In the present study this pattern was expected but could not be unequivocally supported by the findings. (It must be kept in mind that all respondents were seeking help.) Our study suggests that the factors contributing to disturbance in the longer-term group are quite different from those in the recently separated/divorced. The difference between determinants of disturbance in the recent and longer-term group needs to be systematically addressed.

• There have been few attempts to make cross-ethnic comparisons of the phenomena associated with separation and /or divorce. It is possible that there may be important differences between different ethnic groups.

• Future studies should include actual observations of interactions between former spouses. Such observations will minimize distortions that occur when only the reports of spouses are used.

• The question of how important the relationship between former spouses is compared to other relationships, including new partners, friends, and other social supports, is still open. A research design specifically addressed to this question, and differentiating between the recent and longer-term separated/divorced would be valuable.

• *Continued replication of existing studies, even where a consensus has emerged, will remain worthwhile for some time.* We are living in a time of rapid social change, and what is true today may no longer be applicable tomorrow.

REFERENCES

1. Jacobson GF, Portuges SH: Marital separation and divorce: Assessment of and preventive considerations for crisis intervention, in Parad HJ, Resnik HLP, Parad LG (Eds): Emergency and Disaster Management, Bowie, Md., The Charles Press Publishers, 1976
2. Kitson GF, Raschke HJ: Divorce research: What we know; what we need to know. Divorce 4(3):1–37, 1981

Appendix I:
Marginals for Total Sample and the Recently Separated/Divorced (Sub 2)

Table I
Frank Discomfort Scale: Somatic Subscale Item Scores (%)

Variable	Total Sample ($N = 237$)					Recently Separated/Divorced ($N = 105$)				
	1 = No complaint	2 = Slightly distressed	3 = Moderately distressed	4 = Severely distressed		1 = No complaint	2 = Slightly distressed	3 = Moderately distressed	4 = Severely distressed	
Headaches	43.0	32.1	15.2	9.7		48.6	23.8	17.1	10.5	
Pains in the heart and chest	67.9	18.0	10.5	3.0		62.9	21.0	11.4	4.8	
Heart pounding or racing	48.5	32.1	12.7	6.8		41.0	32.4	19.0	7.6	
Trouble getting breath	68.8	18.6	8.4	4.2		64.8	20.0	10.5	4.8	
Constipation	75.3	14.9	6.4	3.4		76.9	13.5	4.8	4.8	
Nausea or upset stomach	48.9	28.3	14.3	8.4		49.5	21.9	19.0	9.5	
Loose bowel movements	68.4	16.0	10.1	5.5		66.7	16.2	10.5	6.7	

Twitching of the face or body	75.1	16.5	5.9	2.5	71.4	21.9	3.8	2.9
Faintness or dizziness	66.7	19.4	8.4	5.5	63.8	18.1	10.5	7.6
Hot or cold spells	62.9	18.1	12.7	6.3	52.4	22.9	16.2	8.6
Itching or hives	78.1	11.8	8.0	2.1	80.0	11.4	7.6	1.0
Frequent urination	62.0	23.6	11.0	3.4	61.9	23.8	9.5	4.8
Pains in the lower part of back	54.0	24.5	16.5	5.1	54.3	24.8	14.3	6.7
Difficulty in swallowing	75.5	18.6	3.8	2.1	73.3	20.0	1.9	4.8
Skin eruptions or rashes	72.0	19.1	6.4	2.5	76.2	17.1	1.9	4.8
Soreness of muscles	57.0	24.5	13.1	5.5	60.0	24.8	9.5	5.7

Table II

Frank Discomfort Scale: Average of Somatic
Subscale Item Scores (%)

Total Sample ($N = 237$)[a]		Recently Separated/Divorced ($N = 105$)[b]
Range	%	
1.000–1.249	25.3	23.8
1.250–1.499	27.9	26.7
1.500–1.749	17.2	19.1
1.750–1.999	11.0	9.6
2.000–2.249	10.1	8.6
2.250–2.499	4.6	5.9
2.500–2.749	1.2	2.0
2.750–2.999	1.6	3.9
3.000–3.249	0.0	0.0
3.250–3.499	.4	0.0
3.500 and above	.4	1.0

Totals do not add up to 100% due to rounding.
Statistics are based on ungrouped data.
[a]Mean = 1.56, median = 1.44, standard error = 0.03, kurtosis = 1.74, standard deviation = 0.46, skewness = 1.22.
[b]Mean = 1.60, median = 1.44, standard error = 0.05, kurtosis = 1.26, standard deviation = 0.51, skewness = 1.16.

Table III
Frank Discomfort Scale: Anxiety Subscale Item Scores (%)

Variable	Total Sample (N = 237)				Recently Separated/Divorced (N = 105)			
	1 = No complaint	2 = Slightly distressed	3 = Moderately distressed	4 = Severely distressed	1 = No complaint	2 = Slightly distressed	3 = Moderately distressed	4 = Severely distressed
Heart racing or pounding	48.5	32.1	12.7	6.8	41.0	32.4	19.0	7.6
Nervousness and shakiness under pressure	26.3	23.7	25.8	24.2	23.1	22.1	26.9	27.9
Sudden fright for no apparent reason	66.7	15.2	10.5	7.6	68.6	7.6	14.3	9.5
Bad dreams	59.9	24.5	8.4	7.2	61.9	21.9	7.6	8.6

Table IV

Frank Discomfort Scale: Average of Anxiety
Subscale Item Scores (%)

Total Sample ($N = 237$)[a]		Recently Separated/Divorced ($N = 105$)[b]
Range	%	
1.000–1.249	15.2	15.2
1.250–1.499	14.8	14.3
1.500–1.749	16.0	13.3
1.750–1.999	12.2	10.5
2.000–2.249	9.7	11.04
2.250–2.499	6.3	5.8
2.500–2.749	10.5	9.5
2.750–2.999	5.5	5.7
3.000–3.249	3.4	5.7
3.250–3.499	3.0	2.9
3.500 and above	3.4	5.7

Totals do not add up to 100% due to rounding.
Statistics are based on ungrouped data.
[a]Mean = 1.87, median = 1.74, standard error = 0.05, kurtosis = .18, standard deviation = 0.72, skewness = 0.84.
[b]Mean = 1.95, median = 1.77, standard error = 0.08, kurtosis = 0.08, standard deviation = 0.80, skewness = 0.78.

Table V
Frank Discomfort Scale: Depression Subscale Item Scores (%)

Variable	Total Sample (N = 237)				Recently Separated/Divorced (N = 105)			
	1 = No complaint	2 = Slightly distressed	3 = Moderately distressed	4 = Severely distressed	1 = No complaint	2 = Slightly distressed	3 = Moderately distressed	4 = Severely distressed
Difficulty in falling asleep or staying asleep	31.2	25.3	21.5	21.9	30.5	22.9	21.9	24.8
Blaming yourself for things you did or failed to do	21.5	30.0	25.7	22.8	21.0	23.8	24.8	30.5
Feeling generally worried or fretful	13.1	23.2	29.5	34.2	13.3	21.0	29.5	36.2
Feeling blue	14.0	21.6	26.7	37.7	13.3	20.0	23.8	42.9
Being easily moved to tears	30.9	25.8	18.6	25.6	24.0	26.0	18.3	31.7
Feeling lonely	19.9	25.4	21.6	33.1	13.5	21.2	23.1	41.3

303

Table VI

Frank Discomfort Scale: Average of Depression Subscale Item Scores (%)

| Total Sample ($N = 237$)[a] | | Recently Separated/Divorced ($N = 105$)[b] |
Range	%	
1.000–1.249	7.2	6.7
1.250–1.499	2.5	1.0
1.500–1.749	11.4	6.7
1.750–1.999	2.5	5.7
2.000–2.249	10.5	10.5
2.250–2.499	7.6	5.7
2.500–2.749	11.4	9.5
2.750–2.999	7.6	9.5
3.000–3.249	11.8	8.6
3.250–3.499	6.7	8.6
3.500 and above	20.6	27.6

Totals do not add up to 100% due to rounding.
Statistics are based on ungrouped data.

[a]Mean = 2.60, median = 2.67, standard error = 0.05, kurtosis = 0.99, standard deviation = 0.84, skewness = 0.18.

[b]Mean = 2.74, median = 2.83, standard error = 0.08, kurtosis = 0.92, standard deviation = 0.84, skewness = 0.33.

Table VII

Social Functioning Rating Scale Item Scores (%) (Total Sample, $N = 233$)

Variable	1 = Not Present	2 = Very Mild	3 = Mild	4 = Moderate	5 = Severe	6 = Very Severe
Low self-concept	30.9	9.0	12.4	24.5	21.5	1.7
Goallessness	67.0	6.4	10.7	8.6	6.9	0.4
Lack of satisfying philosophy or meaning of life	63.5	5.2	15.0	13.3	2.6	0.4
Self-health concern	64.4	6.4	17.2	7.7	3.4	0.9
Emotional withdrawal	68.2	7.7	15.5	6.4	1.7	0.4
Hostility	68.7	10.3	11.6	6.0	3.4	0.0
Manipulation	73.0	10.7	9.4	5.6	1.3	0.0
Overdependency	55.4	9.4	19.3	11.2	4.7	0.0
Anxiety	12.9	6.4	20.2	35.6	23.6	1.3
Suspiciousness	88.8	3.0	4.3	2.6	1.3	0.0
Lack of satisfying relationships with significant persons	77.3	2.6	6.9	9.4	3.4	0.4
Lack of friends/social contacts	76.8	3.4	6.4	10.7	2.1	0.4
Expressed need for more friends/social contacts	48.1	6.4	30.0	12.4	3.0	0.0
Lack of work	67.4	1.3	7.3	12.0	10.3	1.7
Lack of satisfaction from work	59.7	3.0	12.0	17.2	6.4	1.7

(continued)

Table VII *(continued)*

Variable	1 = Not Present	2 = Very Mild	3 = Mild	4 = Moderate	5 = Severe	6 = Very Severe
Lack of leisure-time activities	75.5	4.7	9.0	9.0	1.3	0.4
Expressed need for more leisure, self-enhancing and satisfying activities	51.5	5.6	26.2	15.5	1.3	0.0
Lack of participation in community activities	61.4	4.7	21.5	10.7	1.7	0.0
Lack of interest in community affairs and activities that influence others	72.5	6.4	12.9	7.7	0.4	0.0
Financial insecurity	49.4	10.3	16.7	17.6	5.6	0.4
Adaptive rigidity	63.5	5.6	14.6	14.2	1.7	0.4

Table VIII

Social Functioning Rating Scale Item Scores (%) (Recently Separated/
Divorced, N = 102)

Variable	1 = Not Present	2 = Very Mild	3 = Mild	4 = Moderate	5 = Severe	6 = Very Severe
Low self-concept	26.5	8.8	12.7	25.5	25.5	1.0
Goallessness	68.8	6.9	9.8	8.8	5.9	0.0
Lack of satisfying philosophy or meaning of life	66.7	4.9	16.7	10.8	1.0	0.0
Self-health concern	64.7	11.8	14.7	7.8	1.0	0.0
Emotional withdrawal	67.6	7.8	14.7	7.8	1.0	1.0
Hostility	71.6	7.8	11.8	5.9	2.9	0.0
Manipulation	76.5	5.9	8.8	7.8	1.0	0.0
Overdependency	51.0	4.9	24.5	14.7	4.9	0.0
Anxiety	8.8	9.8	16.7	38.2	24.5	2.0
Suspiciousness	88.2	4.9	2.9	2.0	2.0	0.0
Lack of satisfying relationships with significant persons	79.4	2.9	5.9	8.8	2.0	1.0
Lack of friends/social contacts	79.4	2.9	4.9	10.8	2.0	0.0
Expressed need for more friends/social contacts	48.0	7.8	26.5	15.7	2.0	0.0
Lack of work	69.6	4.9	13.7	10.8	1.0	0.0
Lack of satisfaction from work	62.7	2.9	8.8	19.6	5.9	0.0

(continued)

307

Table VIII *(continued)*

Variable	1 = Not Present	2 = Very Mild	3 = Mild	4 = Moderate	5 = Severe	6 = Very Severe
Lack of leisure-time activities	73.5	3.9	11.8	8.8	2.0	0.0
Expressed need for more leisure, self-enhancing and satisfying activities	49.0	2.9	30.4	15.7	2.0	0.0
Lack of participation in community activities	60.8	3.9	21.6	12.7	1.0	0.0
Lack of interest in community affairs and activities that influence others	70.6	3.9	16.7	7.8	1.0	0.0
Financial insecurity	53.9	6.9	15.7	17.6	5.9	0.0
Adaptive rigidity	65.7	7.8	10.8	14.7	1.0	0.0

Table IX

Average of Social Functioning Rating Scale Item Scores (%)

Total Sample ($N = 233$)[a]		Recently Separated/Divorced ($N = 102$)[b]
Range	%	
1.000–1.249	6.9	6.0
1.250–1.499	15.0	18.6
1.500–1.749	19.6	16.8
1.750–1.999	11.6	11.9
2.000–2.249	11.5	15.7
2.250–2.499	10.9	7.0
2.500–2.749	9.3	9.9
2.750–2.999	6.8	8.9
3.000–3.249	2.9	1.0
3.250–3.499	3.0	3.0
3.500 and above	2.0	3.0

Totals do not add up to 100% due to rounding.
Statistics are based on ungrouped data.

[a]Mean = 2.04, median = 1.95, standard error = 0.04, kurtosis = 0.35, standard deviation = 0.69, skewness = 0.62.

[b]Mean = 2.03, median = 1.95, standard error = 0.06, kurtosis = 0.24, standard deviation = 0.62, skewness = 0.65.

Table X
Brief Psychiatric Rating Scale Item Scores (%) (Total Sample, $N = 233$)

Variable	1 = Not Present	2 = Very Mild	3 = Mild	4 = Moderate	5 = Moderately Severe	6 = Severe	7 = Extremely Severe
Somatic concern	65.2	6.0	13.7	10.3	0.4	3.0	1.3
Anxiety	11.6	6.4	15.5	38.2	16.7	11.6	0.0
Emotional withdrawal	74.2	8.2	11.6	4.7	0.4	0.9	0.0
Conceptual disorganization	91.0	4.7	4.3	0.0	0.0	0.0	0.0
Guilt feelings	37.3	8.2	27.5	25.3	1.3	0.4	0.4
Tension	59.2	15.5	8.2	1.7	0.0	0.0	0.0
Mannerisms and posturing	98.7	0.0	0.9	0.4	0.0	0.0	0.0
Grandiosity	98.3	0.0	1.7	0.0	0.0	0.0	0.0
Depressive mood	13.7	3.9	21.9	38.2	19.7	2.6	0.0
Hostility	67.8	9.4	12.0	7.7	1.7	1.3	0.0
Suspiciousness	90.6	2.1	3.4	2.6	0.4	0.4	0.4
Hallucinatory behavior	97.4	0.0	1.7	0.9	0.0	0.0	0.0
Motor retardation	93.6	4.3	1.3	0.9	0.0	0.0	0.0
Uncooperativeness	96.6	0.9	2.1	0.4	0.0	0.0	0.0
Unusual thought content	97.4	0.0	1.7	0.9	0.0	0.0	0.0
Blunted affect	78.5	6.0	11.2	3.4	0.4	0.4	0.0

Table XI

Brief Psychiatric Rating Scale Item Scores (%) (Recently Separated/Divorced, N = 102)

Variable	1 = Not Present	2 = Very Mild	3 = Mild	4 = Moderate	5 = Moderately Severe	6 = Severe	7 = Extremely Severe
Somatic concern	66.7	8.8	10.8	12.7	0.0	1.0	0.0
Anxiety	9.8	7.8	14.7	40.2	17.6	9.8	0.0
Emotional withdrawal	73.5	12.7	7.8	4.9	1.0	0.0	0.0
Conceptual disorganization	93.1	4.9	2.0	0.0	0.0	0.0	0.0
Guilt feelings	29.4	4.9	30.4	33.3	1.0	1.0	0.0
Tension	51.0	15.7	22.5	10.8	0.0	0.0	0.0
Mannerisms and posturing	100.0	0.0	0.0	0.0	0.0	0.0	0.0
Grandiosity	99.0	0.0	1.0	1.0	0.0	0.0	0.0
Depressive mood	13.7	4.9	14.7	39.2	26.5	1.0	0.0
Hostility	70.6	6.9	12.7	7.8	1.0	1.0	0.0
Suspiciousness	91.2	2.0	2.9	2.9	0.0	1.0	0.0
Hallucinatory behavior	98.0	0.0	1.0	1.0	0.0	0.0	0.0
Motor retardation	94.1	4.9	1.0	0.0	0.0	0.0	0.0
Uncooperativeness	97.1	0.0	2.9	0.0	0.0	0.0	0.0
Unusual thought content	97.1	0.0	2.0	1.0	0.0	0.0	0.0
Blunted affect	81.4	6.9	8.8	2.9	2.9	0.0	0.0

Table XII

Average of Brief Psychiatric Rating Scale Item Scores (%)

Total Sample ($N = 233$)[a]		Recently Separated/Divorced ($N = 102$)[b]
Range	%	
1.000–1.249	8.9	7.5
1.250–1.499	16.3	16.9
1.500–1.749	22.0	33.0
1.750–1.999	24.1	20.8
2.000–2.249	10.7	13.1
2.250–2.499	4.2	2.8
2.500–2.749	2.1	2.0
2.750–2.999	0.0	0.0
3.000–3.249	0.4	0.0
3.250–3.499	0.0	0.0
3.500 and above	0.0	0.0

Totals do not add up to 100% due to rounding.
Statistics are based on ungrouped data.

[a]Mean = 1.68, median = 1.64, standard error = 0.03, kurtosis = 0.45, standard deviation = 0.33, skewness = 0.44.

[b]Mean = 1.70, median = 1.75, standard error = 0.05, kurtosis = 1.20, standard deviation = 0.40, skewness = 0.72.

Table XIII
Average Item Scores of Suicide Potential at Intake (%)[a]

Total Sample (N = 231)[b]		Recently Separated/Divorced (N = 102)[c]
Range	%	
0.0–.999	75.3	71.6
1.000–1.999	1.3	1.0
2.000–2.999	7.3	6.9
3.000–3.999	8.5	10.9
4.000–4.999	5.1	7.0
5.000–5.999	2.0	3.0

[a]Average scores are based on "Suicide Prevention Center, Assessment of Suicidal Potentiality," administered at interview retrospective to time of intake. Persons not considered suicidal on clinical interview were not given the test, and the score was recorded as zero. For all others, the score is the average of the following items, each given with a range of possible scores. Higher scores indicate greater suicidal risk.
Items and range are as follows:

Age and sex (1–9): Higher risks for older men. Symptoms (1–9): Highest risk for severe depression and feelings of hopelessness, helpless, and exhaustion. Stress (1–9): Highest risk for loss of loved person by death, divorce or separation. Acute versus chronic (1–9): Highest risk for sharp, noticeable and sudden onset of symptoms. Suicidal plan (1–9): High rating based on lethality of plan. Resources (1–9): Highest if no support from family, friends, agencies, employment. Prior suicidal behavior (1–7): Higher if one or more prior attempts of high lethality. Medical status (1–7): Higher if chronic debilitating illness. Communication aspects (1–7): Higher if communication broken, with rejection of efforts to reestablish them. Reaction of significant others (1–7): Higher if others have defensive, paranoid, rejecting, or punishing attitude.

[b]Mean = 0.85, median = 0.01, standard error = 0.10, kurtosis = 0.73, standard deviation = 1.56, skewness = 1.49.

[c]Mean = 1.01, median = 0.01, standard error = 0.17, kurtosis = 0.06, standard deviation = 1.68, skewness = 1.25.

Table XIV

Average Item Scores of Suicide Potential at Interview (%)[a]

Total Sample ($N = 232$)[b]		Recently Separated/Divorced
Range	%	($N = 102$)[c]
0.0–.999	83.2	79.4
1.000–1.999	0.9	1.0
2.000–2.999	3.8	6.0
3.000–3.999	8.5	11.0
4.000–4.999	2.1	2.0
5.000–5.999	0.8	1.0

[a]The explanation of the scores is identical to that of footnote a to Table XIII, except that the same test was administered as of the time of interview.

[b]Mean = 0.56, median = 0.01, standard error = 0.09, kurtosis = 2.63, standard deviation = 1.29, skewness = 2.05.

[c]Mean = 0.67, median = 0.01, standard error = 0.14, kurtosis = 1.54, standard deviation = 1.38, skewness = 1.75.

Table XV

Scores on Rater Assessment of Suicide Potential (%)

Total Sample ($N = 233$)[a]		Recently Separated/Divorced
Range	%	($N = 102$)[b]
1.0 (no potential)	80.7	80.4
2.0 (mild potential)	9.9	10.8
3.0 (moderate potential)	9.4	8.8
4.0 (high potential)	0.0	0.0

[a]Mean = 1.29, median = 1.12, standard error = 0.04, kurtosis = 2.52, standard deviation = 0.63, skewness = 2.00.

[b]Mean = 1.28, median = 1.12, standard error = 0.06, kurtosis = 2.72, standard deviation = 0.62, skewness = 2.02.

Appendix II:
Selection of Variables for Regression Equation

This chapter supplements Chapter 11 and discusses further the manner in which variables for inclusion in regression equations were selected. For the most part, we will be concerned with the recently separated/divorced, i.e., those who within the last 13 months have either been separated or have filed for divorce or have obtained a final decree. This group is referred to in this study as Sub 2. Data will be reported for the group as a whole and for men and women separately.

CATEGORIES OF POTENTIAL DETERMINANTS

Previous Studies

Only a limited number of studies exist in which investigators have proposed several categories of determinants of mental health of individuals undergoing separation and divorce, and the variables have been subjected to multivariate analysis. Spanier and Lachman[1] used multivariate analysis to study the separate and combined influence of dating relations, economic stability, health, and social interaction. Economic status and good health were consistently associated with better adjustment. Dating was also positively related to adjustment. However, the frequency of social interaction with relatives and friends was not related to adjustment.

Kitson[2] measured mental health by modification of the subjective distress scale from the Psychiatric Status Schedule.[3] She found that a low positive correlation of female sex with more distress ($r = .14$, $p < .05$) disappears when controls are introduced for seeking mental health help, income, employment, receiving help from the family, and having friends with whom to talk over confidential matters. The association between female sex and distress is increased when controls are introduced for self-esteem and attachment.

Using first-order correlations, distress was associated ($p < .05$) with greater attachment, less expected income in the coming year, more (sic) friends with whom one can discuss confidential matters, greater difficulty in living on one's own, a greater number of difficult adjustments to divorce, felt pressure to divorce and lower self-esteem. Controls were then introduced for attachment, for how long ago divorce was suggested, and for both of these variables. When controls for attachment were introduced, the relationship of more friends and felt pressure to divorce was no longer significant. There were some increases and decreases in p value for other variables, but none gained or lost statistical significance at the $p < .05$ level. When controls for how long ago divorce was suggested were introduced, sex and more friends lost their significant relationship with distress.

Brown et al.[4] investigated attachment, anticipated financial strain, number of children, new friends, frequency of socializing, age of youngest child, and income in relation to a measure of generalized distress as the dependent variable. Using regression analytic techniques, they found that for men and women combined and for women alone, attachment, anticipated financial strain, and fewer children are predictors of generalized distress. In men, attachment and anticipated financial strain are predictors of distress.

Present Study

Variables reported in this book are considered here under three major headings: Basic Demographic and Marital Information, Variables Related to Marital Separation and Divorce, and Variables Predating Separation and Divorce. It should be noted that two variables which are potentially significant in determining mental health—the legal system and custody issues—are not considered in the present study.

APPROACH TO REGRESSION ANALYSIS

Regression analysis was used to help determine which of the variables affect mental health measures when other independent variables are held constant. For readers not familiar with this method, a brief discussion of the meaning of the term "to hold constant" is in order. (This discussion is based on a contribution by Berk.[5]) Take, for example, two variables that may predict anxiety in our subjects: social class and the amount of time spent in memory and fantasy about the spouse. First one determines the amount of anxiety attributable to social class, and then the variation in anxiety that cannot be explained by variation in social class, or the original anxiety "purged" of the impact of social class. Next, one can do parallel calculations with social class again as the independent variable, and with amount of time spent in memory and fantasy about the spouse as the dependent variable. Again, one calculates how much of the variance in time spent in memory and fantasy is not due to social class, or is purged of social class. The last step is to relate the purged memory and fantasy variable to the purged anxiety variable. In other words, we now have the relationship of memory and fantasy about the spouse to anxiety, purged of social class, that is, with social class held constant. Similar logic applies to the simultaneous analysis of three or more variables. In multiple regression, two or more independent variables are held constant simultaneously.

When a regression analysis is undertaken involving a given number of independent variables and a single dependent variable, the F statistic is used to indicate that the group of independent variables as a whole significantly affects the dependent variable; it is also used to address the question of significant impact of each independent variable, with all others held constant, on the dependent variable.

In the present study, significant relationships between independent variables are not uncommon: it is entirely plausible that this should be so, since we are assessing a broad spectrum of aspects of the dissolution situation, which can be expected to be, and are, related to one another, as well as with the dependent mental health measures. This phenomenon is called multicollinearity. Under such circumstances it may happen that, as Berk[5] pointed out, after the residualizing process of holding things constant, very little variance in the independent variable remains with which to explain variance in the dependent variable. There is no ideal solution to this problem. In practice it may be addressed by reducing the number of variables, provided a sound rationale for these reductions exists, to the point where a number of the remaining independent variables are shown to have significant impact on the dependent variable of interest. Such was the course taken in the present study.

The process used in reducing the number of variables through a succession of steps will now be described. Unless otherwise stated, all of these steps apply only to the recently separated and/or divorced (Sub 2). There were 52 variables that were statistically significantly associated with one or more dependent variables in Sub 2 and/or in men and/or women in Sub 2.* Several steps were taken to reduce the number:

• The first step was the grouping of variables into subgroups based on the nature of the variable. These were basic demographic and marital variables, and variables related and not related to separation/divorce. Within these subgroups, variables were included if they showed a Kendall's tau of .200 or above in relation to at least two independent variables. Also, usually variables that were available only for a substantially reduced number of respondents were omitted. These guidelines were generally, but not always rigidly, applied. They were modified at times with regard to the theoretical importance of the variable, or its relationship to a particularly significant dependent variable, such as a suicidal one. This culling resulted in a number of variables still greater than that intended.

• The next step involved carrying out a series of separate regression analyses for the three major categories. The variables most likely to be significant when others in the subgroup were held constant were then selected and a final analysis including representatives of all three variable subgroups was then conducted. In the case of separation/divorce related variables, a preliminary series of regression analyses was carried out, in which variables pertaining to six component aspects of separation/divorce (hostility, attachment, coping, etc.) were analyzed by means of separate regression analyses, and the variables most likely to be significant were selected to represent separation/divorce related variables was a whole.

Pairwise deletion was used throughout. Listwise deletion was also tried, but no substantively meaningful differences emerged. The size of the b's (unstandardized regression coefficients) remained relatively constant. Effects of reduced N (numbers of people) were detectible

---

*For Sub 2 as a whole there were 55 independent variables and 8 dependent variables; thus a total of 440 correlations were possible. Of these, 125 (28.4 percent) were significant at $p = .05$ level.

by loss of significance in some variables, generally one or two in an equation, although the size of the coefficients did not change much.

General Variables

The following basic demographic and marital variables were included in this step of the regression analysis:

- *Sex*. The following dummy variables were used: 0 = female, 1 = male. T-test analysis (Tables 5-1 and 5-3) indicated that for the sample as a whole, females showed significantly more somatic discomfort, anxiety, and depression; however, for Sub 2 (recently separated/divorced) such an association was found only in relation to somatic discomfort.
- *Age,* calculated in years. As previously noted (Chapter 5, p. 96), only rater-assessed suicide potential (ASP) significantly increased with age for the sample as a whole. When the subgroups were separately considered, there were no significant associations with age. For women in the sample as a whole, increasing age predicted higher scores (more impairment) on the BPRS.
- *Socioeconomic status,* determined using the two-factor index of social position.[6] For the sample as a whole all outcome measures except for depression were significantly associated with socioeconomic status. For Sub 2 all mental health measures except the suicidal variables were similarly associated.
- *Length of marriage*. This variable was included because of potential significance, although Kendall's tau showed no significant associations with mental health measures. There were some statistically non-significant trends towards greater suicide potential in persons who had been married for a shorter time in the sample as a whole.
- *Presence or absence of children*. As previously reported, those without children were rated as more suicidal than those with children, for both the sample as a whole and for Sub 2. In addition, for Sub 2 those with children showed significantly less disturbance on the Social Dysfunction Rating Scale (SDRS).

The Pearson correlation matrix for Sub 2 as a whole is shown in Table I. As expected, older respondents are more likely to have chil-

Table I
Pearson Correlation Matrix for Sub 2

	Socio-economic Status	Sex	Age	Presence/Absence of Children	Length of Marriage
Socioeconomic status	1.00	−0.09	0.15	−0.08	0.03
Sex	−0.09	1.00	0.03	−0.07	−0.05
Age	0.15	0.03	1.00	−0.29	0.64
Pres/absence child	−0.08	−0.07	−0.29	1.00	−0.43
Length of marriage	0.03	−0.05	0.64	−0.43	1.00

dren and to be married longer. They also tend to have lower socioeconomic status.

The results of the regression analysis of the five basic demographic and marital variables and the eight dependent mental health measures will be found in Table II, with separate reports for Sub 2 as a whole and for Sub 2 men and women considered separately.

The summary of positive findings for Sub 2 is as follows: The F statistic for the regression equation is significant for somatic discomfort, anxiety, the SFRS, BPRS, SPC 2, and ASP. Individual F values were significant for the following regression coefficients involving combinations of independent and dependent variables: socioeconomic status and somatic discomfort, anxiety, depression, the SFRS, BPRS, and SPC 2; sex and somatic discomfort; age and SPC 2 and ASP; presence or absence of child and SFRS; SPC 1 and SPC 2. *Lower socioeconomic status, female sex, greater age, and absence of child were associated with dysfunction on the reported measures. There were no associations related to length of marriage.*

In regard to women in Sub 2, the F statistic for the regression equation was significant for the SFRS and all three suicidal measures. Individual F values were significant for the following regression coefficients involving combinations of independent and dependent variables: Socioeconomic status and the SFRS; presence/absence of children and SPC 1, SPC 2, and ASP; age and SPC 2 and ASP; and length of marriage and ASP. *Lower socioeconomic status, absence of children, higher age, and briefer marriages were associated with more disturbance in women.*

In regard to men in Sub 2, the F statistic for the regression equation was significant for somatic discomfort, anxiety, depression, SFRS, and BPRS. Individual F values were significant for the follow-

Table II
Demographic Variables, Presence or Absence of Children, and Length of Marriage (Sub 2)

Dependent Variable	Independent Variable	Beta, F			R^2			F			N, Int[c]		
		M	F	M/F	M	F	M/F	M	F	M/F	M	F	M/F
SOMA	Sex	—	—	-.201, 4.43[b]	.279	.067	.153	2.81[b]	1.13	3.48[b]	33, 0.23	67, 1.39	101, 1.17
	Age	.271, 1.41	-0.187, 1.29	-.078, 0.38									
	Socioeconomic status	.538, 10.08[a]	.252, 3.84	.319, 10.96[a]									
	Pres/absence of children	.046, 0.07	.073, 0.28	.044, 0.17									
	Length of marriage	-.252, 1.42	.146, 0.73	.057, 0.18									
ANX	Sex	—	—	-.110, 1.33	.371	.056	.145	4.28[a]	0.93	3.26[a]	33, 0.51	67, 1.31	101, 1.23
	Age	.031, 0.21	-.067, 0.16	-.096, 0.01									
	Socioeconomic status	.610, 14.88[a]	.234, 3.25	.359, 13.72[a]									
	Pres/absence of children	-.020, 0.01	.084, 0.36	.025, 0.06									
	Length of marriage	-.183, 0.69	.088, 0.26	.048, 0.13									
DEP	Sex	—	—	-0.083, 0.69	.306	.019	.070	3.20[b]	0.31	1.45	33, 1.17	67, 2.55	101, 2.32
	Age	.159, 0.50	-.009, 0.00	-0.023, 0.03									
	Socioeconomic status	.558, 11.27[a]	.090, 0.46	0.225, 4.97[b]									
	Pres/absence of children	.035, 0.40	.033, 0.06	0.002, 0.00									
	Length of marriage	-.318, 1.89	-.077, 0.19	-0.097, 0.49									
SOC	Sex	—	—	0.073, 0.68	.500	.240	.288	6.77[b]	4.88[a]	7.52[a]	31, -0.68	66, 0.61	98, 0.31
	Age	.252, 1.63	.290, 3.76	0.220, 3.56									
	Socioeconomic status	.719, 24.21[a]	.279, 5.64[b]	0.423, 22.15[a]									
	Pres/absence of children	.454, 8.99[a]	.238, 3.56	0.278, 8.10[a]									
	Length of marriage	-.151, 0.55	-.219, 1.98	-0.145, 1.39									

(continued)

321

Table II (continued)

Dependent Variable	Independent Variable	Beta, F			R^2			F			N, Int[c]		
		M	F	M/F	M	F	M/F	M	F	M/F	M	F	M/F
BPRS	Sex	—	—	0.146, 2.23	.303	.095	.136	2.93[b]	1.62	2.92[b]	31,.851	66,1.13	98,1.10
	Age	.075, 0.10	.123, 0.57	0.017, 0.18									
	Socioeconomic status	.583, 11.42[a]	.175, 1.88	0.336, 11.50[a]									
	Pres/absence of children	.149, 0.69	.237, 2.97	0.155, 2.08									
	Length of marriage	-.174, 0.52	.063, 0.14	0.037, 0.07									
SPC 1[d]	Sex	—	—	-0.050, 0.25	—	.159	.109	—	2.93[b]	2.28	—	66,-2.07	98,-1.84
	Age	—	.283, 3.26	0.190, 2.14									
	Socioeconomic status	—	.084, 0.46	0.185, 3.39									
	Pres/absence of children	—	.304, 5.25[b]	0.225, 4.23[b]									
	Length of marriage	—	-.178, 1.19	-0.105, 0.59									
SPC 2[d]	Sex	—	—	-0.017, 0.03	—	.155		—	4.40[a]	3.40[a]	—	66,-2.44	98,-2.24
	Age	—	.380, 6.32[b]	0.255, 4.04[b]									
	Socioeconomic status	—	.092, 0.61	0.242, 6.11[b]									
	Pres/absence of children	—	.344, 7.30[a]	0.236, 4.89[b]									
	Length of marriage	—	-.209, 1.77	-0.138, 1.07									
ASP[d]	Sex	—	—	-0.028, 0.08	—	.192	.136	—	3.67[a]	2.93[b]	—	66,.228	98,.138
	Age	—	.378, 6.03[b]	0.296, 5.33[b]									
	Socioeconomic status	—	.030, 0.62	0.170, 2.97									
	Pres/absence of children	—	.260, 3.99[b]	0.211, 3.82									
	Length of marriage	—	-.332, 4.33[b]	-0.211, 2.43									

[a] $p \leq .01$
[b] $p \leq .05$
[c] Int = Intercept (constant)
[d] There were not enough suicidal males to warrant computation of the correlation coefficient.

ing regression coefficients involving combinations of independent and dependent variables: Socioeconomic status and somatic discomfort, anxiety, depression, SFRS, and BPRS; and presence/absence of children and SFRS. *Lower socioeconomic status and absence of children were associated with dysfunction in men.*

In conclusion, *socioeconomic status definitely needs to be included in any further regression analysis. Sex and age, though showing only a few relationships, need to continue to be included because of their general significance. Presence or absence of children will continue to be considered in conjunction with suicidal dependent variables only.* Length of marriage, in spite of one isolated association of shorter marriages with one suicidal measure, will not be further considered.

Separation and Divorce-Related Variables

The next major subgroup selected for regression analysis included variables related to marital separation and divorce. Within this subgroup, regression analyses were at first carried out separately for the following types of variables: hostility, attachment, coping, anger and guilt, new love relationships, and other spouse-related items. The next step was to identify variables representative of marital separation/divorce as a whole.

HOSTILITY VARIABLES

Variables considered for inclusion were discussed in Chapter 8. Two variables were selected on the basis of frequency and extent of correlation with the dependent variables previously reported, and also on the basis of some preliminary regression analyses involving variables representing hostility directed towards the spouse and hostility experienced from the spouse. These preliminary analyses will not be reported here. The two items included are:

• Respondent's answer to the question, Since you seriously discussed separation, did you ever use financial or custody matters to express angry feelings toward your spouse? Answers were scored as yes = 1, no = 2. There were no significant differences in the responses of men and women. Kendall's tau (Table 8-11, p. 188) indicated that for Sub 2 as a whole and for Sub 2 women, there were significant correlations in regard to somatic discomfort, anxiety, depression, and the BPRS. There were no significant correlations in males.

• Respondent's answer to the question, Do you think that your (former) spouse has ever seriously wished you dead? Answers were scored

Table III

Hostility and Mental Health Measures (Sub 2)

Dependent Variable	Independent Variable	Beta, F			R^2			F			N, Int[c]		
		M	F	M/F	M	F	M/F	M	F	M/F	M	F	M/F
SOMA	Finances/custody	−.202, 1.21	−.214, 3.44	−.200, 4.18[b]	.054	.116	.090	0.82	4.39[b]	4.89[b]	31, 1.90	69, 2.32	101, 2.20
	Death wish/spouse	−.084, 0.21	−.222, 3.61	−.189, 3.74									
ANX	Finances/custody	−.263, 2.16	−.170, 2.26	−.193, 4.16[b]	.099	.170	.142	1.60	6.88[a]	8.19[a]	31, 2.73	69, 3.24	101, 3.11
	Death wish/spouse	−.133, 0.55	−.343, 9.18[a]	−.289, 9.27[a]									
DEP	Finances/custody	−.106, 0.32	−.209, 3.16	−.176, 3.17	.012	.108	.069	0.17	4.06[b]	3.64	31, 2.89	69, 3.91	101, 3.61
	Death wish/spouse	−.006, .00	−.216, 3.36	−.163, 2.74									
SOC	Finances/custody	.239, 1.74	−.201, 2.72	−.051, 0.25	.073	.042	.009	1.15	1.48	0.45	31, 1.90	69, 2.45	101, 2.26
	Death wish/spouse	−.176, 0.93	−.019, 0.02	−.070, 0.48									
BPRS	Finances/custody	−.126, 0.52	−.169, 2.01	−.154, 2.51	.149	.077	.091	2.54	2.80	4.99[b]	31, 2.31	69, 1.98	101, 2.07
	Death wish/spouse	−.343, 3.89	−.189, 2.50	−.232, 5.67[b]									
SPC 1[d]	Finances/custody	—	−.050, 0.17	−.071, 0.49	—	.064	.022	—	2.28	1.09	—	69, 2.45	101, 1.95
	Death wish/spouse	—	−.238, 3.90	−.116, 1.32									
SPC 2[d]	Finances/custody	—	−.055, 0.20	−.079, 0.61	—	.062	.017	—	2.23	0.83	—	69, 1.82	101, 1.37
	Death wish/spouse	—	−.233, 3.74	−.087, 0.74									
ASP[d]	Finances/custody	—	.049, 0.16	0.30, 0.09	—	.049	.009	—	1.73	0.45	—	69, 1.58	101, 1.39
	Death wish/spouse	—	−.226, 3.45	−0.10, 0.86									

[a] $p \leq .01$
[b] $p \leq .05$
[c] Int = Intercept (constant)
[d] There were not enough suicidal males to warrant computation of the correlation coefficient.

as yes = 1, no = 2. There were no significant differences in the responses of men and women. Kendall's tau (Table 8-14, p 192) indicated that for Sub 2 as a whole there were significant correlations in regard to somatic discomfort, anxiety, depression and the BPRS. For women there were significant correlations in regard to somatic discomfort, anxiety, depression, the BPRS, and all three suicidal measures. For men there was a significant relationship only with the BPRS.

The Pearson correlation between these two variables was $r = .19$, which is less than the correlation with a number of the dependent variables. The result of the regression analysis involving the two independent hostility variables and the eight mental health measures will be found in Table III, with separate reports for Sub 2 as a whole and for men and women in that group.

In regard to sub 2 as a whole, the F statistic for the regression equation is significant for somatic discomfort, anxiety, and the BPRS. Individual F values were significant for the question, Since you seriously discussed separation, did you ever use financial or custody matters to express angry feelings toward the (former) spouse? and somatic discomfort and anxiety. They were also significant for the question, Do you think that your (former) spouse ever seriously wished you dead? and anxiety and the BPRS.

For women in Sub 2 the F statistic for the regression equation was significant for somatic discomfort, anxiety, and depression. Individual F value was significant for the question, Do you think that your (former) spouse ever seriously wished you dead? and anxiety. In regard to men, the F statistic for the regression equation was never significant, nor were there significant combinations of independent and dependent variables in this regression analysis.

Selection of a variable to represent hostility was based on these findings and on a general inspection of Table III. *The question of whether the respondent thought that the (former) spouse ever wished him or her dead will represent the hostility dimension in further analyses.* It is recognized that while this variable adequately represents Sub 2 as a whole and Sub 2 women, no variable adequately represents men in regard to hostility.

ATTACHMENT AND LOSS

This group will be called, for the sake of brevity, *attachment variables*. Variables considered for inclusion in this group were discussed in Chapter 6 (pp 123–133), Chapter 7 (pp 156–165), and Chapter 9 (pp

203–225). Five items were selected on the basis of frequency and extent of correlation with the dependent variables previously reported. None of the variables from Chapter 6 were included on the basis of these criteria. Those included are:

• Respondent's attitude about reconciliation. This was rated on the basis of the answer to the question addressed to the mental health professional rater, Which of the following statements best characterizes the respondent's attitude towards reconciliation from the spouse? Answers ranged from 1 = definitely does not want to reconcile, to 5 = definitely wants to reconcile. There was a trend for men to seek reconciliation more frequently than women (see p 157). Kendall's tau (Table 7-10, p 162) indicated significant correlations for Sub 2 as a whole and Sub 2 women in regard to somatic discomfort, anxiety, depression, and the BPRS. There was a significant relation to depression in men.

• Discrepancy score reflecting the difference between the extent to which respondent wants a reconciliation and the degree to which he or she believes it is likely. Scores ranged from -1 to $+4$, with higher scores indicating greater discrepancy. A positive score indicates that the respondent's wish for reconciliation was greater than his or her expectation that it would occur; negative scores indicate the reverse. Four respondents had a negative score, 57 a score of zero, and 43 positive scores. There were no significant differences between men and women. Kendall's tau (Table 7-11, p 164) showed that for Sub 2 as a whole and for Sub 2 women there was a significant relation of the variable with somatic discomfort, anxiety, depression, and the BPRS. For Sub 2 as a whole, one suicidal variable, ASP, was significant; the other two suicidal variables approached significance. For men, only depression was significantly associated.

• The respondent's answer to the question, Are you just as happy not being with the spouse? Theoretically possible answers were 1 = yes, 2 = don't know, and 3 = no. In Sub 2, 43.8% of the men ($N = 32$) compared to 27.1% of the women ($N = 70$) answered "no." While the difference did not reach statistical significance ($X_c^2 = 2.77$, 1 df, $p = 0.15$), there appears to be a trend in the direction of men being more likely not to be happy not being with the (former) spouse. Kendall's tau indicated that for Sub 2 as a whole, there were significant correlations of the variable with anxiety, depression, and the BPRS (Table 9-8, p 210). For women, the only significant correlation was with the BPRS. For men, there was a significant correlation with somatic discomfort, anxiety, and depression. This was the only independent variable of the attachment group to be associated with all three discomfort variables in men. For this reason, this variable was chosen for the regression analysis as representing the group of variables dealing with the relationship of feelings towards the spouse to mental health variables (pp 209–215). Being in love with the spouse and missing the spouse were also associated with several dependent variables for women and for Sub 2 as a whole but not for men, and were not chosen for inclusion in the regression analysis.

• The question to the mental health professional rater, Does sadness when it exists [as determined by a prior question] relate to the marital separation? Possible answers ranged from 1 = definitely not, to 5 = definitely yes. There were no significant differences in the responses of men and women in Sub 2. Kendall's tau indicated that for Sub 2 as a whole and for women in that subgroup, there were significant correlations of the variable with anxiety, depression, the BPRS, and one suicidal measure, ASP (Table 9-15, p 220). For women, there was also a significant correlation with SPC 2. There were no significant correlations for men.

• The question to the mental health professional rater, How much time does the respondent spend involving memory or fantasy about the (former) spouse? Possible answers ranged from 1 = none of the time, to 5 = almost all of the time. There were no significant differences in the responses of men and women in Sub 2. Kendall's tau (Table 9-20, p 225) indicated that for Sub 2 as a whole and for women in that subgroup, there were significant correlations of this variable with somatic discomfort, anxiety, depression, the BPRS, SFRS, and SPC 2. In men there was only one significant correlation involving somatic discomfort.

The Pearson correlation matrix involving these five attachment variables showed that the independent variables correlated more highly with each other than any did with the dependent mental health measures, suggesting that they measured a similar phenomenon. The variable indicating response to the question of how much time the respondent was thought to spend involving memory and fantasy regarding the former spouse is of special interest since it had the largest number of significant correlations with the dependent measures for Sub 2 as a whole. That variable correlated with the other four attachment variables at levels ranging from $r = .49$ with a "no" answer to the question of whether the respondent was just as happy not being with the former spouse to $r = .71$ with scores indicating greater degrees of reconciliation wishes. As we will see, however, the phenomena measures, while similar, are probably not identical.

The results of the regression analysis involving the five independent attachment variables and the eight mental health measures will be

Table IV
Attachment and Mental Health Measures (Sub 2)

Dependent Variable	Independent Variable	Beta, F			R^2			F			N, Int[c]		
		M	F	M/F	M	F	M/F	M	F	M/F	M	F	M/F
SOMA	Memory/fantasy	.199, 0.25	.444, 8.00[a]	.372, 6.28[b]	.100	.197	.125	0.53	2.74[b]	2.45[b]	29,1.11	61,1.33	91,1.33
	Discrepancy	.283, 0.31	.114, 0.33	.171, 0.85									
	Not with spouse	.023, 0.01	−.066, 0.22	−.056, 0.21									
	Reconciliation wish	−.314, 0.20	−.059, 0.06	−.205, 0.73									
	Sadness re reconciliation	.194, 0.34	.008, 0.00	.080, 0.36									
ANX	Memory/fantasy	.309, 0.75	.580, 16.32[a]	.530, 14.88[a]	.266	.327	.250	1.73	5.44[a]	5.73[b]	29,1.05	61,1.19	91,1.18
	Discrepancy	−.236, 0.27	.163, 0.81	.175, 1.05									
	Not with spouse	.336, 2.07	.023, 0.03	.089, 0.63									
	Reconciliation wish	.327, 0.27	−.312, 1.87	−.355, 2.55									
	Sadness re reconciliation	−.273, 0.84	.169, 1.53	.108, 0.76									
DEP	Memory/fantasy	−.026, 0.01	.565, 15.75[a]	.460, 11.51[a]	.362	.337	.269	2.72[b]	5.70[a]	6.34[a]	29,2.06	61,2.09	91,2.18
	Discrepancy	.111, 0.07	.199, 1.23	.288, 2.85									
	Not with spouse	.383, 3.09	−.064, 0.25	.048, 0.19									
	Reconciliation wish	.335, 0.32	−.056, 0.06	−.154, 0.49									
	Sadness re reconciliation	−.241, 0.75	−.087, 0.41	−.102, 0.70									
SOC	Memory/fantasy	−.023, 0.00	.333, 4.18[b]	.253, 2.75	.051	.131	.072	0.26	1.70	1.33	29,2.08	61,1.53	91,0.67
	Discrepancy	.345, 0.44	.036, 0.03	.106, 0.31									
	Not with spouse	−.138, 0.27	.050, 0.12	.016, 0.02									
	Reconciliation wish	−.099, 0.02	−.283, 1.20	−.250, 1.02									
	Sadness re reconciliation	.074, 0.05	.225, 2.09	.167, 1.48									

328

					.101	.242	.141	0.54	3.57[b]	2.82[b]	29,1.61	61,1.35	91,1.44
BPRS	Memory/fantasy	.148, 0.20	.264, 3.00	.233, 2.52									
	Discrepancy	−.042, 0.01	.347, 3.26	.275, 2.25									
	Not with spouse	.104, 0.16	.119, 0.76	.114, 0.91									
	Reconciliation wish	.267, 0.14	−.434, 3.22	−.284, 1.42									
	Sadness re reconciliation	−.278, 0.71	.348, 5.74[b]	.148, 1.25									
SPC 1[d]	Memory/fantasy	—	.317, 3.53	.179, 1.31	.069	.037	—	0.83	0.65	—		61,.779	91,0.61
	Discrepancy	—	.106, 0.25	.211, 1.18									
	Not with spouse	—	−.112, 0.55	.007, 0.00									
	Reconciliation wish	—	−.268, 1.00	−.278, 1.21									
	Sadness re reconciliation	—	.061, 0.15	.083, 0.35									
SPC 2[d]	Memory/fantasy	—	.381, 5.79[b]	.229, 2.37	.180	.117	—	2.46[b]	2.28	—		61,.436	91,0.38
	Discrepancy	—	.117, 0.34	.171, 0.85									
	Not with spouse	—	−.045, 0.10	.041, 0.12									
	Reconciliation wish	—	−.376, 2.23	−.331, 1.89									
	Sadness re reconciliation	—	.315, 4.36[b]	.287, 4.58[b]									
ASP[d]	Memory/fantasy	—	.232, 1.88	.072, 0.22	.064	.043	—	0.77	0.78	—		61,1.09	91,1.04
	Discrepancy	—	.133, 0.39	.168, 0.76									
	Not with spouse	—	−.082, 0.30	.011, 0.01									
	Reconciliation wish	—	−.291, 1.17	−.231, 0.85									
	Sadness re reconciliation	—	.186, 1.33	.213, 2.32									

[a] $p \leq .01$
[b] $p \leq .05$
[c] Int = Intercept (constant).
[d] There were not enough suicidal males to warrant computation of the correlation coefficient.

found in Table IV, with separate reports for Sub 2 as a whole and for Sub 2 men and women.

The summary of positive findings for Sub 2 as a whole is as follows: The F statistic for the regression equation is significant for the dependent variables somatic discomfort, anxiety, depression, and the BPRS. Individual F values were significant for the following regression coefficients involving combinations of independent and dependent variables: The question of how much time is spent involving memory and fantasy about the spouse, with somatic discomfort, anxiety, and depression; and the question whether sadness is related to separation, and SPC 2.

The summary of positive findings in regard to women in Sub 2 is as follows: The F statistic for the regression equation is significant for the dependent variables somatic discomfort, anxiety, depression, BPRS, and SPC 2. Individual F values were significant for the following regression coefficients involving combinations of independent and dependent variables: The question of how much time was spent involving memory and fantasy about the spouse, and somatic discomfort, anxiety, depression, SFRS, and SPC 2, and the question whether sadness is related to separation and BPRS and SPC 2.

The summary of positive findings in regard to men in Sub 2 is as follows: The F statistic for the regression equation is significant for the dependent variable depression only. There were no significant individual F values.

The choice of variable for Sub 2 as a whole and for women in that subgroup thus lies between the question of the amount of time the respondent was reported to spend involving memory and fantasy regarding the spouse and the question of the extent to which sadness relates to separation. *The question of the amount of time spent in memory and fantasy involving the spouse was selected on the basis of the larger number of significant individual correlation coefficients for Sub 2 as a whole and for women in that subgroup.* For men in the absence of significant individual correlation coefficients, the choice was made on the basis of Kendall's tau, and *the answer to the question whether respondent is as happy not being with the former spouse was accordingly selected.*

It is clear that *there are gender differences* in the attachment group, both in the correlations and the regression analysis. There are several possible reasons: (1) The number of men in the study is less than half that of women; it is possible that some real relationships were obscured by the small number and may emerge when a larger sample is studied. (2) Attachment variables, singly or in combination, may have less impact on mental health measures in men than they do in women. (3) The attachment measures in this study may more closely represent a single dimension in men than they do in women, which might explain the fact that while three out of the five measures individually correlate significantly with depression in men, and although the overall F value in the regression equation for the attachment group in relation to depression is significant in men, no single independent variable is significant with depression in men in the regression equation. (4) The individual correlations suggest that for men, the variables relating directly to reconciliation wishes (greater wish for reconciliation, greater discrepancy between wish and expectation of reconciliation, and particularly not wanting not to be with spouse) are associated with indicators of disturbance in men, but sadness connected to separation and greater memory/fantasy are less frequently so associated. Inspection of the regression equation reveals that it is possible that the individual F value relating "not with spouse" to depression might become significant in a larger sample. If this is the case, then men may be more likely to respond to specific issues pertaining to their wish to reconcile than to the more subtle emotions of sadness or the presence of memory or fantasy. Such an observation would be compatible with traditional cultural role definitions for men in this society.

An interesting sidelight is the possibility that with a larger sample a relationship of fewer reconciliation wishes to more disturbance might emerge in a regression equation if the other variables previously described were to be held constant. That possibility is suggested by a negative B and an F value of 3.22 relating fewer reconciliation wishes to greater disturbance on the BPRS in women. Should such a phenomenon be found, it is possible that some persons, particularly women, may consciously not wish reconciliation but may nevertheless be preoccupied with memory/fantasy and may show greater disturbance. Perhaps there exists a group of women that is unusually conflicted about the situation.

COPING VARIABLES

Coping in the context of this study is defined as the ability to assess reality relative to the separation, to make and carry out a clear-cut decision regarding separation, and to be consistent about arrangements pertaining to spouse contacts. These variables were selected from those in Chapter 6 (pp 116–123) and Chapter 7 (pp 156–165). They were chosen because they were thought to be indicative of ego function in relation to perception and action. Clinical observation suggests that because of the stress of marital separation, failure to cope effectively in this particular area is common. The three variables are as follows:

- Consistency, defined as the respondent's answer to the question,

Table V
Coping Variables and Mental Health Measures (Sub 2)

Dependent Variable	Independent Variable	Beta, F			R^2			F			N, Int[c]		
		M	F	M/F	M	F	M/F	M	F	M/F	M	F	M/F
SOMA	Vacillation	.006, 0.00	.185, 2.05	.105, 1.03	.218	.223	.205	2.24	4.77[b]	6.68[a]	27,1.07	53,1.31	81,1.23
	Reality testing	.265, 1.69	.063, 0.18	.098, 0.71									
	Consistency	.283, 1.89	.351, 5.48[b]	.359, 9.17[a]									
ANX	Vacillation	.084, 0.22	.191, 1.96	.146, 1.86	.238	.131	.158	2.49	2.51	4.80[a]	27,1.17	53,1.57	81,1.43
	Reality testing	.157, 0.61	.086, 0.30	.083, 0.48									
	Consistency	.377, 3.44	.205, 1.68	.286, 5.48[a]									
DEP	Vacillation	−.064, 0.11	.123, 0.78	.063, 0.32	.089	.093	.088	0.78	1.71	2.50	27,2.34	53,2.39	81,2.35
	Reality testing	.141, 0.41	.117, 0.54	.113, 0.83									
	Consistency	.207, 0.87	.166, 1.05	.201, 2.51									
SOC	Vacillation	−.086, 0.20	−.087, 0.43	−.077, 0.51	.131	.164	.136	1.20	3.26[b]	4.10[b]	27,1.84	53,1.71	81,1.73
	Reality testing	−.182, 0.72	.115, 0.56	.019, 0.03									
	Consistency	.412, 3.60	.346, 4.94[b]	.369, 8.94[a]									

	1	2	3	4	5	6	7	8	9	10	11	12
BPRS Vacillation	.056, 0.08	.033, 0.06	.045, 0.17	.075	.133	.098	0.65	2.56	2.83[b]	27,1.55	53,1.48	81,1.51
Reality testing	.026, 0.01	.027, 0.03	.051, 0.17									
Consistency	.247, 1.21	.339, 4.59[b]	.271, 4.61[b]									
SPC 1[d] Vacillation	—	.220, 2.40	.186, 2.68		.062	.053		1.11	1.44	—	53,0.76	81,0.62
Reality testing		.136, 0.70	.149, 1.37									
Consistency		−.099, 0.36	−.068, 0.28									
SPC 2[d] Vacillation	—	.171, 1.53	.182, 2.74		.102	.108		1.89	3.16[b]	—	53,0.31	81,1.19
Reality testing		.275, 2.99	.282, 5.22[b]									
Consistency		−.066, 0.14	−.056, 0.20									
ASP[d] Vacillation	—	.079, 0.32	.099, 0.79		.064	.079		1.13	2.22	—	53,1.23	81,1.13
Reality testing		.272, 2.81	.279, 4.98[b]									
Consistency		−.115, 0.49	.063, 0.24									

[a] p ≤ .01

[b] p ≤ .05

[c] Int = Intercept (constant).

[d] There were not enough suicidal males to warrant computation of correlations.

How frequently do you say one thing and do another relative to contacts with the (former) spouse? Responses are rated from 1 = almost never, to 5 = almost always. There were no significant differences between the responses of men and women. Kendall's tau (Table 6-4) indicated that for Sub 2 as a whole, there were significant correlations in regard to somatic discomfort, anxiety, depression, SFRS, and BPRS. For Sub 2 women there were significant correlations in regard to somatic discomfort, SFRS, and BPRS. For Sub 2 men there were significant correlations in regard to somatic discomfort and anxiety.

• Vacillation, defined as the respondent's answer to the question, After you and (former) spouse first seriously discussed separation, how often did you decide not to carry it out? Responses ranged from 0 = never, to 6 = 10 or more times. Kendall's tau (Table 7-9) indicated for Sub 2 as a whole there were significant correlations in regard to anxiety and SPC 1 and SPC 2. For Sub 2 women there were significant correlations in regard to somatic discomfort, anxiety, depression, SPC 1, and SPC 2. There were no significant correlations for Sub 2 men.

• Reality testing, defined as the difference between the degree of likelihood of reconciliation as estimated by the respondent on a score of 1 to 5, and by the rater, similarly estimated. Absolute values are used to estimate the difference, regardless of direction. There were no differences in the responses of men and women. Kendall's tau (Table 7-12) indicated that for Sub 2 as a whole there were significant correlations in regard to somatic discomfort, anxiety, depression, BPRS, SPC 1, and SPC 2. For Sub 2 women there were significant correlations in regard to somatic discomfort, depression, SFRS, BPRS, SPC 2, and ASP. There were no significant correlations for men.

The Pearson correlation matrix involving these three variables for Sub 2 as a whole showed $r = .497$ between consistency and reality testing; $r = .230$ between consistency and vacillation, and $r = .130$ between reality testing and vacillation. The results of the regression analysis of the three independent coping variables and the eight dependent mental health measures are found in Table V, with separate reports for Sub 2 as a whole and for men and women in that subgroup.

The summary of positive findings in regard to Sub 2 as a whole is as follows: The F statistic for the regression equation is significant for the dependent variables somatic discomfort, anxiety, the SFRS, BPRS, and SPC 2. Individual F values were significant for the following regression coefficients involving combinations of independent and dependent variables: consistency and somatic discomfort, anxiety, SFRS, BPRS; reality testing and SPC 1 and SPC 2.

The summary of positive findings in regard to Sub 2 women is as follows: The F statistic for the regression equation is significant for the dependent variables anxiety and SFRS. Individual F values were significant for the following regression coefficients involving combinations of independent and dependent variables: consistency and somatic discomfort, the SFRS, and BPRS.

There are no significant F values for the equations for Sub 2 men, nor are there individually significant F values for them. However, a number of regression coefficients approach significance, and the general pattern does not differ greatly from that of women.

On the basis of these findings, *consistency will be included in further regression equations in regard to non-suicidal variables and reality testing in regard to suicidal variables.*

SEPARATION-RELATED ANGER AND GUILT

Several psychological processes relating to separation and divorce have been described in Chapter 9 (p 213). Two of these have been selected for inclusion in this stage of the regression analysis:

• The mental health professional's response to the question: To what extent does the respondent appear to be defending against the feelings of anger associated with the separation from the spouse? Responses range from 1 = not at all, to 5 = extremely great. Kendall's tau (Table 9-18) indicated for Sub 2 as a whole significant correlation existed with SFRS, BPRS, and all three suicidal variables. For Sub 2 women there were significant correlations with SFRS, BPRS, and SPC 2 and ASP. For Sub 2 men there was a significant correlation with ASP.

• The mental health professional's response to the question, Considering the length of the relationship, the recency of the separation and the probability that the separation is permanent, the feelings of guilt are _____? Ratings range from 1 = definitely inappropriate, to 5 = definitely appropriate. Kendall's tau (Table 9-19) indicated that for Sub 2 as a whole, there are significant correlations with all variables except SPC 1. For Sub 2 women, there were significant correlations with anxiety, SFRS, and BPRS. For Sub 2 men, there were significant correlations with depression and SPC 2.

The two variables are highly correlated with each other, $r = .406$ in Sub 2 as a whole, indicating that defense against anger is also associated with inappropriate guilt. For this reason, it was expected that one but not both would be related to dependent variables in a regression equation.

The results of the regression analysis of the two independent anger and guilt variables and the eight dependent mental health measures are

Table VI

Separation-Related Anger and Guilt and Mental Health Measures (Sub 2)

Dependent Variable	Independent Variable	Beta, F			R^2			F			N, Int[c]		
		M	F	M/F	M	F	M/F	M	F	M/F	M	F	M/F
SOMA	Defense against anger	−.117, 0.41	−.089, 0.43	−.132, 1.54	.081	.060	.073	1.27	2.13	3.92[b]	31,1.96	69,2.10	101,2.11
	Inappropriate guilt	−.288, 2.47	−.275, 4.12[b]	−.296, 7.82[a]									
ANX	Defense against anger	−.152, 0.73	−.011, 0.01	−.075, 0.51	.125	.069	.084	2.07	2.46	4.54[b]	31,2.76	69,2.60	101,2.72
	Inappropriate guilt	−.357, 3.99	−.267, 3.92	−.312, 8.79[a]									
DEP	Defense against anger	.126, 0.65	−.049, 0.13	−.032, 0.09	.329	.052	.106	7.11[a]	1.83	5.84[b]	31,3.52	69,3.43	101,3.54
	Inappropriate guilt	−.531, 11.49[a]	−.247, 3.31	−.337, 10.48[a]									
SOC	Defense against anger	−.149, 0.72	.272, 4.46[b]	.123, 1.40	.149	.145	.112	2.53	5.66[a]	6.24[a]	31,2.99	69,2.04	101,2.35
	Inappropriate guilt	−.393, 4.95[b]	−.164, 1.62	−.265, 6.55[b]									
BPRS	Defense against anger	.003, 0.00	.124, 1.04	.104, 1.06	.065	.235	.154	1.02	10.26[a]	9.03[a]	31,2.00	69,1.93	101,1.93
	Inappropriate guilt	−.255, 1.90	−.411, 11.37[a]	−.339, 11.23[a]									
SPC 1[d]	Defense against anger	—	.237, 3.04	.233, 4.39[b]	—	.049	.060	—	1.72	3.19	—	69,0.34	101,0.62
	Inappropriate guilt	—	.039, 0.08	−.047, 0.19									
SPC 2[d]	Defense against anger	—	.427, 11.02[a]	2.78, 7.21[a]	—	.150	.117	—	5.89[b]	6.53[b]	—	69, −0.53	101,0.49
	Inappropriate guilt	—	.107, 0.70	−.116, 1.26									
ASP[d]	Defense against anger	—	.365, 7.77[b]	.276, 7.02[a]	—	.115	.100	—	4.34[b]	5.47[b]	—	69,0.86	101,1.14
	Inappropriate guilt	—	.066, 0.25	−.077, 0.54									

[a] $p \leq .01$
[b] $p \leq .05$
[c] Int = Intercept (constant).
[d] There were not enough suicidal males to warrant computation of the correlation coefficient.

found in Table VI, with separate reports for Sub 2 as a whole and for men and women in that subgroup. In regard to Sub 2 as a whole, the F statistic for the regression equation was significant for all dependent variables. Individual F values were significant for the following regression coefficients involving combinations of independent and dependent variables: Inappropriate guilt and somatic discomfort, anxiety, depression, SFRS, and BPRS; defense against anger and SPC 1, SPC 2,and ASP.

For Sub 2 women, the F statistic for the regression equation was significant for SFRS, BPRS, SPC 2, and ASP. Individual F values were significant for the following regression coefficients involving combinations of independent and dependent variables: inappropriate guilt and somatic discomfort and BPRS; defense against anger and SFRS, SPC 2, and ASP.

For Sub 2 men the F statistic for the regression equation was significant for depression and SPC 2. Individual F values were significant for the following regression coefficients involving combinations of independent and dependent variables: inappropriate guilt and depression, and SFRS.

While there are some differences between men and women, *the overall choice is to include inappropriate guilt in further regression analysis for the non-suicidal variables, and defense against anger for the suicidal variables.*

NEW LOVE RELATIONSHIPS

Two variables were selected for consideration of inclusion in the regression analysis from Chapter 10 (pp 237–254):

• The respondent's answer to the question, Were/are you romantically or sexually involved with someone other than your (former) spouse? The answers were rated as 1 = yes, 2 = no. There were no differences between men and women in Sub 2. However, results need to be interpreted with some caution because 80.4 percent of Sub 2 answered "yes." Kendall's tau (Table 10-7) indicated that for Sub 2 as a whole significant correlations existed with depression, SFRS, and BPRS. For Sub 2 women there were significant correlations with the same items. There were no significant correlations for Sub 2 men. All correlations were in the direction of more disturbance in those who are/were or are not/were not romantically or sexually involved.

• The respondent's answer to the question, How often do you feel sexual satisfaction in your current relationship? This is rated on a scale of 1 = never, to 6 = always. There were no differences in responses by

Table VII
Romantic/Sexual Involvement and Degree of Sexual Satisfaction and Mental Health Measures (Sub 2)

Dependent Variable	Independent Variable	Beta, F			R^2			F			N, Int[b]		
		M	F	M/F	M	F	M/F	M	F	M/F	M	F	M/F
SOMA	Ever involved	−.156, 0.47	.167, 1.11	.088, 0.48	.026	.054	.019	0.25	1.30	0.63	21,1.74	47,1.58	69,1.56
	Frequent sexual satisfaction	−.059, 0.07	−.108, 0.46	−.080, 0.39									
ANX	Ever involved	−.002, 0.00	.145, 0.87	.144, 1.30	.002	.096	.040	0.02	2.40	1.42	21,1.72	47,2.14	69,1.81
	Frequent sexual satisfaction	.040, 0.03	−.221, 2.01	−.104, 0.68									
DEP	Ever involved	.220, 0.96	.204, 1.79	.241, 3.89	.051	.132	.096	0.51	3.43[a]	3.56[a]	21,2.13	47,2.48	69,2.40
	Frequent sexual satisfaction	−.028, 0.02	−.229, 2.25	−.134, 1.20									
SOC	Ever involved	.139, 0.37	.223, 2.20	.229, 3.42	.037	.154	.072	0.36	4.10[a]	2.62	21,1.56	47,2.00	69,1.73
	Frequent sexual satisfaction	.150, 0.44	−.243, 2.61	−.087, 0.50									
BPRS	Ever involved	.062, 0.07	.106, 0.48	.132, 1.09	.040	.122	.025	0.39	3.14	0.87	21,1.49	47,1.79	69,1.59
	Frequent sexual satisfaction	.197, 0.76	−.292, 3.64	−.055, 0.19									
SPC 1[c]	Ever involved	—	.054, 0.12	.080, 0.40	—	.056	.030	—	1.34	1.05	—	47,1.72	69,1.33
	Frequent sexual satisfaction		−.209, 1.73	−.132, 1.09									
SPC 2[c]	Ever involved	—	.119, 0.63	.152, 1.56	—	.157	.097	—	4.20[a]	3.60[a]	—	47,1.40	69,0.79
	Frequent sexual satisfaction		−.332, 4.89[a]	−.228, 3.49									
ASP[c]	Ever involved	—	−.006, 0.00	.055, 0.20	—	.125	.075	—	3.23	2.70	—	47,1.88	69,1.55
	Frequent sexual satisfaction		−.357, 5.44[a]	−.251, 4.12[a]									

[a] $p \leq .05$

[b] Int = Intercept (constant).

[c] There were not enough suicidal males to warrant computation of the correlation coefficient.

gender. Kendall's tau (Table 10-11) indicated that for Sub 2 as a whole significant correlation existed with depression and the ASP. For Sub 2 women there were significant correlations for depression, SFRS, BPRS, SPC 2, and ASP. There was an insufficient number of men available to carry out correlation analysis. All correlations were in the direction of more disturbance being associated with less frequent sexual satisfaction.

The two variables for Sub 2 as a whole are correlated at $r = -.310$. Respondents who are/were or had been romantically/sexually involved tended, unsurprisingly, to have a greater frequency of sexual satisfaction than those not so involved. The correlation is not greater because respondents may have been involved prior to but not at time of interview, may be romantically but not sexually involved, or may be sexually involved and not have sexual satisfaction.

The results of the regression analysis of the two variables representing new love relationships and the eight dependent measures will be found on Table VII, with separate reports for Sub 2 as a whole and for Sub 2 men and women.

The summary of positive findings in regard to Sub 2 as a whole is as follows: The F statistic for the regression equation is significant for depression and for SPC 2. Individual F value is significant only for the combination of frequency of sexual satisfaction and ASP.

The summary of positive findings in regard to Sub 2 women is as follows: The F statistic for the regression equation is significant for depression, SFRS and SPC 2. Individual F values were significant for the following regression coefficients involving combinations of independent and dependent variables: frequency of sexual satisfaction and SPC 2 and ASP. There were no significant values for the regression equation nor individual F values in men.

Based on the above analysis, the variable of *frequency of sexual satisfaction was selected for inclusion in further regression analysis.*

OTHER SPOUSE-RELATED VARIABLES: INITIATION AND TRIANGLES

Two other variables related to the (former) spouse were considered for inclusion in the regression analysis. They are:

• The respondent's answer to the question, Who initiated the last separation? Possible scores were 1 = self, 2 = spouse, 3 = mutual decision, 4 = don't know, 5 = other. Only scores of 1 = self and 2 = spouse were considered for inclusion in the regression analysis. This will be called the "initiation" variable. There were no significant differences in Sub 2 (recently separated/divorced) between males and females as reported initiators, though for the sample as a whole men reported spouse-initiated separation more often than women. Kendall correlation analysis indicates that for Sub 2 as a whole (Table 7-5) there were significant correlations with depression, the SFRS, the BPRS, and SPC 2. For Sub 2 women (Table 7-6) there were significant correlations with somatic discomfort, anxiety, depression, the SFRS, and the BPRS. There were no significant correlations for Sub 2 men. In all cases, disturbance was greater when spouse rather than self was reported to be the initiator.

• The respondent's answer to the question, In regard to the (former) spouse's romantic/sexual involvement, how involved are you? Responses were rated on a four-point scale from 1 = not involved at all, to 4 = very much involved. This will be called the "triangles" variable. Kendall correlation analysis indicates that for Sub 2 as a whole (Table 10-8) there were significant correlations with depression and the BPRS. For Sub 2 women there were significant correlations with somatic discomfort, anxiety, depression and the BPRS. There was an insufficient number of men for correlation analysis.

The correlation between these two variables is low: $r = .069$.

The results of the regression analysis will be found in Table VIII with separate reports for Sub 2, the recently separated/divorced, as a whole, and for men and women in that subgroup. The summary of positive findings in regard to Sub 2 is as follows: The F statistic for the regression equation is significant for depression and the BPRS. Individual F values were significant for the regression coefficients involving initiation and depression and the BPRS.

The summary of positive findings in regard to Sub 2 women is as follows: The F statistic for the regression equation is significant for somatic discomfort, anxiety, depression, and the BPRS. Individual F values were significant for regression coefficients involving triangles and somatic discomfort, anxiety and depression; and initiation and depression and the BPRS.

There were no statistically significant positive findings in regard to Sub 2 men. While this is in part due to the small number (17), men appear to show no relation between triangles and mental health measures, and this finding seems to result in the failure of this variable to significantly impact somatic discomfort, anxiety and depression in Sub 2 as a whole in spite of significant associations in women.

On the strength of the findings in Sub 2 as a whole, *initiation was chosen to represent these variables in further regression analysis,* but triangles also appear to be of importance in Sub 2 women.

Table VIII

Initiation and Triangles and Mental Health Measures (Sub 2)

Dependent Variable	Independent Variable	Beta, F			R^2			F			N, Int[c]		
		M	F	M/F	M	F	M/F	M	F	M/F	M	F	M/F
SOMA	Initiation	.027, 0.01	.232, 2.76	.079, 0.39	.018	.196	.060	0.14	5.01[b]	1.88	17,1.54	43,1.06	61,1.28
	Triangles	−.140, 0.28	.378, 7.31[a]	.277, 3.21									
ANX	Initiation	.048, 0.03	.252, 3.21	.123, 0.96	.007	.189	.068	0.05	4.76[b]	2.17	17,1.81	43,0.99	61,1.36
	Triangles	−.082, 0.10	.355, 6.36[b]	.222, 3.11									
DEP	Initiation	.197, 0.58	.339, 5.90[b]	.255, 4.39[b]	.065	.203	.132	0.52	5.23[a]	4.50[b]	17,1.97	43,1.54	61,1.77
	Triangles	.117, 0.20	.299, 4.61[b]	.243, 3.99									
SOC	Initiation	.159, 0.36	.273, 3.49	.219, 3.05	.024	.126	.076	0.18	2.97	2.42	17,1.78	43,1.33	61,1.47
	Triangles	−.032, 0.02	.229, 2.47	.152, 1.47									
BPRS	Initiation	.083, 0.10	.367, 6.87[b]	.264, 4.59[b]	.015	.196	.109	0.12	5.01[b]	3.62[b]	17,1.57	43,1.22	61,1.32
	Triangles	.072, 0.07	.250, 3.20	.181, 2.18									
SPC 1[d]	Initiation	—	.113, 0.54	.069, 0.29	—	.025	.022	—	0.53	0.66	—	43,0.24	61,0.30
	Triangles		.111, 0.52	.126, 0.95									
SPC 2[d]	Initiation	—	.209, 1.98	.201, 2.55	—	.094	.070	—	2.13	2.21	—	43,−.060	61,−0.50
	Triangles		.226, 2.31	.158, 1.58									
ASP[d]	Initiation	—	−.031, 0.04	.011, 0.01	—	.026	.025	—	0.54	0.74	—	43,1.19	61,1.09
	Triangles		.156, 1.04	.156, 1.46									

[a] $p \leq .01$

[b] $p \leq .05$

[c] Int = Intercept (constant).

[d] There were not enough suicidal males to warrant computation of the correlation coefficient.

VARIABLES REPRESENTING SEPARATION AND
DIVORCE AS A WHOLE

As previously indicated, variables were selected from each of the
subgroups of variables related to separation and divorce discussed
above, and subjected to further regression analysis. The variables,
termed key separation/divorce related variables, and the subsection
from which they were derived, are as follows:

- From the hostility subsection: Respondent's answer to the question, Do you think that (former) spouse has ever seriously
  wished you dead? This variable will be referred to as "death
  wish by spouse."
- From the attachment subsection: The answer to the question to
  the mental health professional rater, How much time does the
  respondent spend involving memory or fantasy about the (former) spouse? This variable will be referred to as "memory/fan-
  tasy." In men, the following variable was substituted: The respondent's answer to the question, Are you just as happy not
  being with the spouse? This variable will be referred to as "not
  with spouse."
- From the coping variables subsection: Consistency, defined as
  the respondent's answer to the question, How frequently do you
  say one thing and do another relative to contacts with the (former) spouse? This variable will be referred to as "consistency."
- From the separation-related anger and guilt subsection: The
  mental health professional's response to the question, Considering the length of the relationship, the recency of the separation
  and the probability that the separation is permanent, the feelings
  of guilt are (appropriate to inappropriate)? This variable will be
  referred to as "inappropriate guilt."
- From the section on new love relationships: The respondent's
  answer to the question, How often do you feel sexual satisfaction in your current relationship? This variable will be referred to
  as "frequency sexual satisfaction."
- From the subsection on other spouse-related variables: The respondent's answer to question, Who initiated the separation?
  This variable will be referred to as "initiator."

Correlation analysis (Pearson correlation coefficient) is shown in
Table IX. As expected, there are moderately high correlations between
the various separation/divorce-related variables. The largest number of
higher correlations are found in regard to memory/fantasy, with four of
five possible correlations above .200 and one above .300. In women

Table IX

Key Separation/ Divorce-related Variable	Death Wish by Spouse	Memory/ Fantasy	Consis- tency	Inappro- priate Guilt	Frequency of Sexual Satisfaction	Initiator
Death wish by spouse	1.00					
Memory/fantasy	−.096	1.00				
Consistency	−.232	.211	1.00			
Inappropriate guilt	−.097	−.260	−.224	1.00		
Frequency of sexual satisfaction	.035	−.218	−.171	.147	1.00	
Initiator	.111	.376	.093	.253	.175	1.00

these correlations are still higher: memory/fantasy correlates with frequency of sexual satisfaction at $-.442$, and with the initiator at $.412$. For Sub 2 as a whole, inappropriate guilt has the next highest number of correlations above $.200$, with the other variables having fewer correlations in that range.

Persons spending more time in memory and fantasy about the (former) spouse were somewhat more likely (1) to report that the spouse had wished him/her dead; (2) to be inconsistent in regard to spouse contacts; (3) to be reported to feel inappropriate guilt; (4) to have less frequent sexual satisfaction; and (5) to report that the separation or divorce was spouse-initiated.

Persons reported to feel inappropriate guilt (lower scores) are somewhat more likely (1) to have said that the (former) spouse did not wish him/her dead; (2) to have spent more time in memory/fantasy about the (former) spouse; (3) to have been inconsistent in regard to (former) spouse contacts; (4) to have experienced less frequent sexual satisfaction; and (5) to have reported self- rather than spouse-initiation of the separation/divorce.

Thus memory/fantasy and inappropriate guilt are related to each other, and both are related to greater inconsistency and less frequent sexual satisfaction. However, they differ in regard to reported spouse death wishes with memory/fantasy being associated with the presence of such wishes, but inappropriate guilt with their absence, though the correlations are relatively low. Insofar as they are meaningful, they suggest that inappropriate guilt is linked with self-blame and therefore lack of viewing the spouse as hostile. The other difference is in regard to initiation: not surprisingly, those inappropriately guilty are more likely to have initiated the separation, while those high in memory/fantasy are more likely to report spouse initiation.

The results of the regression analysis will be found in Table X, with separate reports for Sub 2 and for Sub 2 men and women.

The summary of positive findings in regard to Sub 2 as a whole is as follows: The F statistic for the regression equation was significant for somatic discomfort, anxiety, depression, and the BPRS. Individual F values were significant for regression equations involving consistency and somatic discomfort; death wish by spouse and anxiety and the BPRS; memory/fantasy and anxiety and depression; and inappropriate guilt and the BPRS. In regard to Sub 2 women, the F statistic for the regression equation was significant for somatic discomfort, anxiety, depression, and the BPRS. Individual F values were significant for memory/fantasy and anxiety and depression, as well as for inappro-

Table X

Key Separation/Divorced-Related Variables and Mental Health Measures (Sub 2)

Dependent Variable	Independent Variable	Beta, F			R^2			F			N, Int[c]		
		M	F	M/F	M	F	M/F	M	F	M/F	M	F	M/F
SOMA	Death wish by spouse	−.102, 0.14	−.133, 0.68	−.137, 1.15	.261	.332	.278	0.71	2.41[b]	3.15[b]	18,1.86	35,1.95	55,1.54
	Memory/fantasy[d]	.162, 0.41	.326, 3.08	.237, 2.98									
	Consistency	.358, 1.82	.324, 3.76	.327, 6.22[b]									
	Inappropriate guilt	−.254, 0.93	−.090, 0.29	−.134, 1.04									
	Frequent sexual satisfaction	−.100, 0.16	.118, 0.45	.018, 0.02									
	Initiator	−.147, 0.28	.069, 0.16	−.041, 0.90									
ANX	Death wish by spouse	−.172, 0.55	−.274, 3.24	−.259, 4.73[b]	.470	.402	.375	1.77	3.26[b]	4.89[a]	18,2.21	35,2.06	55,2.21
	Memory/fantasy[d]	.403, 3.51	.424, 5.81[b]	.378, 8.72[a]									
	Consistency	.355, 2.52	.093, 0.35	.184, 2.27									
	Inappropriate guilt	−.313, 1.96	−.137, 0.75	−.176, 2.07									
	Frequent sexual satisfaction	−.026, 0.01	.013, 0.01	−.006, 0.00									
	Initiator	−.135, 0.33	.031, 0.04	−.037, 0.09									
DEP	Death wish by spouse	−.181, 0.86	−.146, 0.86	−.169, 1.85	.630	.361	.324	3.41[b]	2.73[b]	3.91[a]	18,3.51	35,2.22	55,2.83
	Memory/fantasy[d]	.504, 7.86[b]	.418, 5.28[b]	.340, 6.55[b]									
	Consistency	.055, 0.09	.083, 0.26	.097, 0.59									
	Inappropriate guilt	−.571, 9.37[a]	−.051, 0.10	−.197, 2.40									
	Frequent sexual satisfaction	−.111, 0.39	−.042, 0.06	−.067, 0.30									
	Initiator	.049, 0.06	.133, 0.64	.091, 0.49									

(continued)

Table X (*continued*)

Dependent Variable	Independent Variable	Beta, F			R²			F			N, Int[c]		
		M	F	M/F	M	F	M/F	M	F	M/F	M	F	M/F
SOC	Death wish by spouse	−.214, 0.59	.046, 0.07	−.044, 0.11	.242	.260	.216	0.64	1.70	2.25	18,2.60	35,1.78	55,1.97
	Memory/fantasy[d]	−.024, 0.01	.069, 0.13	.056, 0.15									
	Consistency	.208, 0.60	.029, 2.78	.273, 4.01									
	Inappropriate guilt	−.336, 1.58	−.118, 0.45	−.205, 2.23									
	Frequent sexual satisfaction	.080, 0.10	−.160, 0.75	−.045, 0.12									
	Initiator	.118, 0.17	.149, 0.69	.128, 0.83									
BPRS	Death wish by spouse	−.456, 3.10	−.166, 1.16	−.268, 4.59[b]	.348	.390	.313	1.07	3.09[b]	3.73[a]	18,2.12	35,1.84	55,1.86
	Memory/fantasy[d]	.183, 0.58	.065, 0.13	.124, 0.86									
	Consistency	.102, 0.17	.179, 1.26	.141, 1.21									
	Inappropriate guilt	−.289, 1.36	−.334, 4.37[b]	−.305, 5.65[b]									
	Frequent sexual satisfaction	.124, 0.27	−.094, 0.32	.040, 0.10									
	Initiator	.150, 0.33	.207, 1.61	.176, 1.80									
SPC 1[e]	Death wish by spouse	—	−.247, 1.77	−.143, 0.96	—	.119	.064	—	0.65	0.56	—	35,3.12	55,2.52
	Memory/fantasy[d]		.037, 0.03	.076, 0.24									
	Consistency		−.112, 0.34	−.050, 0.11									
	Inappropriate guilt		−.034, 0.03	−.120, 0.64									
	Frequent sexual satisfaction		−.196, 0.94	−.123, 0.73									
	Initiator		.053, 0.07	.018, 0.01									

SPC 2[c]	Death wish by spouse	—	−.191, 1.20	−.110, 0.64	.214	.156	—	1.32	1.51	—	35,1.75	55,1.62
	Memory/fantasy[d]		.123, 0.37	.127, 0.73								
	Consistency		−.045, 0.06	−.006, 0.00								
	Inappropriate guilt		.029, 0.03	−.152, 1.14								
	Frequent sexual satisfaction		−.302, 2.52	−.205, 2.25								
	Initiator		.102, 0.30	.103, 0.49								
ASP[e]	Death wish by spouse	—	−.202, 1.29	−.087, 0.38	.182	.108	—	1.08	0.99	—	35,2.67	55,2.16
	Memory/fantasy[d]		.019, 0.01	.038, 0.06								
	Consistency		−.119, 0.41	−.003, 0.00								
	Inappropriate guilt		−.078, 0.18	−.170, 1.35								
	Frequent sexual satisfaction		−.362, 3.48	−.244, 3.03								
	Initiator		−.133, 0.50	−.068, 0.21								

[a] $p \leq .01$

[b] $p \leq .05$

[c] Int = Intercept (constant).

[d] "Not with spouse" was used in place of "Memory/fantasy" for males.

[e] There were not enough suicidal males to warrant computation of the correlation coefficient.

priate guilt and the BPRS. For Sub 2 men the F statistic for the regression equation was not significant in any instance. Individual F values were significant for "not with spouse" and depression and for inappropriate guilt and depression.

The following variables were selected on this basis to represent separation/divorce-related variables in the final overall regression equation: *Death wish by spouse* and *memory/fantasy*, each of which was significant in relation to two mental health measures for the group as a whole, and *consistency*, which was significant for one mental health measure and closely approached significance for a second. For men, *not with spouse* will continue to be substituted for memory/fantasy.

Variables Not Related to Separation/Divorce

It is self-evident that factors other than marital separation and divorce affect the mental health of individuals undergoing marital dissolution. Some of the literature in the field takes the position that separation and divorce is often the result of a preexisting impairment of mental health. Bergler[7] believed that an unhappy marriage is usually the symptom rather than the cause of neurotic difficulty. Briscoe and Smith[8] stated that "three quarters of the divorced women and two thirds of the divorced men have . . . psychiatric disease," of which "definite unipolar affective disease" is the most common form.[8] Rogers et al.[9] stated that persons seeking help with their marriage have lower scores on emotional stability than non-help-seekers. (The authors stated that they made no attempt to determine causality.) Overall[10] believed that marital discord is part of a depressive spectrum disorder, though not necessarily based on heredity.

Hunt[11], however, saw the contemporary consensus of professionals as being that "only a minority of divorces can be explained as a neurotic answer to a neurotic problem." Bernard[12] believed that earlier work such as Bergler's has tended to increase the feelings of shame of those divorcing by emphasizing pathology, and that more current research by deemphasizing such "causes" has been in the general direction of relieving such feelings of shame.

A number of writers hold the view that disturbance in those undergoing marital dissolution is caused by multiple factors. Fisher[13] stated that the divorced "range from those with enough ego strength . . . to cope with ordinary life situations to those whose neurotic pattern does not allow for much autonomy and intimacy, to those whose pathology is such as not to permit them to assume . . . adult roles such as those demanded in marriage." Similarly, Bloom et al.[14] stated that "the most appropriate interpretation of the research and conceptualization reviewed is that an unequivocal association between marital dissolution and physical and emotional disorder is demonstrated. Furthermore, this association suggests at least two interdependent components: First, illness (physical or emotional) can precede and likely precipitate marital disruption, and second, marital disruption can serve to precipitate physical and psychiatric difficulties in persons who might otherwise not have developed such problems."

In the present study, the question was asked whether the inclusion of variables independent of separation and divorce could contribute to the overall understanding of the marital dissolution process. It was decided to include such items and to compare their contribution to mental health measures with those related to separation and divorce.

To this end, a list of childhood stress factors was taken from the Social Assets Scale designed by Luborsky et al.[15] as a potential predictor of physical and psychological symptoms. The items in question, provided they are accurately reported, are by definition independent of marital dissolution, since they refer to an earlier period of time. They were originally derived from Langner and Michael's work.[16]

Eight such pre-adult stress factors are noted: parents' poor physical health, parents' poor mental health, childhood economic deprivation, childhood poor physical health, childhood broken homes, parents' character negatively perceived, parents' quarrels, and disagreements with parents.[16]

In the present study, seven of the eight factors, as represented in the Social Assets Scale, were related to dependent mental health measures by Kendall's tau. One item, disagreement with parents, was not represented in the Social Assets Scale. Three other items either failed to show significant correlation with any dependent mental health measures, or correlated significantly with no more than one. These were childhood broken homes due to either death or divorce, parents' character negatively perceived, and parents' quarrels. It is not clear why correlations with mental health were minimal or non-existent in the present study; however, since this was the case they were omitted from further analysis.

Four of the Langner and Michael items included in the Social Assets Scale showed Kendall correlations at the $p = .05$ level, one-tailed test, with two or more dependent mental health measures:

• Parents' poor physical health, as measured by the score of the response to the question, When you were growing up, were either of your parents in poor health? Answers were scored as follows: 10 =

yes, all of the time; 20 = yes, frequently, 30 = yes, but rarely, 35 = no, never. The following was the distribution of responses for Sub 2 (N = 106). 10, 8.5 percent; 20, 15.1 percent; 30, 27.4 percent; 35, 49.1 percent. Kendall's tau showed significant associations of poorer parental health with greater somatic discomfort (τ = $-.252$, p ≤ .01, N = 105) and with more anxiety (τ = $-.236$, p ≤ .01, N = 105). Association with more depression approached significance (τ = $-.142$, p ≤ .10, N = 105) as did association with higher score on the BPRS (τ = $-.139$, p ≤ .10, N = 105).

• Parents' poor mental health as represented, according to Langner and Michael[16] by the combined scores of answers to the question, Did your father or mother ever have any of the following conditions (arthritis, asthma, bladder trouble, colitis, diabetes, hay fever, heart condition, high blood pressure, neuralgia or sciatica, nervous breakdown, epilepsy, stomach trouble, or skin condition)? Each condition was rated as 20 if checked, 30 if blank. The following is the distribution of responses for the Sub 2 (N = 105): 24.62, 1.0 percent; 25.39, 1.0 percent; 26.15, 3.8 percent; 26.92, 8.6 percent; 27.69, 11.4 percent; 28.46, 19.0 percent; 29.23, 28.6 percent; 30.00, 26.7 percent. Note that the scores are the average of the scores on the 13 individual illness items. The range of scores is rather narrow, and most of the respondents' parents did not have many of the listed illnesses.

Kendall's tau showed significant associations of poorer parental mental health with greater respondent somatic discomfort (τ = $-.185$, p ≤ .05, N = 104) and with more anxiety (τ = $-.154$, p ≤ .05, N = 104). Association with greater suicide potential at interview (SPC 2) approached significance (τ = $-.144$, p ≤ .10, N = 101).

• Childhood poor physical health. In the present study two or more correlations were found only in relation to the question, My health between the ages of 16 and 20 years was _____? Answers were scored as 40 = good, 30 = fair, 10 = poor. The following was the distribution of responses for Sub 2 (N = 106): 10, 7.5 percent; 30, 18.9 percent; 40, 73.6 percent. Kendall's tau showed significant association of poorer childhood (adolescent) health with greater somatic discomfort (τ = $-.160$, p ≤ .05, N = 105), with greater suicide potential at entry, SPC 1 (τ = $-.262$, p ≤ .01, N = 102), with greater suicide potential at interview, SPC 2 (τ = $-.245$, p ≤ .01, N = 102), and with greater rater-assessed suicide potential, ASP (τ = $-.252$, p ≤ .01, N = 102). None or one significant correlation was found for questions about health for ages 1–5, 6–10, or 11–15, and these questions were not further considered.

• Childhood economic deprivation as indicated by response to the question, When I was growing up, my parents had trouble finding money for necessities _____? The answers were scored as 00 = always, 10 = often, 20 = sometimes, 30 = rarely, 40 = never. The following was the distribution of responses for Sub 2 (N = 102): 00, 13.7 percent; 10, 14.7 percent; 20, 24.5 percent; 30, 20.6 percent; 40, 26.5 percent. Kendall's tau showed significant association of economic deprivation with greater somatic discomfort (τ = $-.148$, $p \leq .05$, N = 101) and greater anxiety (τ = $-.196$, $p \leq .05$, N = 101).

Parents' poor physical health, parents' poor mental health, childhood (adolescent) poor physical health, and childhood economic deprivation were included in a preliminary regression analysis for Sub 2 as a whole and for Sub 2 men and women separately. The results were as follows: Childhood economic deprivation did not show any significant individual F values and was dropped from further consideration. It was decided in advance to reduce the remaining three variables to two to be included in further regression analysis, in order to limit the total number of variables. For this reason, the variable of parents' poor mental health was dropped, since it had the lowest number of individually significant F values. The other two variables had the following significant individual F values for Sub 2 as a whole: parents' poor physical health and somatic discomfort, anxiety, and the BPRS; and childhood (adolescent) poor physical health and somatic discomfort and all three suicidal variables. For this reason, *parents' poor physical health and childhood (adolescent) poor physical health were selected to represent non-separation/divorce-related variables in further regression analyses.* While both of these relate to parents' or respondents' physical health, they do not measure the same phenomenon for Sub 2 as a whole, since the Pearson correlation between them is r = .177. It is r = .012 in women. It is quite high in men: r = .641; however, in men only childhood (adolescent) poor physical health and not parents' poor physical health showed significant F values in relation to any mental health measures.

FACTORS ASSOCIATED WITH MENTAL HEALTH: AN OVERVIEW

Further analyses were carried out to obtain an overview of the impact of independent variables on the dependent mental health measures. These can be found in Chapter 11, which discusses (1) a general regression equation for Sub 2, (2) a regression equation including independent variables significantly related to the suicidal dependent measures, and (3) regression analyses pertaining to Sub 1 and Sub 3.

Another analysis was run including a variable representing the three divisions of Sub 2: separated but not filed, filed but not final, and final decree, each within 14 months previous to interview. That variable was used instead of either "financial" or "friends." The variable was not significant in relation to any dependent measures nor did it substantially affect other relationships.

REFERENCES

1. Spanier GB, Lachman ME, cited in Spanier GB, Fleer S: Factors sustaining marriage: Factors in adjusting to divorce, in Corfman E (Ed): Families Today: A Research Sampler on Families and Children. US Dept of Health Education and Welfare, 1979, pp 205–231
2. Kitson GC: Attachment to the spouse in divorce: A scale and its application. J Marriage Family 44:379–393, 1982
3. Spitzer RL, Endicott J, Fleiss J, et al: The psychiatric status schedule: A technique for evaluating psychopathology and impairment in role functioning. Arch Gen Psychiatry 23:41–55, 1970
4. Brown P, Felton BJ, Whitman V, et al: Attachment and distress following marital separation. J Divorce 3(4):303–316, 1980
5. Berk RA: An introduction to applications of the general linear model, in Rossi P (Ed): Review of Survey Research. New York, Academic Press, 1981
6. Myers JK, Bean LL: A Decade Later: A Follow-up of Social Class and Mental Illness. New York, John Wiley & Sons, 1968
7. Bergler E: Divorce Won't Help. New York, Harper Bros, 1970
8. Briscoe W, Smith JB: Psychiatric illness, marital units and divorce. Arch Gen Psychiatry 29:811–817, 1973
9. Rogers LS, Young HH, Cohen IH, et al: Marital stability, mental health and marital satisfaction. J Clin Consul Psychol 35(3):342–348, 1970
10. Overall JE, Henry BW, Woodward A: Dependence of marital problems on parental family history. J Abnormal Psychology 83(4):446–450, 1974
11. Hunt M, Hunt B: The Divorce Experience. New York, McGraw-Hill, 1977
12. Bernard J: No news, but new ideas, in Bohannan P (Ed): Divorce and After. New York, Doubleday,1970
13. Fisher EO: Divorce: The New Freedom. New York, Harper & Row, 1974
14. Bloom BL, White SW, Asher, SJ: Marital disruption as a stressful life event, in Levinger G, Moles OC (Eds): Divorce and Separation: Context, Causes and Consequences. New York, Basic Books, 1979
15. Luborsky L, Todd TC, Katcher A: A self-administered social assets scale for predicting physical and psychological illness and health. J Psychosom Res 17:109, 120, 1973
16. Langner TS, Michael ST: Life Stress and Mental Health. Glencoe, Ill, The Free Press, 1963

Index